BECKER-SHAFFER'S
DIAGNOSIS AND THERAPY
OF THE GLAUCOMAS

BECKER-SHAFFER'S

DIAGNOSIS AND THERAPY OF THE GLAUCOMAS

ALLAN E. KOLKER, M.D.

Professor of Ophthalmology and Associate Director of the
Glaucoma Center, Department of Ophthalmology,
Washington University School of Medicine,
St. Louis, Missouri

JOHN HETHERINGTON, Jr., M.D.

Associate Clinical Professor of Ophthalmology and Associate
Director of the Glaucoma Center, University of California
Medical Center, San Francisco, California

with 448 illustrations and 8 color plates
21 stereoscopic views in full color on 3 View-Master® reels

FOURTH EDITION

The C. V. Mosby Company

Saint Louis   1976

FOURTH EDITION

Copyright © 1976 by The C. V. Mosby Company

Previous editions copyrighted 1961, 1965, 1970

Printed in the United States of America

Distributed in Great Britain by Henry Kimpton, London

Library of Congress Cataloging in Publication Data

Becker, Bernard.
    Becker-Shaffer's diagnosis and therapy of the
glaucomas.

    First-2d ed. by B. Becker and R. N. Shaffer
published under title: Diagnosis and therapy of
the glaucomas.
    Includes bibliographies and indexes.
    1. Glaucoma. I. Shaffer, Robert N., joint
author. II. Kolker, Allan E., 1933-
III. Hetherington, John, 1930-   IV. Title.
V. Title: Diagnosis and therapy of the glaucomas.
[DNLM: 1. Glaucoma—Diagnosis. 2. Glaucoma—
Therapy. WW290 B395d]
RE871.B4 1976   617′.741   76-4591
ISBN 0-8016-2720-6

CB/CB/B 9 8 7 6 5 4 3

PREFACE

We again have placed Becker and Shaffer's names in the book title because of our high regard for these two men who have provided the stimulus, suggestions, and final review of changes in this edition. The basic outline and much of the written material are still theirs.

Current developments have demanded a more extensive revision than originally planned. New electron microscopic techniques and studies on aqueous outflow provided additional material on the pathophysiology of the anterior segment. Data on visual fields and optic discs have added clinically useful information. The glaucoma surgery chapters required further description and illustrations of new techniques. Numerous additions and a moderate number of deletions were made in almost every subject to update the book. Of particular value was the addition of the stereoscopic gonioscopy supplement, obtained through the courtesy of Dr. Shaffer. Much of the material on tonography was maintained, although considerable revisions were made in its interpretation. It is hoped that this will still permit use of the book as a reference on the subject for residents and clinicians while placing its importance in clinical management of glaucoma in proper perspective.

It is important to realize that the information presented in this book is a guide to better patient care, based on our review of the literature and our own personal experiences. The physician's judgment in any given case is most important and may take precedence, even if it deviates from these guidelines.

We wish to especially thank Dr. H. Dunbar Hoskins, Laurie McBride, and Joan Waddell for their help and patience with this revision.

Allan E. Kolker

John Hetherington, Jr.

CONTENTS

COLOR PLATES

SECTION **I**

CLASSIFICATION

CHAPTER **1**

Classification of the glaucomas

Glaucoma is an eye disease in which the complete clinical picture is characterized by increased intraocular pressure, excavation and degeneration of the optic disc, and typical nerve fiber bundle damage, producing defects in the field of vision. Any or all of these signs may be present at a given examination. The rate of aqueous production by the ciliary body and the resistance to the outflow of aqueous humor at the angle of the anterior chamber determine the height of the intraocular pressure. The true intraocular pressure in the completely undisturbed eye is difficult to determine, for the methods of measurements alter it. Clinically, this pressure is estimated by tonometry. A definite diagnosis of glaucoma cannot be made unless the increased intraocular pressure has produced damage to the optic nerve. However, every effort of the good clinician is bent toward the early recognition of the conditions that will almost inevitably lead to such damage.

The primary glaucomas are genetically determined bilateral diseases. The term *secondary glaucoma* refers to pressure rises caused by some known antecedent or concomitant ocular disease. The common denominator in both primary and secondary glaucoma is an intraocular pressure increased sufficiently to threaten damage to the optic nerve.

As knowledge of etiology becomes more exact, it grows easier to classify the glaucomas by the mechanism responsible for the increased intraocular pressure. The etiology of acute angle-closure glaucoma is well known, and every day we are learning more and more about the pathogenesis of open-angle (chronic simple) glaucoma. Since neither one is associated constantly with other recognized ocular disease, it seems appropriate to continue using the time-honored term *primary glaucoma*. The anatomic basis for classification, which has proved so useful for diagnosis and management of the primary glaucomas, may also be applied to the secondary glaucomas. Although this is not conventional, it places emphasis on mechanism and permits a number of practical simplifications and generalizations. Furthermore, as the mechanisms of the various glaucomas become better understood, the subclassifications within anatomic categories can be modified more read-

3

ily. In general, the primary glaucomas are bilateral, whereas the secondary glaucomas are often unilateral.

It will be noted that this classification divides the glaucomas into four major divisions: (1) the angle-closure glaucomas, subdivided into those that are and those that are not caused by pupillary block, (2) the open-angle glaucomas, subdivided into those produced by resistance to aqueous outflow in and beyond the trabecular meshwork and those caused by hypersecretion or increased venous pressure, (3) a group of glaucomas in which both angle-closure and trabecular mechanisms may be contributory, and (4) the congenital glaucomas, in which some anomaly of the anterior segment is present at birth.

Unfortunately any classification is arbitrary, and individual cases will be found that do not fit neatly into any one part of the framework. Furthermore, when knowledge is inexact or incorrect, the classification will require correction. It is hoped that the majority of the glaucomas can be classified conveniently and usefully and that knowledge of the basic mechanisms responsible for elevations of intraocular pressure will help to guide the clinician in the proper choice of therapy.

  I. Angle-closure glaucoma (Figs. 1-1 and 1-2)

    A. With pupillary block

      This glaucoma occurs typically in hyperopic, narrow-angled eyes, which usually have small anterior segments and shallow anterior chambers. Tension elevation tends to occur abruptly, causing acute symptoms.

      1. Primary angle-closure glaucoma

        a. Prodromal or intermittent

        b. Acute

        c. Chronic

      2. Secondary angle-closure glaucoma

        a. Miotic-induced

        b. Swollen lens—acute unilateral angle-closure glaucoma

        c. Posterior synechias to lens—iris bombé

        d. Lens subluxation into either anterior chamber or vitreous humor

        e. Following panretinal photocoagulation

        f. Following scleral buckling procedures

        g. Posterior synechias to vitreous humor in aphakic eye

        h. Epithelial ingrowth

        i. Ciliary block glaucoma (malignant glaucoma)

    B. Without pupillary block

      In this type of glaucoma the trabecular meshwork is covered by the iris root, but a pupillary block is not responsible for holding the iris against the meshwork.

      1. Primary plateau iris

        In this type of primary angle closure there is an insignificant amount of pupillary block. The angle is mechanically blocked by the last roll of the iris if the pupil is dilated. Iridectomy may not be curative, for it only bypasses the pupillary block.

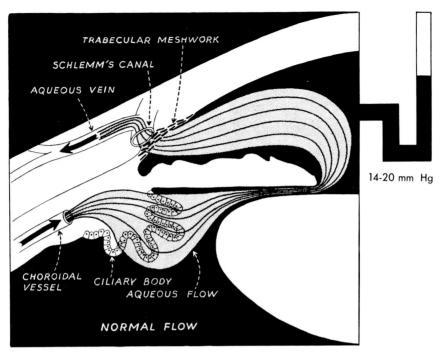

Fig. 1-1. Diagrammatic cross section of anterior segment of the eye, demonstrating aqueous humor formation and flow and outflow pathways in the normal eye.

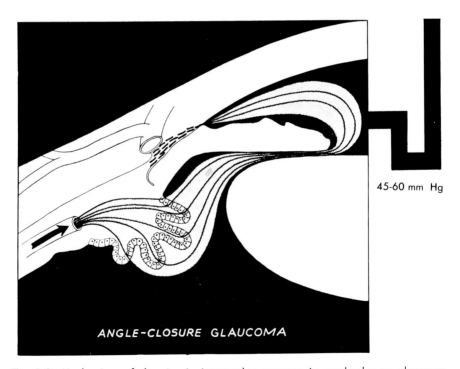

Fig. 1-2. Mechanism of the rise in intraocular pressure in angle-closure glaucoma.

2. Secondary angle closure by iris
   Peripheral anterior synechias are caused by the iris becoming permanently attached to the trabecular meshwork. In the absence of pupillary
   block, a chronic form of glaucoma results.
   a. Previous pupillary block
   b. Flat anterior chamber
   c. Tumors or cysts
   d. Inflammation
   e. Neovascular glaucoma (rubeosis iridis)
   f. Essential iris atrophy
II. Open-angle glaucoma (Fig. 1-3)
   A. With decreased facility of aqueous outflow
      In open-angle glaucoma the iris is not in apposition to the trabecular mesh-
      work. The decreased facility of outflow is caused by interference with
      aqueous flow through the outflow passages to the venous system. Symp-
      toms are usually negligible until extensive ocular damage has occurred.
      1. Primary open-angle glaucoma
         a. Chronic simple glaucoma
         b. Open-angle glaucoma with low tension

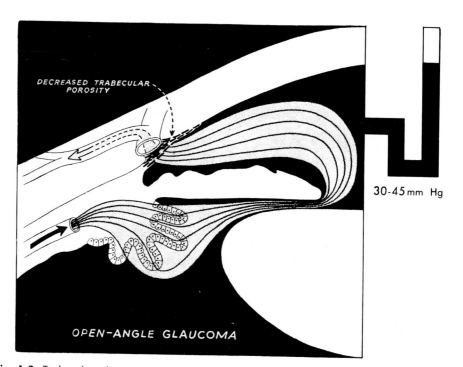

Fig. 1-3. Trabecular obstruction as the mechanism of rise in intraocular pressure in open-angle glaucoma.

    2. Secondary open-angle glaucoma
      a. Corticosteroid induced
      b. Secondary to inflammation
      c. Lens induced
      d. Traumatic
      e. Alpha-chymotrypsin induced
      f. Associated with tumors
      g. Secondary to epithelial ingrowths
      h. Neovascular glaucoma (rubeosis iridis)
      i. Secondary to retrobulbar pressure
      j. Secondary to epidemic dropsy
      k. Prostaglandins
    3. Open-angle glaucoma associated with ocular abnormalities or diseases
      a. High myopia
      b. Retinal vein occlusion
      c. Krukenberg's spindle and marked trabecular pigment band
      d. Diabetes mellitus
      e. Exfoliation syndrome (pseudoexfoliation)
      f. Retinal detachment
      g. Fuchs' dystrophy
      h. Retinitis pigmentosa

B. With normal outflow facility

This rare group of cases demonstrates increased intraocular pressure resulting in field defects. However, at all times the eyes have open angles and normal facilities of outflow.

    1. Hypersecretion glaucoma
    2. Glaucoma with increased episcleral venous pressure

III. Combined mechanisms

This category includes various combinations of angle-closure and open-angle glaucoma.

IV. Congenital glaucoma

Although the primary glaucomas are, at least in part, genetically determined, this category refers only to those cases in which anomalies of the anterior segment are present at birth. The glaucoma may be present at birth or may appear in the first four decades of life.

A. Primary congenital, or infantile, glaucoma

B. Glaucoma associated with congenital anomalies

    1. Late-developing infantile glaucoma
    2. Aniridia
    3. Sturge-Weber syndrome (oculofacial angiomatosis)
    4. Neurofibromatosis (von Recklinghausen's disease)
    5. Marfan's syndrome (arachnodactyly)
    6. Pierre Robin syndrome (microgenia and glossoptosis)

   7. Homocystinuria
   8. Goniodysgenesis (iridocorneal mesodermal dysgenesis; Rieger's anomaly, Axenfeld's syndrome, Peter's syndrome)
   9. Lowe's syndrome (oculocerebrorenal syndrome)
   10. Microcornea
   11. Spherophakia (Marchesani syndrome)
   12. Rubella
   13. Chromosome abnormalities
   14. Broad thumb syndrome (Rubinstein-Taybi syndrome)
   15. Persistent hyperplastic primary vitreous
C. Secondary glaucoma in infants
   1. Retrolental fibroplasia
   2. Tumors
      a. Retinoblastoma
      b. Juvenile xanthogranuloma
   3. Inflammation
   4. Trauma

SECTION **II**

GONIOSCOPY

Gonioscopy is a method of biomicroscopic examination of the angle of the anterior chamber of the eye where aqueous humor gains access to Schlemm's canal. By its use, the glaucomas are classified into two main groups, angle-closure and open-angle glaucomas. Gonioscopy is helpful diagnostically, prognostically, and therapeutically, particularly in angle-closure glaucoma.

CHAPTER 2

Methods of gonioscopy

EQUIPMENT

Because of the radius of curvature of the cornea, light rays coming from the far peripheral iris, from the angle recess, and from the trabecular meshwork undergo total internal reflection (Fig. 2-1), which prevents the clinician from examining these structures without the use of a contact lens to eliminate the corneal curve. The most commonly used gonioscopic contact lenses are the Goldmann, the Zeiss, and the Koeppe (Fig. 2-2).

Goldmann and Zeiss lenses (indirect method)

The Goldmann and Zeiss lenses are termed indirect gonioscopic lenses because they have mirrors by which the angle is examined with reflected light (Figs. 2-3 and 2-4). The patient can be examined with the light and magnification of the slit lamp and corneal microscope. The magnification obtained is dependent on the power of the microscope and should be at least 20×.

Koeppe lens (direct method)

The Koeppe lens is a direct lens through which the observer looks directly at the angle under observation (Fig. 2-5). The curvature of this lens adds 1.5× to the magnification of the angle image. The 16 mm lens is the preferred size. Light-

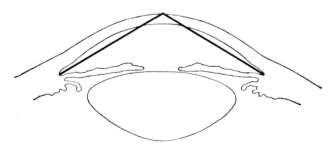

Fig. 2-1. Diagram of rays of light originating at the anterior chamber angle. These rays undergo total internal reflection by the cornea.

11

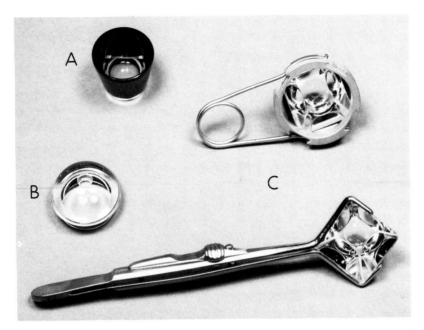

Fig. 2-2. Gonioscopic contact lenses. **A**, Goldmann. **B**, Koeppe. **C**, Zeiss with two different holding mounts.

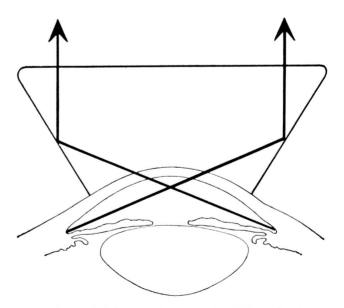

Fig. 2-3. Diagram of rays of light emerging through a Zeiss indirect gonioscopic lens.

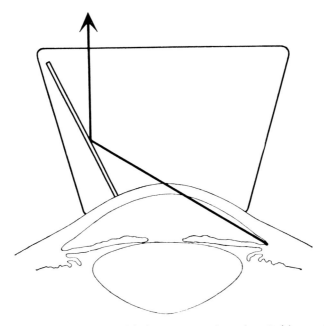

Fig. 2-4. Diagram of rays of light emerging through a Goldmann lens.

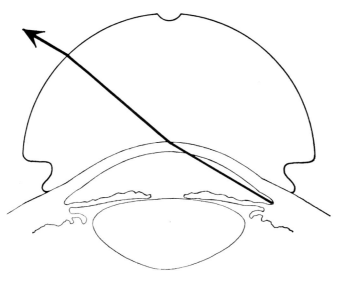

Fig. 2-5. Diagram of rays of light from the angle, emerging through a Koeppe lens.

ing is usually obtained by a Barkan hand illuminator, and magnification by a supported, counterbalanced microscope having 1.6× objective lenses and 10× oculars. With the 1.5× magnification of the Koeppe lens itself, a 24× magnification of the trabecular area is obtained. A hand-held microscope may be used for less exacting gonioscopy, but without support, the depth of focus is too critical at a magnification above 16×. Therefore 6× oculars should be used for hand-held instruments.

TECHNIQUE

Indirect gonioscopic lenses (Figs. 2-6 to 2-9)

The patient should sit upright at the slit lamp with his head firmly against the headrest. When the Goldmann lens is used, a drop of 1% methylcellulose is placed in the corneal curve of the lens. With the patient looking up, one edge of the lens is positioned in the lower fornix. The upper lid is elevated, the patient is instructed to look straight ahead, and the lens is rotated against the eye (Fig. 2-6). With the Zeiss lens the precorneal tear film is employed, and no methylcellulose solution is necessary. The Zeiss lens may be mounted on the slit lamp with a rubber-band

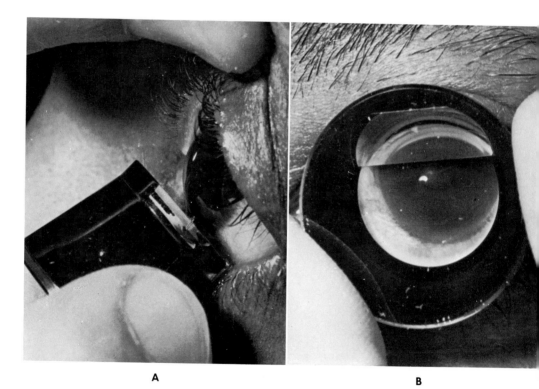

A   **B**

Fig. 2-6. Goldmann lens indirect gonioscopy. **A,** Method of inserting lens. **B,** Lens in position.

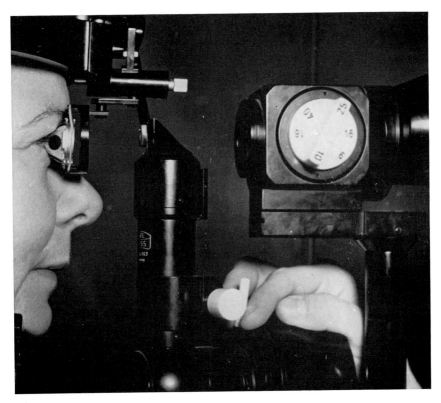

Fig. 2-7. Zeiss indirect gonioscopy.

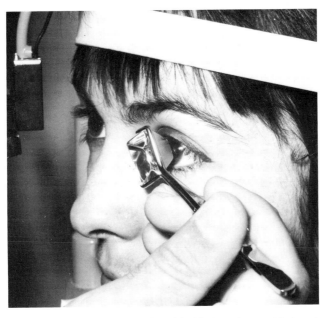

Fig. 2-8. Slit-lamp gonioscopy position of hand-held Zeiss lens, with hand resting against the cheek for maximum control.

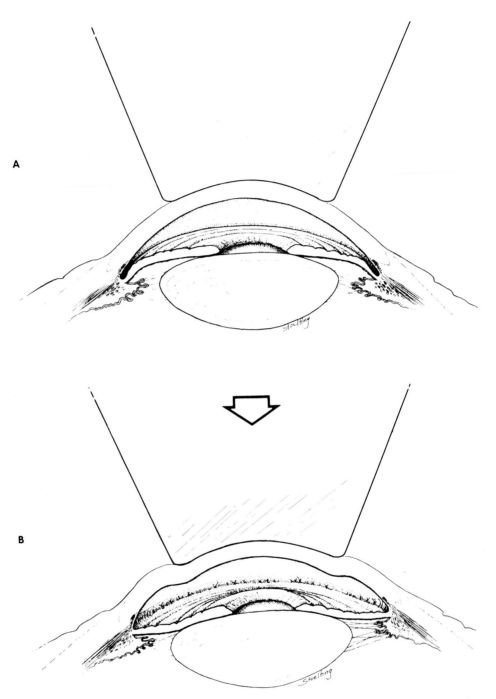

Fig. 2-9. Pressure gonioscopy. Demonstration of the manner in which pressure on the cornea displaces iris to widen a narrow or closed anterior chamber angle. This maneuver exposes additional anatomic landmarks and is useful in determining the presence or absence of peripheral synechias. Anterior synechias, if present, can sometimes be separated. **A,** Without pressure. **B,** With pressure.

support (Fig. 2-7). Using this attachment, the physician merely advances the lens to the point of contact with the cornea of the eye to be examined while the opposite eye follows the fixation light. Both hands of the examiner are free for manipulation of the microscope and slit beam. By varying the amount of pressure applied to the cornea with the contact lens, the physician is able to observe the effects of pressure on angle width. Increased pressure indents the central cornea and displaces fluid into the angle, thereby tending to open the angle more widely. A holding fork has been devised for mounting the same goniolens (Fig. 2-8), which has the convenience of requiring less manipulation in applying the lens. It has the disadvantages of occupying one hand to hold the lens and of having less control of pressure applied to the cornea. With proper experience, however, this lens can be used to observe the effects of varying pressure on angle width (Fig. 2-9). A Koeppe lens has been modified by Kitazawa for direct compression gonioscopy. The corneal contact surface of the lens has a small diameter for central corneal indentation.

Direct gonioscopic lens (Figs. 2-10 to 2-13)

The patient lies comfortably supine with the head turned toward the examiner and the eyes looking at the examiner's nose. The Koeppe lens is held at the equator between the thumb and index finger of the right hand for the right eye

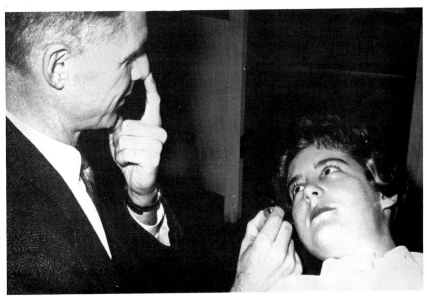

Fig. 2-10. Koeppe lens direct gonioscopy. The patient's head is turned toward the examiner. For insertion, the Koeppe lens should be held between the thumb and forefinger of the right hand for the right eye and of the left hand for the left eye. This permits rotation of the lens. The patient is asked to look steadily at the examiner's nose. By appropriate movements of the examiner's head, the patient's eyes can then be turned upward as the lens is inserted under the lower lid and downward before rotating the lens under the upper lid.

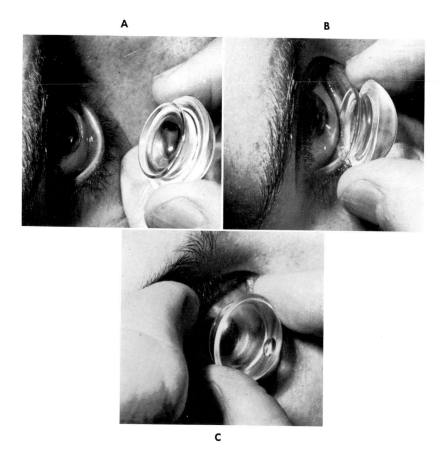

Fig. 2-11. A, With the lens pivoted between the thumb and forefinger or the third finger, the opposite hand is used to pull down the lower lid. **B,** With the upper pole pivoted away from the upper lid lashes until it is almost at right angles to the eye, the lower pole of the lens is pressed into the inferior cul-de-sac. **C,** The hand holding down the lower lid now lifts the upper lid. The contact lens is pivoted back against the eye.

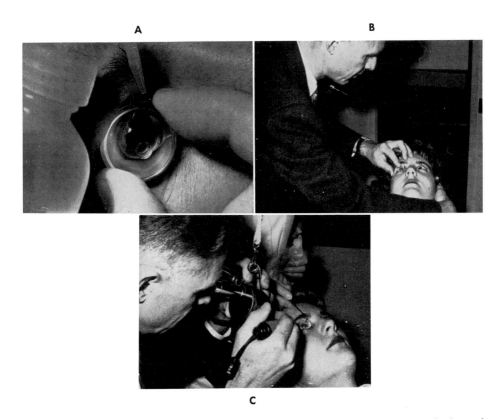

Fig. 2-12. A, While the examiner is still holding the lens equator in line with the palpebral aperture, the nasal edge of the lens is lifted away from the eye so that the lens can be filled with 0.2 ml of isotonic sodium chloride solution. The index finger of the hand holding the upper lid is placed on the dimple of the contact lens and pushes directly back toward the pupil. This displaces excess isotonic sodium chloride solution, which should be caught by gauze held at the temple. The relative vacuum helps to hold the lens on the eye and to prevent bubbles. **B,** The patient's head is turned upright. The examiner should bend over the patient in this maneuver so that the patient's eyes will maintain forward fixation. It is desirable to have an assistant steady the lens with a muscle hook or an applicator. **C,** Direct gonioscopy is performed with a supported microscope and a Barkan illuminator.

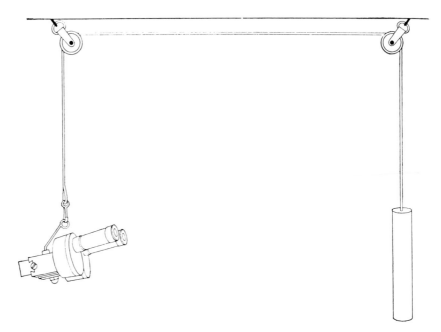

Fig. 2-13. Diagram of a gonioscopic microscope supported by nylon rope pulleys and counterbalanced by a stainless steel container weighted with sufficient lead pellets. The Barkan gonioscopic light should be hand-held to provide flexibility in illuminating narrow angles.

and between the thumb and index finger of the left hand for the left eye and is inserted between the lids. After the lens is filled with isotonic sodium chloride solution, it is desirable to have an assistant steady it with a muscle hook or applicator. There is less need for this assistance if the more viscous 1% methylcellulose is used instead of isotonic sodium chloride solution.

CHAPTER 3

Gonioscopic and microscopic anatomy of the angle of the anterior chamber of the eye

GROSS ANATOMY

Anatomic features of normal eyes

The most important anatomic factors in regulation of intraocular pressure are contained in the anterior segment of the eye, as diagrammed in Fig. 3-1. Behind the rounded apex of the angle is seen the ciliary body, which plays an important role in accommodation, in production of aqueous humor, and probably in the control of its ease of outflow. The position of the lens and its overlying iris determine the depth of the anterior chamber. The contour of the iris as it wraps around the lens, its point of insertion upon the ciliary body, and the pupillary size determine the width of the chamber angle and the area of contact with the lens. Finally, there is the corneoscleral trabecular meshwork through which aqueous humor percolates to reach Schlemm's canal, the collector channels, and the anterior ciliary veins of the limbal area. This region is not only the site of the prime pathologic changes responsible for increased pressure of glaucoma but also the focus of most of the medical and surgical procedures designed to alleviate the increased intraocular pressure.

The size and shape of an eyeball are characteristics that are genetically determined. The deep-chambered eye almost always has a wide open angle, whereas the angle contour of the shallow-chambered eye tends to be narrow. However, occasionally a moderately deep anterior chamber is seen with a narrow angle. When the angle formed between the iris and the surface of the trabecular meshwork is between 20° and 45°, the eye is said to have a wide angle. Angles smaller than 20° are termed narrow angles (Fig. 3-2). The narrower the angle, the closer the iris comes to the meshwork, and the more probable angle closure becomes. The major contribution of gonioscopy is distinction of open-angle from angle-closure glaucoma.

In the deep-chambered, wide-angled eye, such as shown in Plate 1, *A* and *E*, and Reel I-1, the lens is held by the zonular ligaments more or less centered in the ring made by the ciliary body. The iris originates at the inner anterior border of the ciliary body and lies with minimal contact on the anterior lens surface of such an eye. An increase in intraocular pressure in such an eye must be due to an increase in resistance to outflow, as shown in Fig. 1-3, or to an increase in the rate of aqueous production.

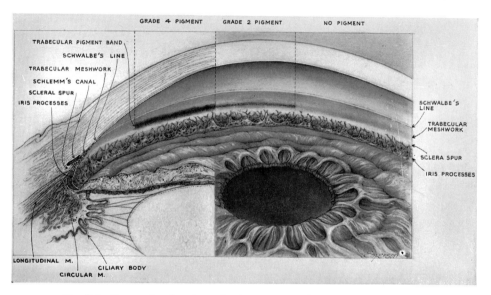

Fig. 3-1. Composite drawing of microscopic and gonioscopic anatomy.

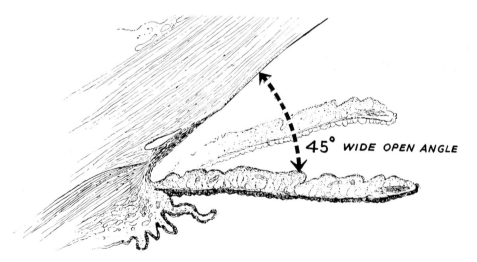

Fig. 3-2. Narrow angles, 0° to 20°. Wide open angles, 20° to 45°. (From Shaffer, R. N.: Trans. Amer. Acad. Ophthal. **64:**112, 1960.)

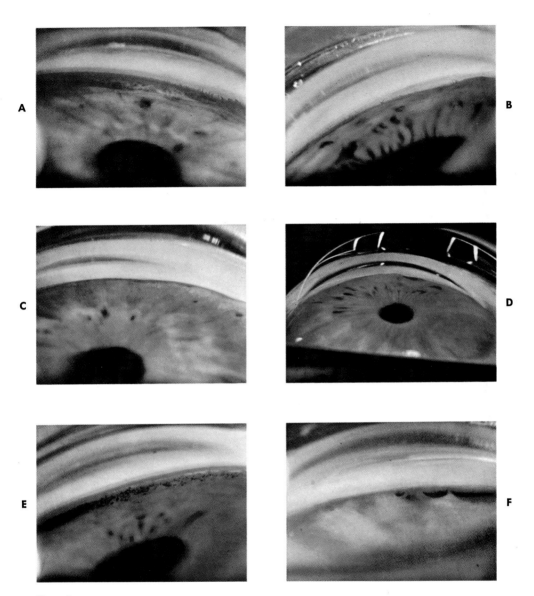

Plate 1

A, Wide open angle, Grade 4, with brown iris processes extending to the scleral spur.
B, Narrow angle, Grade 2, in a 25-year-old man. Father had acute glaucoma at 50 years of age.
C, Grade 1 or slitlike angle.
D, Closed angle.
E, Iris processes with blood in Schlemm's canal—wide open angle, Grade 4.
F, Peripheral anterior synechias formed during a period of anterior chamber collapse.

Anatomic features of narrow-angled eyes

By contrast, the lens of the shallow-chambered, narrow-angled eye is well anterior to the ciliary body ring, and the iris is held more snugly against a much larger area of its anterior surface (Plate 1, *C* and *D,* Fig. 12-2, and Reels I-2 and I-4). There results a physiologic or relative pupillary block. In such an eye a somewhat higher pressure is required in the posterior chamber to push aqueous humor through this tight iris-lens apposition than past the looser apposition of the wide-angled eye. An exaggeration of this block is the chief cause of angle-closure (acute) glaucoma. The slight excess aqueous pressure in the posterior chamber lifts the iris root forward. If the angle is sufficiently narrow and the iris base sufficiently distensible, the iris is forced against the surface of the trabecular meshwork, blocking aqueous flow into Schlemm's canal, and an acute attack of angle-closure glaucoma may ensue.

GONIOSCOPIC ANATOMY AND MICROSCOPIC INTERPRETATION
Pupil and iris

It is best to start gonioscopy by looking at the pupil for rapid orientation. The anterior lens surface can be observed for *Glaukomflecken* and for posterior synechias. This is also an excellent position to see the white dandrufflike flecks on the pigment at the posterior edge of the pupil, which are typical of lens exfoliation. Iridodonesis is present to a small degree, even in some normal eyes, and is easily observed if of pathologic degree. The examiner's gaze should pass over the plane of the iris, noting its flatness when the anterior chamber is deep and its convexity in eyes with shallow anterior chambers. Neovascularization, hypoplasia, atrophy, and polycoria should be noted. The final iris roll can be seen at the beginning of the angle recess just central to the thinned iris at its point of union with the anterior ciliary body.

Ciliary body, iris processes, and synechias

Beyond the final iris roll is the angle recess. At birth this recess is incompletely developed. By the age of 1 year the recess has formed a concavity into the anterior surface of the ciliary body. The anterior iris stroma wraps around this surface. Irregular, threadlike thickenings of these fibers branch and coalesce and sometimes bridge the angle recess. This tissue, called the uveal meshwork, and its individual tendrils, known as iris processes, probably represent the vestigial remains of the pectinate ligament of lower animals. Gonioscopically, the processes usually seem to terminate near the spur, but some may extend in front of Schlemm's canal, occasionally running as high as Schwalbe's line. These represent an incomplete embryologic cleavage of the angle, which is seen in exaggerated form in the pathologic congenital syndrome of mesodermal dysgenesis. Most of the fibers lose their pigment at the scleral spur and then continue up to Schwalbe's line as the innermost of the trabecular fibers, often called the uveal meshwork.

In blue eyes the iris processes are light gray in color and can be seen with difficulty, but in brown eyes the pigmented processes stand out prominently against the light background of the scleral spur. The neophyte gonioscopist may misinterpret these processes as synechias. They do not interfere in any way with outflow of aqueous humor (Plate 1, *A* and *E,* and Reel I-1).

True synechias are formed when the peripheral iris becomes attached to the trabecular wall. There are several clues that are used to distinguish iris processes from peripheral anterior synechias. Iris processes are irregular cords or sheets that closely follow or bridge the concavity of the angle recess. Peripheral anterior synechias are adhesions of actual iris tissue that cover up variable amounts of the angle from the recess up as high as Schwalbe's line. Often normal angle structures can be seen in one area, only to be concealed by the synechias in others. Synechias can form only when the iris is pushed against the trabecular meshwork as in angle-closure glaucoma or when iris is pulled up onto the meshwork as the result of the shrinkage of inflammatory products or fibrovascular membranes attached to both iris and meshwork. In the area of a synechia, peripheral iris tissue butts flat against the trabecular surface. It does not wrap around the angle recess as does an iris process (Fig. 3-3, Plate 1, *F,* and Reel I-3).

Scleral spur (posterior border ring)

The most anterior projection of the sclera internally is the scleral spur. In wide-angled eyes it is seen gonioscopically as a gray-white line of varying width

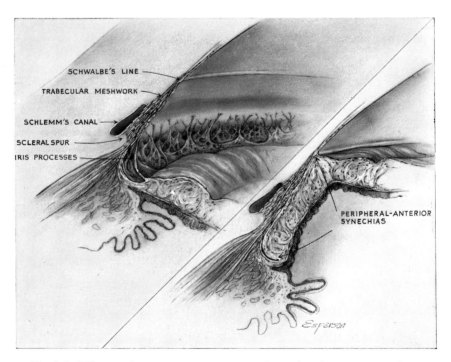

Fig. 3-3. Difference between iris processes and peripheral anterior synechias.

at the outer end of the angle recess and is the point of attachment of the ciliary body and the point of termination of most of the iris processes. If blood can be seen in Schlemm's canal, the band is just anterior to the spur.

The spur forms the posterior concavity of the scleral sulcus. Schlemm's canal is held in the sulcus by the corneoscleral trabecular sheets that form an inner wall to the sulcus. The majority of these fibers insert at the spur. The spur is also the insertion point for most of the longitudinal muscle fibers of the ciliary body whose action may alter the facility of aqueous outflow (Fig. 3-1).

Schwalbe's line (anterior border ring)

The important gonioscopic landmark, Schwalbe's line, marks the most anterior extension of the meshwork and the termination of Descemet's membrane of the cornea. By slit-lamp examination of normal eyes it can often be seen somewhere in the limbal circumference as a hazy zone of the inner corneal surface. With an indirect contact lens, the corneal parallelepiped of the slit-lamp beam comes together at this point. With the use of the Koeppe contact lens, Schwalbe's line is seen as a translucent or white ledge projecting slightly into the anterior chamber, or it may be only a vague line of demarcation between the smooth surface of Descemet's membrane covering the inner cornea and the less transparent rough texture of the meshwork. The line itself is composed of a bundle of collagenous connective tissue fibers running circumferentially around the eye at the end of Descemet's membrane. Here the corneal radius of curvature changes to the larger radius of the sclera. This change in curvature and the beginning roughness of the surface give a lodging place for the pigment granules that may be carried down over the posterior cornea by the aqueous convection currents. Consequently they tend to deposit in the lower portion of the inner cornea. Such pigmentation is rare in healthy young eyes but becomes increasingly common in diseased or aged eyes.

Trabecular meshwork and trabecular pigment band

Between Schwalbe's line and the scleral spur stretch the perforated layers of connective tissue sheets of the trabecular meshwork through which aqueous humor flows to Schlemm's canal. The innermost fibers, known as the uveal portion, run on the trabecular surface and then curve around the angle recess in a thin layer continuous with the longitudinal muscle of the ciliary body. The outer fibers, the corneoscleral meshwork, insert in the scleral sulcus and the spur. Iris processes are continuous with the anterior iris stroma.

Gonioscopic anatomy

Gonioscopically, the trabecular meshwork has an irregularly roughened surface, which in childhood is glistening and translucent like semitransparent gelatin with a stippled surface. With increasing age its transparency gradually decreases. The roughness of its surface is due to the large 40 to 60 μm openings of its inner sheets. It should be stressed that the viewer's gaze should parallel the iris as nearly as possible when he looks at the trabecular surface. Otherwise the obliquity of both the angle wall and the observer's line of vision prevents adequate visualization. In the narrow-angled eye, the convex plane of the iris forces this oblique visualization, giving a foreshortened appearance to the meshwork.

Just anterior to the scleral spur is the effective filtering portion of the meshwork lying in front of Schlemm's canal. In aging and disease processes, pigment from the iris is carried by the aqueous flow and deposited in varying amounts and depths in the meshwork, giving rise to the trabecular pigment band, which tends to be more dense in the lower angle (Fig. 3-1).

Microscopic anatomy (Figs. 3-4 to 3-20)

Microscopically, the meshwork is made up of layers of superimposed perforated sheets between the anterior chamber and Schlemm's canal. The surface of the innermost trabecular sheet is largely covered by a netlike structure of interconnecting bands, comprising the uveal meshwork (Fig. 3-7). Traditional light microscopy shows the trabecular meshwork to be a series of cords extending from Schwalbe's line to the scleral spur and the ciliary body. Investigations with the use of tangential, tilted-frontal, and electron microscopic sections clearly show that these cords are actually cross sections of connective tissue sheets running parallel to Schlemm's canal the whole way around the inner corneal periphery.

Anteriorly, the uveal meshwork bands insert obliquely into the termination of Descemet's membrane to form Schwalbe's line. Posteriorly, they originate from

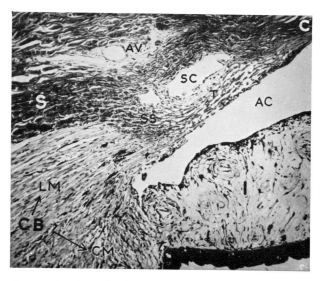

Fig. 3-4. Photomicrograph of angle. *I*, iris; *C*, cornea; *S*, sclera; *AC*, anterior chamber; *SC*, Schlemm's canal; *CB*, ciliary body; *LM*, longitudinal muscle; *CM*, circular muscle; *AV*, aqueous vein; *SS*, scleral spur; *T*, trabecular meshwork. (Courtesy Dr. L. E. Zimmerman, Washington, D. C.; AFIP collection.)

the ciliary body and iris root. The corneoscleral portion of the meshwork consists of five to nine fenestrated sheets, which are attached to the corneal stroma just beneath Descemet's membrane. Each succeeding lamella is located farther posterior, so that the last one is attached to scleral tissue near the anterior extremity of Schlemm's canal. Posteriorly, two thirds of the corneoscleral lamellas blend with the scleral spur. One third is continuous with the tendinous extension of the longitudinal muscle of the ciliary body.

The trabecular sheets contain oval perforations through which aqueous humor can flow in random tortuous passages from the anterior chamber to Schlemm's canal. The perforations near the anterior chamber measure 40 to 60 μm and can be shown experimentally and mathematically to contribute little to the resistance to aqueous outflow in the normal eye. These inner trabecular sheets with their large pores are characterized by a central core of collagen with a periodicity of 640 Å

Text continued on p. 32.

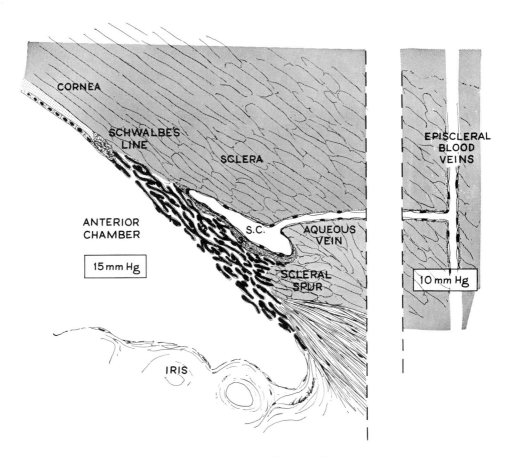

Fig. 3-5. Diagram of corneoscleral meshwork of a normal human eye, showing pressure differential of approximately 5 mm Hg between the anterior chamber and the episcleral veins. SC, Schlemm's canal. (Courtesy L. Feeney, San Francisco.)

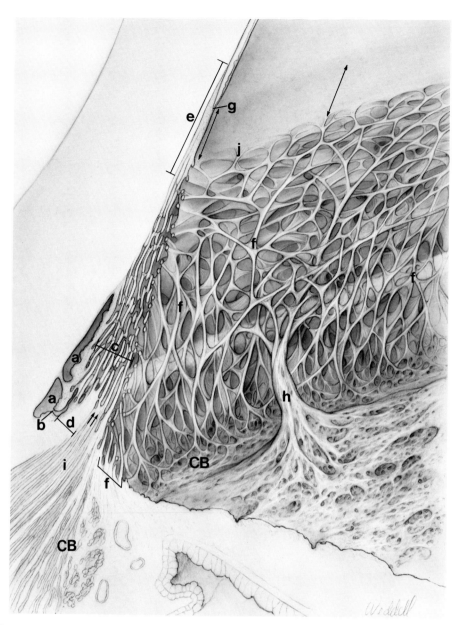

Fig. 3-6. Drawing of the aqueous outflow apparatus and adjacent tissues. Schlemm's canal, a, is divided into two portions. An internal collector channel (Sondermann's canal), b, opens into the posterior part of the canal. The sheets of the corneoscleral meshwork, c, extend from the corneolimbus, e, posteriorly to the scleral spur, d. The ropelike components of the uveal meshwork, f, occupy the inner portion of the trabecular meshwork; they arise in the ciliary body, CB, near the angle recess and end just posterior to the termination of Descemet's membrane, g. An iris process, h, extends from the root of the iris to merge with the uveal meshwork at about the level of the anterior part of the scleral spur. The longitudinal ciliary muscle, i, is attached to the scleral spur but has a portion that joins the corneoscleral meshwork (arrows). Descemet's membrane terminates within the deep corneolimbus. The corneal endothelium becomes continuous with the trabecular endothelium at j. A broad transition zone (double-headed arrows) begins near the termination of Descemet's membrane and ends where the uveal meshwork joins the deep corneolimbus. (From Hogan, M. J., Alvarado, J., and Weddell, J. E.: Histology of the human eye, an atlas and textbook, Philadelphia, 1971, W. B. Saunders Co.)

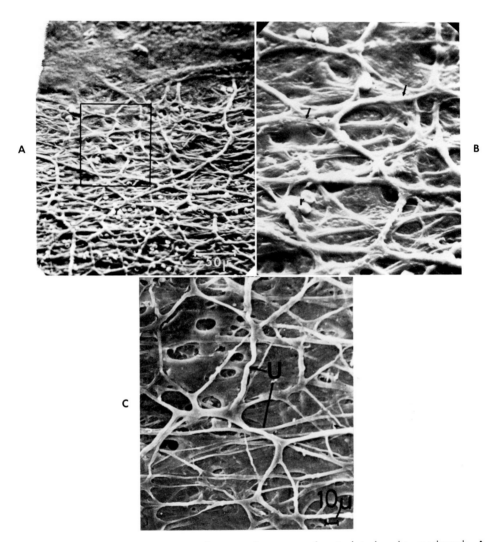

Fig. 3-7. Whole mount scanning electron microscopy of apical trabecular meshwork. **A** and **B,** Patient is 90 years old. **A,** Individual uveal and trabecular bands interconnect in a random manner and cover most of the surface of the underlying trabecular sheets. The interband spaces are very large. A smooth zone is located at the transition between corneal endothelium and trabecular endothelium. Ropelike uveal bands insert into the limbal zone at the posterior border of the smooth zone. (×300.) **B,** Enlargement of area outlined in **A.** The uveal trabecular bands average 3 to 4 μm in diameter. They are covered by an endothelial sheath, which extends between adjacent bands in some areas (arrows). Red blood cells (r) lie on the trabecular endothelium which envelops the trabecular bands. (×1400.) **C,** Detail of corneoscleral meshwork. The attached uveal meshwork has been stripped away to give a view of the first corneoscleral sheet. The oval openings in the trabecular sheet are clearly visible. Magnification same as in **B.** (**A** and **B** from Spencer, W. H., Alvarado, J., and Hayes, T. L.: Invest. Ophthal. **7:**651, 1968; **C** from Bill, A., and Svedbergh, B.: Acta Ophthal. **50:**295, 1972.)

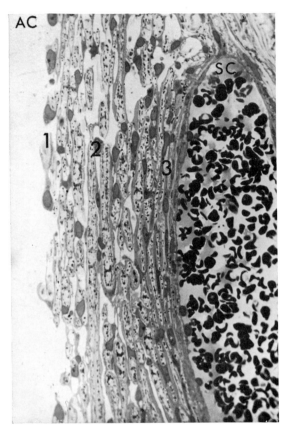

Fig. 3-8. Light micrograph of a portion of the trabecular meshwork and Schlemm's canal. Endothelial cells with prominent nuclei and dark-staining cytoplasm surround the rounded profiles of the uveal lamellas facing the anterior chamber at left. The 5 to 9 lamellas of the corneoscleral trabecular meshwork appear as interrupted segments of connective tissue covered by cytoplasm of the endothelial cell. Trabecular spaces (aqueous humor spaces) separate the segments and successive lamellas. The dark dots in the segments are long-spacing collagen plaques and elastic tissue. The collagen cores of these segments are lightly stained. Near the canal the successive corneoscleral sheets appear to be fused together and to share their endothelial covering with the neighboring, deeper lamellas. The trabecular spaces are indiscernible, and the nuclei of the cells in this region are flattened. These features, together with the disappearance of the dark-staining dots, mark the beginning of the juxtacanalicular meshwork. The matrix of the meshwork appears to stain more deeply than collagen but less deeply than the long-spacing plaques. The inner wall of the canal is lined by endothelial cells with protruding nuclei, whereas the outer wall endothelium has flattened nuclei. The lumen of the canal is filled with blood cells and plasma. *AC,* Anterior chamber; *SC,* Schlemm's canal; *1,* uveal meshwork; *2,* corneoscleral trabecular meshwork; *3,* juxtacanalicular tissue. (Richardson's stain; ×650.) (Courtesy L. Feeney, San Francisco.)

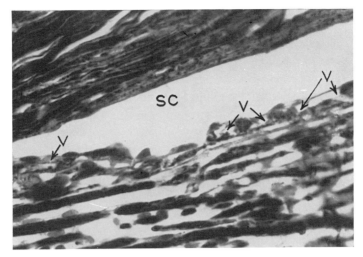

Fig. 3-9. Photomicrograph of trabecular tissue sectioned in the meridional plane. Note "vacuoles" on inner wall of canal, V. SC, Schlemm's canal. (From Garron, L., and Feeney, L.: Arch. Ophthal. **62:**966, 1959.)

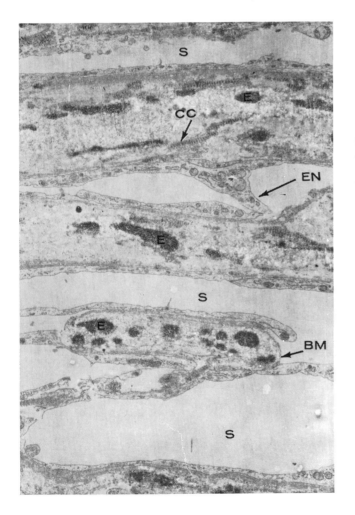

Fig. 3-10. Typical section of trabecular meshwork at survey magnification, showing several trabecular sheets. The cores of the sheets are surrounded by endothelial cells, *EN,* or at least their basement membranes, *BM.* The sheets often contain heavy-banded, 1000 Å, or curly collagen, *CC;* a more dense material, *E,* having the stained characteristics of elastic material; and much regular collagen whose banding cannot be distinguished at this magnification. *S,* Intratrabecular spaces. (×7000.) (Courtesy Dr. J. Kayes, St. Louis.)

as shown by electron microscopy. Surrounding this core is a homogeneous matrix containing loosely arranged fibers and clumps with a periodicity of 1000 Å. A layer of endothelial cells covers the trabecular sheets and is separated from the underlying collagen core and its surrounding ground substance by a thin basement membrane. The size of the perforations in the sheets decreases progressively as Schlemm's canal is approached. Particulate matter larger than 1 μm has great difficulty in passing through the meshwork. This size opening is not found except in the juxtacanalicular tissue of the outer meshwork near Schlemm's canal. These openings should not be confused with Sondermann's canals, which are probably outpocketings of Schlemm's canal and are 10 μm or more in diameter.

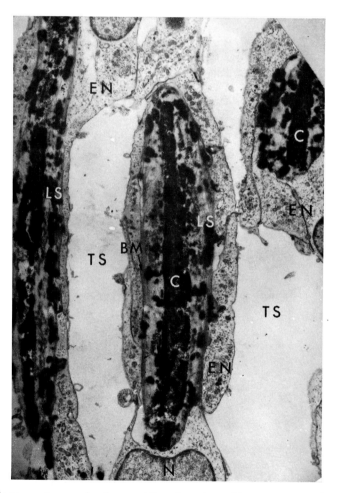

Fig. 3-11. Electron micrograph of a meridional section of human corneoscleral trabecular meshwork (neurofibroma of the orbit of patient 39 years of age). *TS,* Trabecular space; *EN,* endothelial cell; *N,* nucleus of endothelial cell; *BM,* basement membrane; *LS,* long-spacing collagen; *C,* collagen core. (×11,000.) (Courtesy L. Feeney, San Francisco.)

The outer or juxtacanalicular portion of the corneoscleral meshwork contains an amorphous ground substance. Long-spacing collagen is seen infrequently. The collagen bundles are smaller and less well organized than in the corneoscleral meshwork. In some regions the juxtacanalicular tissue is only 1 or 2 μm in width, consisting of a layer of endothelial cells facing the trabecular spaces, a zone of fine fibrils, and the endothelial cells facing the lumen of Schlemm's canal.

The endothelial cells lining Schlemm's canal on the scleral side have a well-developed basement membrane, whereas on the anterior chamber side the membrane is quite tenuous or absent. Pinocytotic vesicles are seen in the endothelial cells on both surfaces, but only in the trabecular side are large vesicles seen. In

Text continued on p. 38.

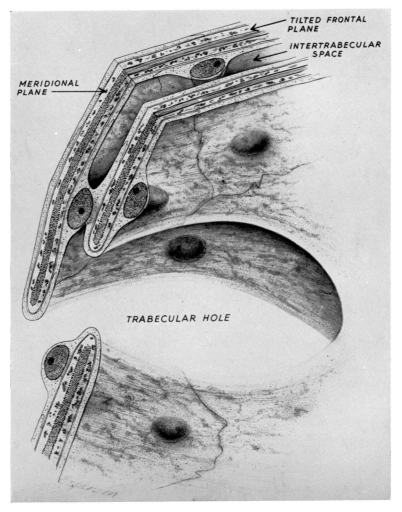

Fig. 3-12. Diagrammatic representation of portions of two adjacent corneoscleral trabecular sheets, showing appearance of cut sections in meridional and tilted frontal planes. (From Garron, L., and Feeney, L.: Arch. Ophthal. **62:**966, 1959.)

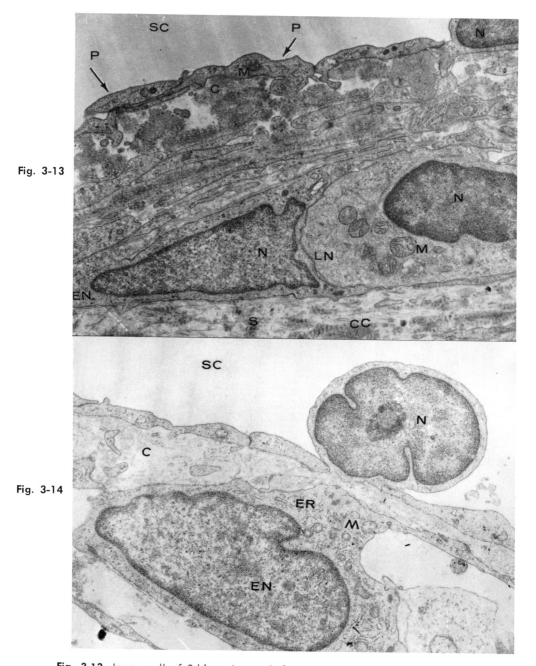

Fig. 3-13

Fig. 3-14

Fig. 3-13. Inner wall of Schlemm's canal shows great variability, most often seen as a single layer of cells with scattered collagen fibers, *C*, only partly filling the spaces toward the anterior chamber. Occasionally a cell nucleus, *N*, is seen. Here part of a trabecular sheet, *S*, with its surrounding endothelial cells, *EN*, can be seen. A few pinocytotic vesicles, *P*, can be seen even at this magnification. *CC*, 1000 Å-banded collagen; *LN*, lymphocyte; *M*, mitochondria; *SC*, Schlemm's canal. (×10,500.) (Courtesy Dr. J. Kayes, St. Louis.)

Fig. 3-14. In the light microscope the inner wall of Schlemm's canal often shows irregularities. One cause of this is probably a nucleus, *N*, jutting into the canal, *SC*. Loose fibrils, *C*, are seen. An underlying endothelial cell, *EN*, is noted with its mitochondria, *M*, and endoplasmic reticulum, *ER*. (×11,000.) (Courtesy Dr. J. Kayes, St. Louis.)

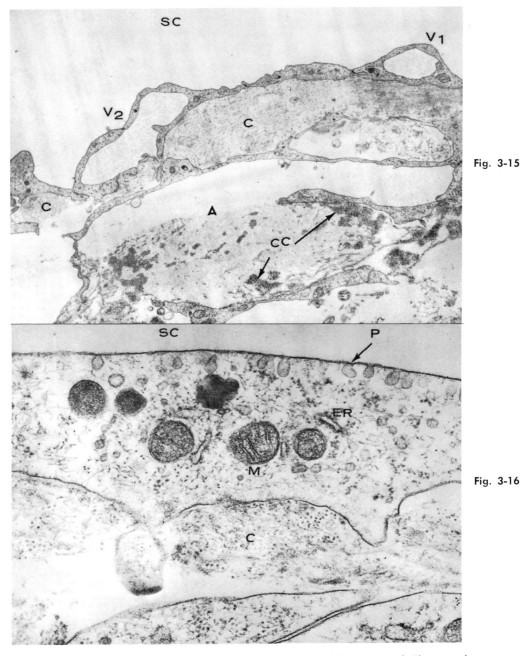

Fig. 3-15

Fig. 3-16

Fig. 3-15. In some areas vacuoles appear in the lining of Schlemm's canal. The vacuole wall consists of one cell, as in V_1, or two or more cells, as in V_2. Scattered collagen, C, is usually found near these cells, whereas the heavier-banded collagen, CC, lies farther from the canal, SC. It is these vacuoles that are shown in serial section to connect the trabecular spaces with the lumen of Schlemm's canal. (×7520.) (Courtesy Dr. J. Kayes, St. Louis.)

Fig. 3-16. Higher-power magnification of cell lining Schlemm's canal, SC. Scattered fibrils, C, are seen outside the cell. Mitochondria, M, and endoplasmic reticulum, ER, are seen within the cell, as well as other cell particles and fibrils. A number of pino-cytotic vesicles, P, are seen. They are often seen on both cell surfaces. (×40,050.) (Courtesy Dr. J. Kayes, St. Louis.)

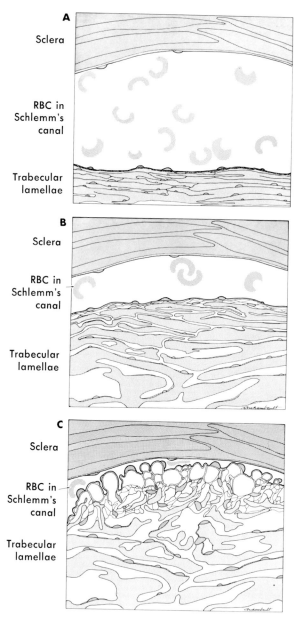

Fig. 3-17. Composite schematic drawing of the trabecular meshwork and Schlemm's canal of the human eye. **A,** With intraocular pressure less than episcleral venous pressure. **B,** With equal intraocular and episcleral venous pressures. **C,** With intraocular pressure 30 to 40 mm Hg greater than episcleral venous pressure. (From Johnstone, M. A., and Grant, W. M.: Amer. J. Ophthal., **75:**380, 1973.)

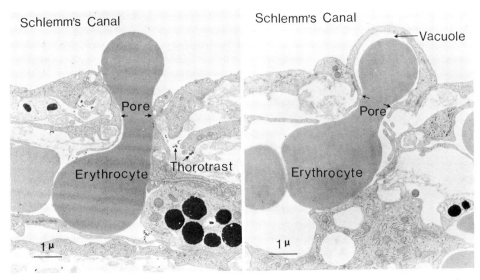

Fig. 3-18. Electron micrographs of the trabecular surface of Schlemm's canal (cynomolgus monkey), showing erythrocytes passing from the trabecular meshwork into Schlemm's canal. One erythrocyte is entering the canal directly; the second is presumably about to do so but is located in a vacuole. The eye was perfused at normal intraocular pressure with a suspension of the monkey's own erythrocytes in Ringer's solution. (Courtesy Drs. H. Inomata, A. Bill, and G. K. Smelser, New York; cover illustration, Invest. Ophthal. **8:** Aug., 1969.)

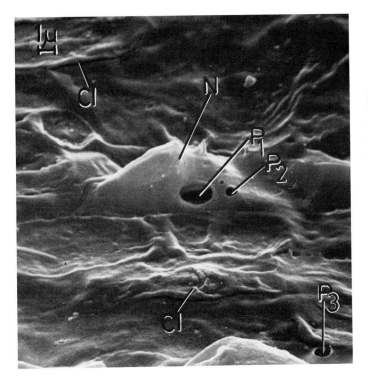

Fig. 3-19. Detail of the inner wall of Schlemm's canal. A partly collapsed bulging structure has two openings, P_1 and P_2. Part of the nucleus, N, can be seen through one opening. Structures most probably representing collapsed invaginations, C_1, are seen at several places. P_3 is also a pore. Scanning electron micrograph, freeze-dried preparation. (From Bill, A., and Svedbergh, B.: Acta Ophthal. **50:**295, 1972.)

serial electron microscopic sections Holmberg found them to be intraendothelial channels connecting the trabecular spaces to Schlemm's canal and opening as pores in the inner canal wall. The ultimate pore size in fixed tissues was found to measure 0.5 to 1.5 μm, in excellent agreement with values predicted by calculations from perfusion of particles. It is of interest that 1200 pores, 2 μm in size, could take care of the entire outflow of aqueous humor from the eye.

Holmberg's findings have been confirmed by many other investigators. The exact nature of the vacuoles, however, and their possible role in glaucoma remains in dispute. Calculations based on scanning electron microscopy suggest that as many as 20,000 pores may be present in the inner wall of Schlemm's canal. If all these pores exist in vivo, this pathway contributes only a small fraction of the total resistance to outflow. This suggests that the main resistance to outflow is located in the outer part of the trabecular meshwork and the juxtacanalicular tissue. Experimental studies indicate that such tissue contributes at least three fourths of the resistance to aqueous outflow in the normal eye. Pathologic changes in this area may well be responsible for primary open-angle glaucoma (Chapter 6).

Johnstone and Grant, in a remarkable study on monkey eyes in vivo and enucleated human eyes, demonstrated striking pressure-induced changes in the trabecular meshwork and inner wall of Schlemm's canal. When intraocular pres-

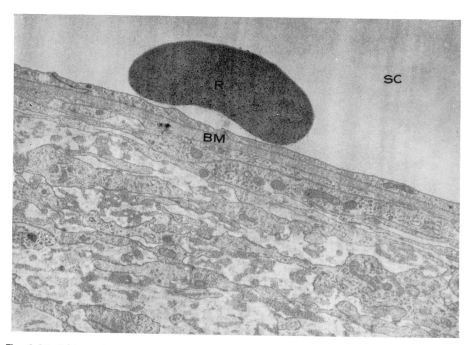

Fig. 3-20. Schlemm's canal on the scleral side, *SC*, showing the thick basement membrane, *BM*, beneath the lining cell. These thin cells contain many pinocytotic vesicles. *R*, Red blood cell. (×10,000.) (Courtesy Dr. J. Kayes, St. Louis.)

sure was near zero, the trabecular sheets and endothelium were compressed together, and only a few vacuoles seen. With increasing intraocular pressure, the trabecular sheets became distended. The endothelium developed progressively larger and more numerous vacuoles, and the inner wall of the canal expanded to approach the outer wall, thereby partially occluding the lumen. The changes occur in vivo, can be induced several hours after enucleation, and are reversible. The system appears to act as a one-way valve, with compression of the trabecular sheets and endothelium preventing reflux of blood from Schlemm's canal into the anterior chamber. Structural alterations in the ability to form vacuoles could lead to outflow impairment and glaucoma. The lumen of Schlemm's canal is maintained, in part, by septae which cross from the anterior to the posterior walls. A change in the structural components of these septae could lead to collapse of the canal and occlusion of the lumen with resultant decrease in outflow.

Within the vesicles and the trabecular spaces, a ground substance is often found that is, at least in part, a hyaluronidase-sensitive acid mucopolysaccharide. It probably corresponds to the hyaluronidase-sensitive material that is responsible

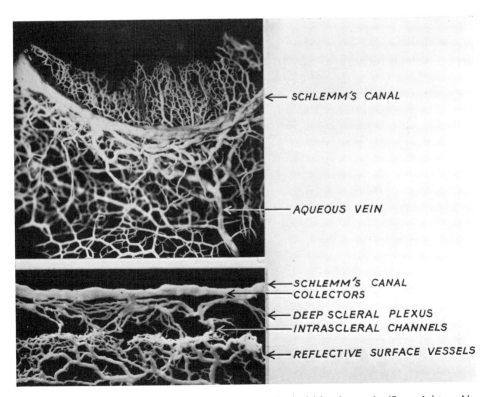

Fig. 3-21. Neoprene casts of Schlemm's canal and limbal blood vessels. (From Ashton, N.: In Duke-Elder, S., editor: Glaucoma: A symposium, Oxford, 1955, Blackwell Scientific Publications, Ltd.)

for approximately half of the perfusion resistance to outflow in the normal eyes of several species of experimental animals and in some fresh normal human eyes.

Schlemm's canal

Schlemm's canal lies in the scleral sulcus just anterior to the scleral spur at the junction between the middle and posterior thirds of the trabecular meshwork. Gonioscopically, it can sometimes be seen as a faint gray line and at others as a pink-red line that intensifies or wanes, depending on the blood content of the aqueous humor in the canal. Blood is often seen in normal or congested eyes when intraocular pressure is normal or low. When tension is high, blood is seldom seen in the canal. It is unusual to see blood in the canal in chronic simple open-angle glaucoma even when the tension is normal (Plate 1, *E*).

Aqueous veins (Figs. 3-21 and 3-22)

Arising from the outer circumference of the canal are the external collector channels that drain almost entirely into episcleral and conjunctival venous plex-

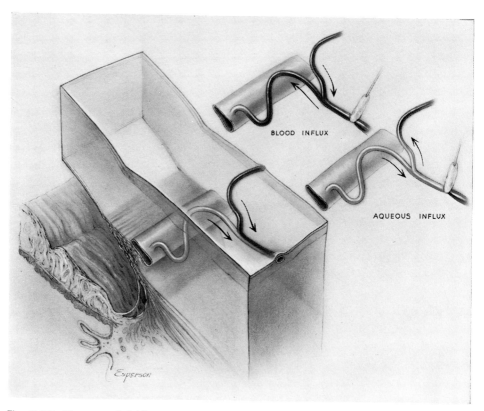

Fig. 3-22. Diagram of Schlemm's canal and a collector channel, illustrating blood influx and aqueous influx phenomena.

uses. There are twenty-five to thirty-five of these vessels. When one of them connects directly with surface veins, it can be seen by biomicroscopy and is termed an aqueous vein. The junction point resembles a clear stream emptying into the muddy water of a river, blood and aqueous flowing in a laminar pattern for some distance before mixing. In most normal eyes the aqueous vein pressure is higher than the venous pressure, so that aqueous humor displaces blood in the channel if the vein is blocked by pressure of an applicator or pressure on the lid. This is called an aqueous influx phenomenon. If the venous pressure is higher, blood fills the aqueous vein and flows back toward Schlemm's canal. This is called a blood influx phenomenon. It is a typical finding in open-angle glaucoma in which there is an increased resistance to aqueous outflow.

CHAPTER 4

Clinical interpretation of gonioscopic findings

GRADING OF ANGLE WIDTH (Fig. 4-1)

Both primary and secondary glaucomas are divided into two major classifications based on the gonioscopic observation of an open angle or of a potential or actual angle closure. The widest angles are characteristically seen in myopia and aphakia. Such eyes have a deep chamber and a flat iris plane that makes an angle of about 45° with the trabecular surface. As the chamber depth shallows, the angle narrows. There is both increasing relative pupillary block and increasing danger of angle closure as the angle becomes smaller than 20°.

For one to compare different angles, it is convenient to have a grading system. The following descriptive classification includes numerical grades of angles for convenience in recording on office charts. The most widely open angle is a Grade 4, and a closed angle is Grade 0 (Reels I-1, I-2, I-4, and I-5). There are some very narrow angles in which it is impossible to decide whether or not an opening exists between the iris root and the trabecular surface. Such angles are labelled "slit," which does not commit the examiner to an interpretation that iris apposition is necessarily responsible for the increased tension if it is present (Plate 1, C).

Angle grade	Numerical grade	Implied clinical interpretation
Wide open angle	3-4	Closure impossible
Narrow angle, moderate	2	Closure possible
Narrow angle, extreme	1	Closure probable, eventually
Narrow angle, complete or partial closure	0	Closure present or imminent

Angle width can also be estimated at the time of a routine slit-lamp examination. By directing the slit-lamp beam adjacent to the limbus, one can use the peripheral anterior chamber depth to indicate angle width. This procedure is helpful when corneal clouding reduces visualization with the goniolens. The rela-

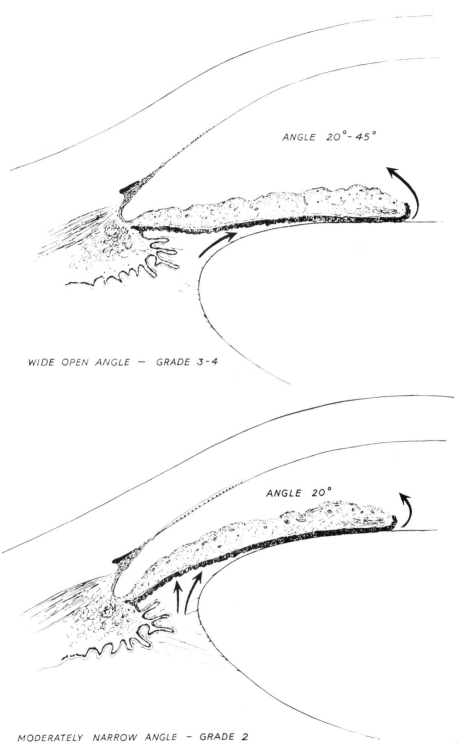

ANGLE 20°-45°

WIDE OPEN ANGLE — GRADE 3-4

ANGLE 20°

MODERATELY NARROW ANGLE — GRADE 2

Fig. 4-1. Grading of angles by name and number.

Continued.

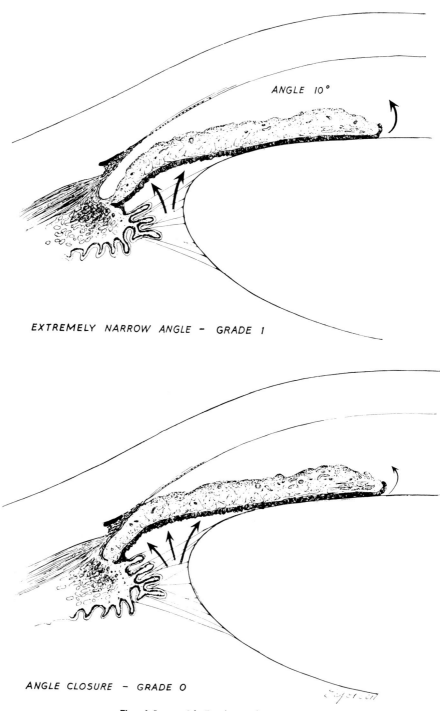

ANGLE 10°

EXTREMELY NARROW ANGLE - GRADE 1

ANGLE CLOSURE - GRADE 0

Fig. 4-1, cont'd. For legend see p. 43.

tionship between peripheral anterior chamber depth and corneal thickness determines angle width as follows:

Grade 4 angle: AC depth = corneal thickness
Grade 3 angle: AC depth = ¼ to ½ corneal thickness
Grade 2 angle: AC depth = ¼ corneal thickness
Grade 1 angle: AC depth = less than ¼ corneal thickness
Slit angle: AC depth = slitlike (extremely shallow)
Closed angle: Absent peripheral anterior chamber

In some eyes the iris root is attached anteriorly on the ciliary body near the scleral spur. This forms a V-shaped angle recess with the peripheral iris close to the filtering portion of the trabecular meshwork. Such an eye can develop angle-closure glaucoma, and yet the anterior trabeculum can easily be seen gonioscopically. It is obvious that the various angle grades merge into one another, and therefore the usefulness of this or any other classification will depend on the skill and experience of the observer in judging which angles are capable of occlusion and which angles are actually occluded and not merely extremely narrow.

DIAGRAMMING OF ANGLE WIDTH, SYNECHIAS, AND PIGMENTATION

Figs. 4-3 and 4-4 show a method of diagramming the angles and recording angle width and position of synechias. The density of the trabecular pigment band can also be recorded. In the diagram, the cornea is opened out to place Schwalbe's line outside the angle recess so that synechias can be diagrammed as continuous

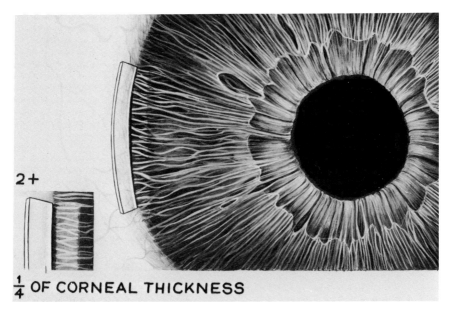

2+

¼ OF CORNEAL THICKNESS

Fig. 4-2. Slit-lamp estimation of angle width—example of a Grade 2 angle. Angle width can be estimated with the slit lamp by comparing the anterior chamber depth to the corneal thickness. (From Van Herick, W.: Amer. J. Ophthal. **68:**626, 1969.)

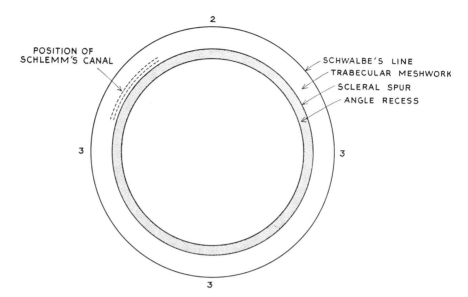

Fig. 4-3. Diagram of the method of numbering the angle width in different quadrants. This Grade 3 angle would be considered incapable of closing. As is usual, the angle is narrower above than below. If it were a Grade 1 above and a Grade 2 below, the observer would judge it capable of occlusion.

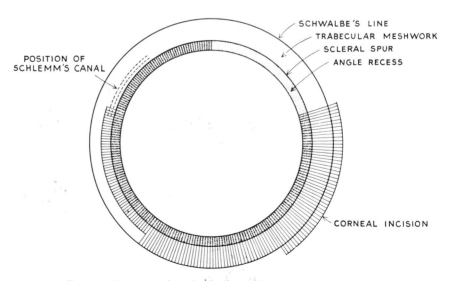

Fig. 4-4. Diagram of method of recording height of synechias.

with the peripheral iris stroma. Synechias as high as the scleral spur would not directly block outflow. Conceivably they could interfere with the pull of the ciliary body on the trabecular meshwork, decreasing the facility of aqueous outflow. In the presence of normal outflow channels there is a qualitative relationship between the extent of synechia formation and the decrease in facility of outflow (Plate 1, *F*, and Reels I-6 and I-7).

TRABECULAR PIGMENT BAND

In the normal eye of youth it is unusual to see any trabecular pigment band. This is because no loose pigment has been filtered out by the trabecular meshwork as aqueous flows through it toward Schlemm's canal. The presence of such a band denotes either aging or a disease process. The pigment band is usually most prominent in the lower chamber angle. For convenience in recording, the dense dark band of pigmentary glaucoma is recorded as Grade 4, and slight pigmentation as Grade 1.

Some allowance must be made for the color of the individual eye. Thus a Grade 1 pigment band in a brown eye would be considered a Grade 2 band in a blue eye. It should be remembered that extensive brown iris processes are normal structures and do not represent pigmentation of the angle. The two abnormal conditions in which the pigment band is most prominent are pigmentary glaucomas and exfoliation of the lens capsule (Fig. 3-1 and Reel II-6). To a less extent it is seen in many intraocular disease processes including open-angle glaucoma, trauma, iritis, and diabetes.

DIFFICULTIES AND ARTIFACTS IN GONIOSCOPY

In performing gonioscopy with any gonioscopic lens, one should be sure to realize that certain artifacts may be induced by the method and lens used. Angles tend to look somewhat wider with the Koeppe lens. The Koeppe lens and early models of the Goldmann lens are made with a scleral lip. This lip can press on the outer sclera and indent it toward the iris, thereby narrowing the angle (Fig. 4-5). Rotating the lens away from the portion of angle under observation and avoiding any pressure on the lens reduce this error. Excessive pressure by the Zeiss lens on the central cornea can artifactually widen the angle by displacing aqueous peripherally. Such pressure frequently produces folds in Descemet's membrane, which obscure the view of the angle. For proper gonioscopy the pressure on the lens should be just sufficient to permit a capillary fluid level between the lens and cornea without inducing folds in Descemet's membrane. When the lens is properly adjusted, slight reduction in pressure causes intrusion of an air bubble under the lens. Errors in gonioscopy most often result from misinterpretation of structures poorly visualized.

The mirror in the Goldmann lens is closer to the center of the cornea than are the mirrors of the Zeiss lens. This permits better visualization into the angle recess in some eyes with markedly narrowed angles. It also creates a slightly different

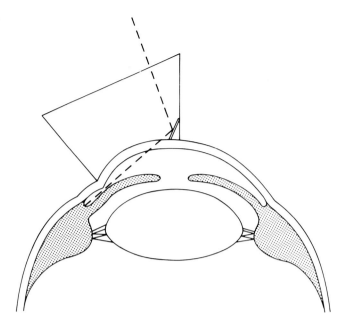

Fig. 4-5. Left edge of goniolens has indented cornea, creating an artificially narrow angle. (From Hoskins, H. D. Jr.: Invest. Ophthal. **11:**97, 1972.)

view of the angle topography when the same eye is examined with different gonioscopic lenses. In the vast majority of cases this is of little clinical importance. In a few instances, however, inexperience with a particular lens can lead to false interpretation of the gonioscopic findings. Awareness that such differences may exist and acquisition of sufficient clinical experience with one technique of gonioscopy will largely eliminate these problems. Changing the position of the indirect lens will help one see the angle depths (Fig. 4-6). In confusing circumstances, the continuity of the slit-lamp beam of light often helps the gonioscopist interpret angle findngs. Fig. 4-7 illustrates this.

When Koeppe gonioscopic lenses are used, tiny air bubbles sometimes adhere to the inner surface. This means that oily secretions have formed a film on the surface and should be removed by soap and water. Similar residues of methylcellulose or secretions may collect on the Goldmann and Zeiss lenses and cloud the appearance of the angle.

With the Koeppe lens the patient's nose sometimes prevents adequate visualization of the upper temporal angle. Gonioscopy can be accomplished by having the patient look up and temporally. With any of the indirect gonioscopic lenses it is difficult to remain binocular when examining the horizontal areas of the angle. Accurate centering of the mirror or prism will be helpful.

When high intraocular pressure produces edema of the epithelium, the use of oral glycerol can improve visualization by lowering the pressure. Dehydration of the corneal edema can also be accomplished by using 100% glycerol drops topically. It is sometimes necessary to remove the hazy edematous corneal epithelium by curettage, as is done in surgery for infantile glaucoma.

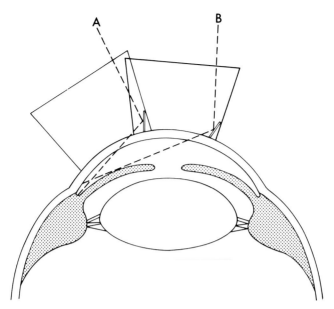

Fig. 4-6. With goniolens centered on cornea, line of sight, *B*, does not reach depths of angle. Lens must be rotated toward angle, *A*. (From Hoskins, H. D., Jr.: Invest. Ophthal. **11:**97, 1972.)

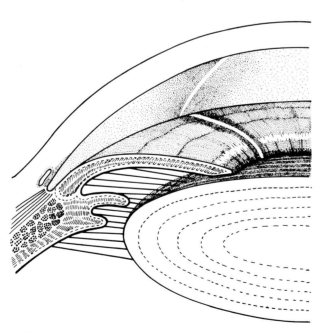

Fig. 4-7. Failure of slit-lamp beam crossing iris to meet beam coming down from cornea indicates that point of iridocorneal junction is not being viewed. (From Hoskins, H. D.:, Jr.: Invest. Ophthal. **11:**97, 1972.)

Endothelial dystrophy or even mild cornea guttata decreases the clarity of the angle image. Focusing on the cornea during gonioscopy provides an oblique view of the defective endothelium, which has a pebbled, shagreen appearance against the white background of the scleral tissue. The diagnosis of cornea guttata is often easier by this method than by direct slit-lamp microscopy.

CLINICAL USEFULNESS OF GONIOSCOPY
Aid in diagnosis of type of glaucoma

By means of gonioscopy alone, one can determine which eyes are in critical danger of angle closure and which are completely safe from closure. This finding forms the basis for classifying eyes into angle-closure and open-angle types.

In an open-angle glaucoma, gonioscopy may reveal inflammatory or fibrovascular membranes, or it may reveal a tumor that is covering or invading the trabecular meshwork. Such a case would be classified as a secondary glaucoma. If no obstruction can be seen, the block to outflow must be beyond the trabecular surface. After the occlusion of the central retinal vein or long-standing diabetic retinopathy, the first sign of impending neovascular glaucoma (rubeosis iridis) may be a network of blood vessels growing anteriorly on the trabecular wall. Generally a similar network appears around the pupil at approximately the same time. The angle vessels extend as high as Schwalbe's line. When the accompanying fibrous tissue shrinks, peripheral anterior synechias and ectropion uveae are produced.

With the patient lying on his back for Koeppe gonioscopy, mild iridodonesis can be seen in some normal eyes, particularly if they are myopic. It is especially prominent in eyes with pigmentary glaucoma. Although a marked trabecular pigment band is diagnostic of this condition, considerable pigmentation is also seen in cases with capsular exfoliation. The exfoliated material is often best seen under the edge of the pupil against the contrasting dark pigment of the iris pigment layer.

The cause of secondary glaucoma is occasionally revealed by finding a foreign body in an angle, by seeing holes in the peripheral iris caused by the passage of an intraocular foreign body, by noting a traumatic angle recession, or by seeing keratic precipitates on the trabecular surface.

Evaluation of symptoms

When a patient comes to the ophthalmologist complaining of halos around lights, this symptom should suggest episodes of angle-closure glaucoma if the angles are found to be critically narrowed. However, if the angles are wide open, the risk of sudden, catastrophic tension elevation by angle closure is virtually nonexistent, and the history of halos requires other explanation.

Use of drugs

If an angle is found to be wide open, it is safe to use strong miotics, to dilate the pupil, or to use sympathomimetic drugs freely. Such use might be disastrous with a narrow angle because of the risk of precipitating angle closure. If weak miotics should be necessary for the management of narrow-angle glaucoma, the angle should be reevaluated after therapy is initiated. Occasionally miotics further narrow the angle as a result of increased pupillary block.

Preoperative examination

Particularly in eyes with narrow angles, the choice of surgery may rest largely on the gonioscopic findings. If pressure is elevated at a time when the angle is definitely open, even though narrow, iridectomy will probably not cure the glaucoma.

When planning intraocular surgery, one should be sure to note the position of peripheral anterior synechias and large blood vessels. Avoiding such areas may prevent serious complications.

Operative examination

At the time of surgery for the correction of angle-closure glaucoma, gonioscopy can be used to determine the extent and permanence of synechias (Chapter 23). This can be done after iridectomy or by deepening the anterior chamber through a paracentesis before the iridectomy. Gonioscopic control is essential for safe goniotomy (Chapter 26).

Postoperative examinations

The success of iridectomy in opening an angle and of cyclodialysis in producing a suprachoroidal cleft can be promptly evaluated. Reasons for failure can often be detected and guarded against in subsequent operations. After filtering procedures the inner opening can often be seen gonioscopically. If failure of filtration is threatened, the presence of such an opening will encourage an attempt to restore the bleb by plastic procedures on the conjunctiva.

Conditions other than glaucoma

The diagnosis of peripheral tumors or cysts can often be made by gonioscopy. Operability can be determined by an accurate view of the extent to which the iris and ciliary body are involved. Foreign bodies in the angle and holes in the peripheral iris from penetrating foreign bodies may occasionally be discovered. Inflammatory and traumatic conditions such as keratic precipitates covering the meshwork, iridodialysis, etc. can be visually evaluated (Chapter 15).

When a portion of the cornea is hazy, it may be possible by gonioscopy to look through a clear portion of cornea to see the reason for the haze. Tears in Descemet's membrane, epithelial downgrowths, and areas of vitreous adhesions can be diagnosed in this way.

Gonioscopic examples are given in Chapter 30 of the Appendix and the stereo reels.

Summary of important gonioscopic techniques

In clinical practice unusual situations can arise. The following special techniques can be used to arrive at a correct diagnosis.

1. *Flashlight test* (Fig. 12-1). In the absence of slit-lamp or gonioscopic equipment the shallow chamber of the narrow-angled eye can be identified by shining a flashlight across the eye. The iris-lens diaphragm bows forward and produces a shadow on the side opposite the light.

2. *Slit lamp* (Fig. 4-2). The slit-lamp estimation of the angle is helpful in screening patients and is an advantage when contact lens visualization of the angle is poor through a cloudy cornea.

3. *Bilateral gonioscopy* (Fig. 17-5). Comparison of corresponding areas of the angles of the two eyes is facilitated by placing a contact lens on each eye simultaneously. Subtle differences such as unusual iris processes, angle anomalies, peripheral anterior synechias, and areas of angle recession are best identified by this comparison.

4. *Gonioscopy of the fellow eye.* When conditions prevent accurate gonioscopy of the affected eye, examination of the fellow eye may aid in the diagnosis.

5. *Compression gonioscopy* (Figs. 2-7 to 2-9). Indentation of the central cornea with a Zeiss lens widens the peripheral angle. This is useful in a narrow-angled eye to distinguish between areas of iris apposition and permanent periph-

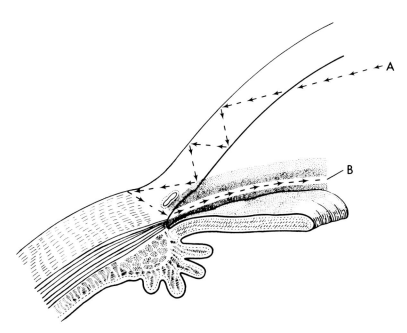

Fig. 4-8. Light directed from point *A* strikes the cornea anterior to the angle and is internally reflected within the cornea and sclera. The pigment in the trabecular meshwork and ciliary body prevents the light from entering the angle. The scleral spur, *B*, lights up brightly. (From Hoskins, H. D., Jr.: Invest. Ophthal. **11**:97, 1972.)

eral anterior synechias. It also helps the examiner estimate the anterior width of a narrow angle, because the additional anatomic structures are exposed and improve orientation.

6. *Management of corneal edema.* Epithelial edema can be reduced by lowering the intraocular pressure, particularly by the use of hyperosmotic agents intravenously, orally, or topically. Mechanical removal of the edematous epithelium is effective and is of particular value in infantile glaucoma.

7. *Retroillumination of the angle structures.* By the use of scleral scatter as in Fig. 4-8, angle structures can sometimes be seen and identified more accurately than with direct illumination.

PROBLEMS FOR CONSIDERATION

Although the anatomic abnormalities in the trabeculum of eyes with open-angle glaucoma can be studied histologically, clinical examination of such changes is not possible at present. Efforts should be made to develop better methods of in vivo examination of the angle, perhaps utilizing techniques of vital staining of ocular tissues. Such methods would enable the clinician to identify defective structures and correlate the findings with impairment of function.

References—Section II

Allen, L., Burian, H. M., and Braley, A. E.: A new concept of the anterior chamber angle, Arch. Ophthal. **62:**966, 1959.

Ashton, N.: Anatomical study of Schlemm's canal and aqueous veins by means of neoprene casts. I. Aqueous veins, Brit. J. Ophthal. **35:**291, 1951.

Ashton, N., Brini, A., and Smith, R.: Anatomical studies of the trabecular meshwork of the normal human eye, Brit. J. Ophthal. **40:**257, 1956.

Barkan, O., Boyle, S. F., and Maisler, S.: On the genesis of glaucoma: an improved method based on slitlamp microscopy of the angle of the anterior chamber, Amer. J. Ophthal. **19:**209, 1936.

Becker, S. C.: Unrecognized errors induced by present-day gonioprisms and a proposal for their elimination, Arch. Ophthal. **82:**160, 1969.

Bill, A., and Svedbergh, B.: Scanning electron microscopic studies of the trabecular meshwork and the canal of Schlemm; an attempt to localize the main resistance to outflow of aqueous humor in man, Acta Ophthal. **50:**295, 1972.

Burian, H. M., Braley, A. E., and Allen, L.: Visibility of the ring of Schwalbe and the trabecular zone, Arch. Ophthal. **53:**767, 1955.

Busacca, A.: Éléments de gonioscopie normale, pathologique, et expérimentale, Saõ Paulo, Brazil, 1945, Tipografia Rossolillo.

Flocks, M.: The anatomy of the trabecular meshwork as seen in tangential section, Arch. Ophthal. **56:**708, 1956.

Forbes, M.: Gonioscopy with corneal indentation; a method for distinguishing between appositional closure and synechial closure, Arch. Ophthal. **76:**488, 1966.

François, J.: La gonioscopie, Louvain, 1948, Editions Fonteyn.

François, J.: In Duke-Elder, S., editor: Glaucoma: a symposium, Springfield, Ill., 1955, Charles C Thomas, Publisher.

François, J., Neetens, A., and Collette, J. M.: Microradiographic study of the inner wall of Schlemm's canal, Amer. J. Ophthal. **40:**491, 1955.

Garron, L. K., and Feeney, M. L.: Electron microscopic studies of the human eye, Arch. Ophthal. **62:**966, 1959.

Gorin, G., and Posner, A.: Slit lamp gonioscopy, Baltimore, 1957, The Williams & Wilkins Co.

Hogan, M. J., Alvarado, J. A., and Weddell, J. E.: Histology of the human eye, Philadelphia, 1971, W. B. Saunders Co.

Hogan, M. J., and Zimmerman, L. E.: Ophthalmic pathology: an atlas and textbook, ed. 2, Philadelphia, 1962, W. B. Saunders Co.

Holmberg, A. S.: The fine structures of the inner wall of Schlemm's canal, Arch. Ophthal. **60:**58, 1959.

Holmberg, A. S.: Our present knowledge of the structure of the trabecular meshwork. In Leydhecker, W., editor: Glaucoma, Tutzing Symposium, Basel, 1967, S. Karger.

Hoskins, H. D., Jr.: Interpretive gonioscopy in glaucoma, Invest. Ophthal. **11:**97, 1972.

Inomata, H., Bill, A., and Smelser, G. K.: Unconventional routes of aqueous humor outflow in cynomolgus monkey *(Macaca irus);* an electron microscopic study, Amer. J. Ophthal. **73:**760, 1972.

Jocson, V. L., and Sears, M. L.: Channels of aqueous outflow and related vessels, Arch. Ophthal. **80:**104, 1968.

Johnstone, M. A., and Grant, W. M.: Pressure-dependent changes in structures of the aqueous outflow system of human and monkey eyes, Amer. J. Ophthal. **75:**365, 1973.

Kayes, J.: Pore structure of the inner wall of Schlemm's canal, Invest. Ophthal. **6:**381, 1967.

Kimura, R.: Color atlas of gonioscopy, Tokyo, 1974, Igaku Shoin, Ltd.

Kupfer, C.: Gonioscopy in infants and children in diagnostic procedures in pediatric ophthalmology, International Ophthalmology Clinics, vol. 3, Boston, 1963, Little, Brown & Co.

Nakamura, Y., and Kitazawa, Y.: A new goniolens for corneal indentation gonioscopy, Acta Ophthal. **49:**964, 1971.

Raviola, G.: Effects of paracentesis on the blood-aqueous barrier, Invest. Ophthal. **13:**828, 1974.

Rohen, J. W.: Electron microscopic studies on the trabecular meshwork in two cases of corticosteroid glaucoma, Exp. Eye Res. **17:**19, Oct., 1973.

Salzmann, M.: The anatomy and histology of the human eyeball (translated by E. V. L. Brown), Chicago, 1912, University of Chicago Press.

Shaffer, R. N.: Stereoscopic manual of gonioscopy, St. Louis, 1962, The C. V. Mosby Co.

Spencer, W. H., Alvarado, J., and Hayes, T. C.: Scanning electron microscopy of human ocular tissues: the trabecular meshwork, Invest. Ophthal. **7:**651, 1968.

Sugar, H. S.: Concerning the chamber angle; gonioscopy, Amer. J. Ophthal. **23:**853, 1940.

Sugar, H. S.: The glaucomas, ed. 2, New York, 1957, Hoeber Medical Division, Harper & Row, Publishers.

Troncoso, M. U.: A treatise on gonioscopy, Philadelphia, 1947, F. A. Davis Co.

Van Beuningen, E. G. A.: Die Bedeutung der spaetlampen Gonioskopie für die Diagnose des primar chronischen Glaukoms, Graefe Arch. Ophthal. **156:**35, 1954.

van Herick, W.: Estimation of width of angle of anterior chamber, Amer. J. Ophthal. **68:**626, 1969.

Vegge, T.: The fine structure of the trabeculum cribriforme and the inner wall of Schlemm's canal in the normal human eye, Z. Zellforsch. **77:**267, 1967.

Zuege, P., Boyd, T. A. S., and Stewart, A. G.: Angle pigment in normal and chronic open angle glaucomatous eyes, Canad. J. Ophthal. **2:**271, 1967.

TONOMETRY AND TONOGRAPHY

The elevated intraocular pressure that characterizes the glaucomas almost always results from impaired outflow of aqueous humor. Tonometry permits the recognition of the abnormal pressure, and tonography affords the opportunity to evaluate the ease of aqueous outflow.

PROBLEMS FOR CONSIDERATION

CHAPTER 5

Intraocular pressure

NORMAL INTRAOCULAR PRESSURE

The intraocular pressure of the nonglaucomatous population approximates a normal (Gaussian) distribution and may be described in statistical terms. By applanation tonometry, mean values of 15.4 ($\sigma \pm 2.5^*$) mm Hg (sitting) and 16.5 ($\sigma \pm 2.6$) mm Hg (reclining) have been obtained. Schiøtz tonometry reveals a mean of 16.1 ($\sigma \pm 2.8$) mm Hg. These values should be considered only approximations, since the actual frequency distribution of intraocular pressures in the population is skewed toward the higher levels. This skewness is the result of several statistically different subpopulations (glaucoma relatives, people of different ages, etc.) that comprise the general population. Each of these subpopulations has its own characteristics of mean intraocular pressure and pressure distribution.

Mean intraocular pressure increases with age and is slightly higher in women than men over the age of 40 years. Pressures measured in the morning are usually higher than those measured in the afternoon or evening. Mean intraocular pressure also increases with elevation of systolic blood pressure.

Definition of glaucoma

Glaucoma may be defined for the individual eye as that intraocular pressure which produces damage to the optic nerve. Because of variations in susceptibility to such damage of optic nerves of different individuals, or perhaps of the same individual at different times, it is impossible to define glaucoma for all eyes in terms of absolute pressure values.

Statistically, an intraocular pressure over 21 mm Hg (mean + 2σ) should occur in less than 2.5% of the normal population, and a pressure of over 24 mm Hg (mean + 3σ) in less than 0.15% of the normal population. Thus, using these values, one can describe a normal range, an abnormal range, and an intermediate twilight zone of suspicious values. It is important to realize, however, that in the

---

*σ is the standard deviation.

individual eye, in the absence of damage to the optic nerve, an abnormal pressure is not necessarily synonymous with impending glaucomatous damage. Furthermore, a "normal" intraocular pressure is merely a statistical concept, and one cannot define glaucoma by the presence of an arbitrary value of intraocular pressure. The concept is useful, however, in identifying the levels of intraocular pressure at which glaucoma is more likely to develop.

Intraocular pressures should be measured in all patients old enough to tolerate the procedure, and values over 21 mm Hg (Schiøtz scale reading: 4.0 with 5.5-gram weight or 6.25 with 7.5-gram weight) should be considered suspicious and a reason for further evaluation. The term *ocular hypertension* has become increasingly more popular in describing such patients. At the present time it is impossible to separate benign ocular hypertension from glaucoma on the basis of measurement of intraocular pressure. Fortunately the opportunity is available to recheck periodically the suspicious pressures as well as the appearance and functional status of the optic nerve. It is extremely important to follow these patients closely, for ultimately, ophthalmoscopy and visual field testing provide the only absolute estimate now available of the pressure a given eye will tolerate. It is hoped that more precise methods will become available for determining the susceptibility of individual optic nerves to pressure damage. Until such time, statistical methods and close observation remain the bases for clinical diagnosis.

MAINTENANCE OF INTRAOCULAR PRESSURE

As postulated by Goldmann, the intraocular pressure (P_0 in mm Hg) varies directly with the rate of secretion of aqueous humor (F in μl/min) and inversely with the facility of aqueous outflow (C)

$$P_0 = F/C + P_V \qquad (1)$$

where P_V = episcleral venous pressure (mm Hg).

Normal intraocular pressure

In the normal eye, variations in aqueous secretion related to diurnal fluctuations, aging, endocrine disturbances, hydration, drugs, surgery, etc. result in alterations in intraocular pressure. However, these are usually of small magnitude and are accompanied by what appear to be compensatory adjustments in outflow facility so as to maintain relatively constant intraocular pressure.

Variations in the volume of blood in the eye can alter intraocular pressure rapidly and markedly. Thus the individual pulse beats produce changes in intraocular pressure, and the variations in blood pressure associated with Traube-Hering waves are recorded in the eye. Acute changes in systemic or carotid blood pressure are reflected in the intraocular pressure. Respiration produces oscillations of intraocular pressure. External pressure, traction of muscles on the globe, forceful lid closing, etc. may result in rapid and large changes in intraocular pressure.

Glaucoma

In most eyes with open-angle glaucoma the outflow facilities are not only reduced but also much less adaptable. This results in a rise in pressure and in greater fluctuations of intraocular pressure with alterations in aqueous secretion. From Equation 1 it is obvious that variations in episcleral venous pressure alter intraocular pressure millimeter for millimeter, but in the absence of impairment of outflow facility, they are only rarely of clinical significance (e.g., mediastinal tumor or carotid-cavernous fistula).

MEASUREMENT OF INTRAOCULAR PRESSURE (METHODS AND ERRORS)

The clinical measurement of intraocular pressure depends on subjecting the eye to a force that indents or flattens it. Either the effect of a particular force or the force for a given effect is measured.

There are two methods in common use for the estimation of intraocular pressure—Schiøtz tonometry and applanation tonometry.

Schiøtz tonometry (Fig. 5-1)

Schiøtz tonometry determines intraocular pressure by applying a carefully standardized instrument to the cornea and measuring the depth of indentation of the cornea by the plunger while it is loaded with a given weight. The scale of Schiøtz tonometers is calibrated in such fashion that each scale unit represents 0.05 mm protrusion of the plunger. The units of indentation may be magnified by

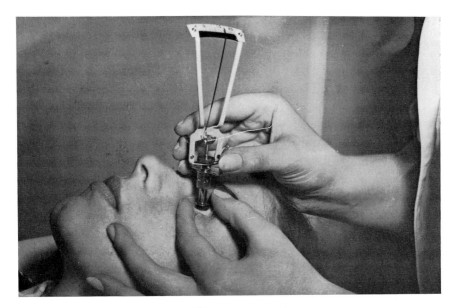

Fig. 5-1. Schiøtz tonometer in use.

mechanical or electronic means. The mechanical tonometer has the advantages of relatively simple construction, extensive clinical use, portability, ease of application, and relatively low cost. The electronic instruments provide larger magnification and an opportunity to obtain continuous readings and permanent records, as in tonography.

Errors in Schiøtz tonometry

Schiøtz tonometry is subject to a number of sources of error. These stem from the use of nonstandard, defective, or dirty instruments or from improper application of the tonometer to the eye (e.g., tilting or pressing on the eye). Also inherent in this type of measurement is the application of a 16.5-gram tonometer to the eye, which causes a large alteration in the intraocular pressure. Although it is just this artificial increase in pressure by the Schiøtz tonometer that is exploited in tonography, the assumption is made in tonometry that all eyes behave in similar fashion when a weight is applied to them. The calibration tables depend on measurements, estimations, and approximations derived from mean values for normal eyes. Unfortunately the indentation of an eye and the pressure elevation so induced depend not only on the weight applied but also on the distensibility of the individual eyes. This distensibility varies from eye to eye and even in the same enucleated eye from one hour to the next. Furthermore, the scale reading of the standard tonometer will vary with the curvature of the cornea.

Because of the difficulty and inconsistency of measurement of the intraocular pressure before the tonometer is placed on the eye (P_0, closed stopcock readings), open manometer measurements were chosen as a basis for calibration. Open manometer calibrations provide accurate estimates of intraocular pressure (P_t) with the tonometer resting on the cornea. These are not much influenced by ocular rigidity and are useful not only in tonometry but also in tonography. The volume of corneal indentation during tonometry (V_c) has been estimated on excised corneas. It varies with corneal curvature, corneal thickness, and plunger weight.

Ocular rigidity

Friedenwald postulated from empirical data that change in ocular volume (ΔV_s) varied as a log function of intraocular pressure in the living human eye. For tonometry, when P_0 is raised to P_t by applying the tonometer, the volume of corneal indentation (V_c) is assumed equal to the distention of the sclera (ΔV_s):

$$\log \frac{P_t}{P_0} = E\Delta V_s = EV_c$$

where E = coefficient of ocular rigidity

or
$$\log P_t = \log P_0 + EV_c \qquad (2)$$

Thus, if $\log P_t$ is plotted against V_c as in the Friedenwald nomogram, straight lines are obtained. The coefficient of ocular rigidity, E, is the slope of the line, and P_0 is the Y intercept. It should be emphasized that this formulation neglects such factors as intraocular blood volume and the expulsion of blood from the eye by the tonometer. It also fails to provide for posterior indentation of the globe by pressure against the orbit and retrobulbar tissues. Such indentation would lead to false overestimates of E. Furthermore, both blood expulsion and the posterior indentation might not be proportional to $\log P_t$ and very likely would vary from one patient to another. In spite of its theoretical limitations, the apparent ocular rigidity remains a usable concept.

Calibration nomograms

With log P and V as coordinates, Friedenwald constructed calibration nomograms, using the experimental data for P_t and V_c for each plunger weight (Fig. 5-2). Curves were obtained that expressed the volume of corneal indentation (V_c) and P_t for each scale reading

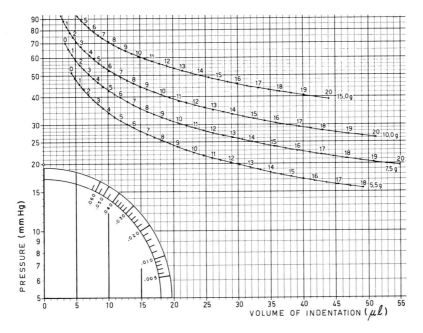

Fig. 5-2. Friedenwald nomogram.

(marked along the curves). Measurements with different plunger weights provide points through which a line can be drawn, giving estimates of E and P₀. Unfortunately the errors in tonometer readings and the relatively small separation of the two points obtained make estimations of ocular rigidity by this method subject to large inaccuracies unless repeated paired measurements are made. The combined use of applanation and Schiøtz tonometry affords better estimates because greater differences in volumes and pressures are utilized for a better definition of the rigidity line.

The tonometry tables for P_0 are calculated from the volume of indentation and P_t values corresponding to a given scale reading, using a mean value for E of 0.0215. If E deviates from this value, the true P_0 may be calculated from Equation 2, found in Tables 28-8 and 28-9, or estimated graphically using the Friedenwald nomogram (Figs. 5-2, 28-1, and 28-2).

It is now apparent that more accurate estimates of P_t values and V_c are possible. Furthermore, in the enucleated eye E as formulated may not be independent of intraocular pressure. Since E is constant with pressure as measured by injections in the living human eye, questions have been raised as to the variable role of blood expulsion and posterior indentation of the globe in tonometry. Much more calibration data are needed on the cannulated living human eye with the use of the newer and more accurate methods. Recent findings merely confirm the prediction of Friedenwald about calibration tables, that "there can never be a final and absolutely correct tonometer calibration" and his anticipation of "further revisions as additional data are obtained." However, at this writing the 1955 scales appear consistent and a close approximation to the truth. It is wise, however, to record Schiøtz readings as scale reading and weight used (e.g., 4.0/5.5 or 6.5/10), for these findings remain meaningful and independent of calibration revisions.

Footplate hole

It has been found that an additional important source of error, particularly in electronic tonometers of the Schiøtz variety, stems from an abnormally large footplate hole. Under these circumstances the cornea protrudes into the hole in the footplate at small indentations of the plunger (low-scale readings). This results in an overestimation of intraocular pressure in tonometry and a tonographic tracing falsely resembling hypersecretion. The error is best avoided by insisting on scale readings greater than "four"—that is, using sufficient weight to produce at least an indentation of four scale units.

Applanation tonometry

Applanation tonometry provides a simple and reliable method for measuring intraocular pressure. In the tonometer devised by Goldmann, pressure is measured directly as the force required to flatten a standard area of cornea (3.06 mm diameter). Since the applanation tonometer does not displace much fluid (approximately 0.5 μl) or increase the pressure in the eye significantly, this method is almost independent of ocular rigidity (Fig. 5-2). Furthermore, when applanation readings are compared with Schiøtz readings, the best available estimates of the ocular rigidity coefficient, E, are obtained (Figs. 28-1 and 28-2). In addition, the method is little influenced by variation in corneal curvature.

Method of applanation tonometry (Fig. 5-3)

Applanation tonometry may be carried out with the Goldmann applanation tonometer mounted on a Haag-Streit, Zeiss, or other slit lamp. In this ingeniously devised instrument the force is supplied by a calibrated coil spring or by a weight, and the area of contact is accurately obtained by a double prism. After administration of drops of 0.5% proparacaine (Ophthaine), 0.4% benoxinate (Dorsacaine), or similar topical anesthetic (but not tetracaine [Pontocaine]), the tear fluid is made fluorescent by a sterile fluorescein paper strip moistened with isotonic sodium chloride solution or distilled water. It is best not to use anesthetic solutions to wet the paper strip, for they tend to quench the fluorescence. Fluress, a combination of benoxinate anesthetic and fluorescein may also be used. The patient and examiner sit in the usual positions at the slit lamp. The prism is cleaned with distilled water. The blue filter is placed in front of the open slit beam, and the beam is aimed at the black line on the prism from a wide (60°) angle. With the patient looking straight ahead, the instrument under low power (10×), and the drum set at 1.0 gram, the prism is moved forward with the control stick until it just makes contact with the eye. At this point the limbus is illuminated. If necessary, the lids may be retracted manually but with care to avoid pressure on the globe. Two semicircles are seen through the right ocular (6×). The microscope is raised or lowered until the two semicircles are equal in size.

It is possible to center the mires before touching the cornea. As the tip of the prism nears the cornea, two blue semicircles can be seen through the ocular. When these are centered, no further adjustment of the yellow-green semicircles will be needed after contact with the cornea. The tonometry can be completed more quickly and with a minimum of corneal trauma. The method is particularly helpful in small children and in eyes with nystagmus or defects in the corneal epithelium. The spring knob is turned until the semicircles interlock, the inner edge of the upper overlapping the inner edge of the lower symmetrically with each

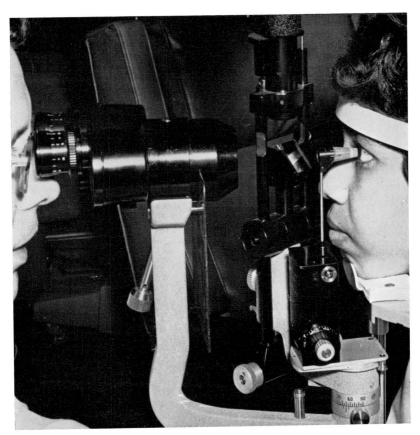

Fig. 5-3. Applanation tonometry with Haag-Streit model 900 slit lamp.

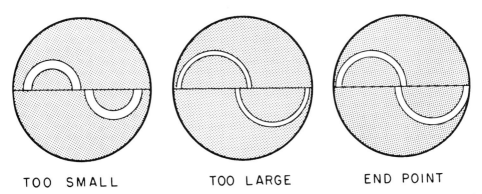

TOO SMALL   TOO LARGE   END POINT

Fig. 5-4. Pattern as seen through the microscope. The arcs are fluorescein-stained tear fluid and are light green against a blue background.

pulsation of the eye (Fig. 5-4). The reading on the drum at this point multiplied by 10 is an estimate of intraocular pressure in mm Hg. If the semicircles cannot be made to overlap, the whole instrument is too far away. If the semicircles cannot be separated, the instrument is too far forward. If there is marked corneal astigmatism, it is recommended that the prism be rotated so that the dividing line is at a 43° angle to the major axis. This is easily done by setting the red line on the prism holder at the major axis on the prism scale.

Horizontal applanation tonometry

Several modifications of the applanation tonometer have been devised to permit its use with the patient in the horizontal position.

The two most successful of these are the Draeger applanation tonometer (Fig. 5-5) and the Perkins applanation tonometer (Fig. 5-6). These hand-held, self-illuminated, portable instruments have a counterweight that balances the tonometer in any position. This permits accurate applanation tonometry completely independent of the position of the patient or eye. The area of cornea applanated is the same as in the Goldmann instrument (3.06 mm diameter). The force is applied by means of a built-in electric motor (Draeger) or spring (Perkins), and the readings are read directly from a scale projected into the eyepiece. Overlapping semicircles are aligned as in the Goldmann applanation tonometer, and measurements between the instruments correlate well. These tonometers are valuable additions, especially for the examination of supine patients and children under general anesthesia.

Halberg has recently developed a hand-held applanation tonometer that seems reliable and easy to use. With the use of a carrier, a 5-gram applanating cylinder is lowered onto the surface of the cornea. The area applanated is accurately measured by a built-in millimeter scale, and the measurement translated into mm Hg of intraocular pressure by use of a conversion table. The instrument is almost maintenance-free, and results correlate well with the Goldmann tonometer.

The Mackay-Marg electronic tonometer provides another method for applanation tonometry in the horizontal patient. Readings are automatically recorded on a continuous running tape, and the results appear accurate when the tonometer is used with topical anesthesia. Multiple measurements can be rapidly made, and a permanent record is obtained. The instrument is expensive and has not received wide acceptance by ophthalmologists. It is a useful instrument for animal research and is used by many optometrists because the rapidity of the measurement permits its use without anesthesia. Unfortunately such readings are not as accurate as those obtained with topical anesthesia. In eyes with corneal edema Mackay-Marg measurements are said to be more accurate than Goldmann applanation readings.

Noncontact applanation tonometry

An applanation tonometer has recently been developed that measures intraocular pressure without contact between the instrument and the eye. Applanation

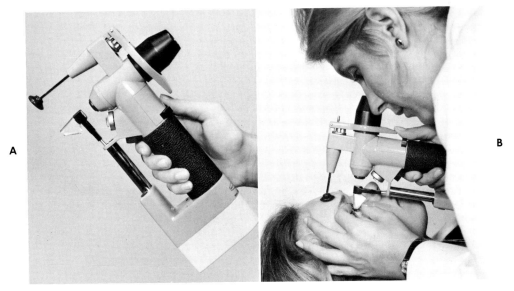

A

B

Fig. 5-5. A, Draeger applanation tonometer. **B,** Tonometer in use on a reclining patient.

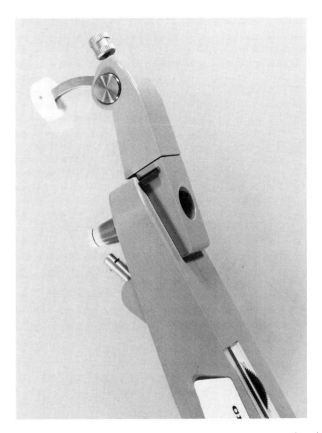

Fig. 5-6. Perkins hand-held tonometer. This tonometer is as accurate but less costly than most other hand-held applanation tonometers.

of the cornea is produced by a controlled air pulse of linearly increasing force. A monitoring system senses light reflected from the corneal surface and records a maximal signal at the instant of applanation. The interval of time required for the air pulse to produce applanation is proportional to intraocular pressure, and the reading is achieved within a few milliseconds. The instrument is calibrated against the Goldmann applanation tonometer, and clinical results appear to correlate well except at very high levels of intraocular pressure. It is, however, expensive. Also, vision must be adequate to fixate a target, and the corneal surface must be clear enough to provide a reflex for recording.

Errors in applanation tonometry

Sources of error in applanation tonometry stem largely from poor technique and inadequate experience of the examiner. Other errors include failure to calibrate the instrument, squeezing by the patient, permitting the lids to touch the prism, and various types of corneal irregularities due to edema, scars, etc.

Another important source of error in applanation tonometry results from the use of inadequate concentrations of fluorescein in the tear fluid. Furthermore, topical anesthetic solutions quench the fluorescence of fluorescein. Under these circumstances the lack of visibility of the tear fluid edge (apex of wedge of meniscus) results in an overestimation of the area of applanation and thus an underestimation of the intraocular pressure.

Sterilization of tonometers

The problem of tonometer sterility has been a most difficult one. Ultraviolet lamps and heat devices greatly delay use of the instrument and are far from foolproof. Chemical sterilization with such agents as benzalkonium chloride (Zephiran) fails to destroy viruses and spores. Most ophthalmologists have resolved the problem for the mechanical Schiøtz tonometer by cleaning all parts of the disassembled tonometer with alcohol and ether. For the electronic tonometer, water and Kimwipes are usually used. The use of sterile disposable latex covers (Tonofilms) has been demonstrated to be effective for both mechanical and electronic Schiøtz tonometers and to produce only insignificant changes in the estimates of intraocular pressure or outflow facility. Similar latex covers are used for the Mackay-Marg tonometer. It is common practice merely to wash off the Goldmann applanation tip with a sterile sponge moistened with sterile water or benzalkonium chloride. Unfortunately such practice does not produce complete sterilization of the tip, and use of the applanation tonometer in infected eyes should be avoided. In a two-part study, Corboy and associates found mechanical rinsing and wiping to be as effective as prolonged germicidal immersion in dealing with bacteria and virus particles. Spread of ocular infection from the hands of medical personnel is considered the greater hazard by some.

CHAPTER $\bigcirc$

Outflow facility

The volume of fluid per unit of time that will flow out of the eye is proportional to the pressure gradient across the trabecular meshwork

$$F \propto (P_0 - P_V)$$

where F = rate of aqueous flow (μl/min)
         P_0 = intraocular pressure in the undisturbed eye (mm Hg)
         P_V = episcleral venous pressure (mm Hg)

or $$F = C(P_0 - P_V)$$ (3)

where C = proportionality coefficient (outflow facility)

METHODS OF MEASUREMENT
Flow and pressure measurements

From these equations it is apparent that the coefficient of outflow facility may be computed from measurements of intraocular pressure, episcleral venous pressure, and rate of aqueous flow by the use of the following equation:

Outflow facility = Outflow per minute/pressure gradient
$$C = F/(P_0 - P_V)$$ (4)

Fluorescein method

The only methods of measurement of flow that have been applied clinically in this fashion are those that involve the turnover in the anterior chamber aqueous humor of intravenously administered fluorescein. This method is tedious, requires elaborate instrumentation, and is subject to serious errors, but it permits determinations on the relatively undisturbed eye. Careful measurements have resulted in outflow facility values averaging 0.33 in normal human eyes. Most importantly these measurements established that the outflow facility is decreased in most of the glaucomas. As will be demonstrated presently, other methods for measurement of flow have been devised. Some of these have been applied to animal eyes and provide estimates of outflow facility from the previous equations.

Perfusion at constant pressure

A more direct method of measuring outflow facility is to perfuse the eye either in vitro or in vivo. Under these circumstances a volume of fluid (I in μl/min) is forced through the

69

eye under a given pressure head (P_I in mm Hg), and outflow facility (C) in vivo is measured from the equation

$$C = I/(P_I - P_0) \qquad (5)$$

where P_0 = intraocular pressure in the undisturbed eye. In vitro, $P_0 = 0$ and the equation is simplified to the following:

$$C = I/P_I \qquad (6)$$

In practice, it is easiest to perfuse at different pressure levels and to plot inflow pressure P_I (mm Hg) against inflow I ($\mu l/min$). From the slope of such plots a measure of C may be obtained; P_0 may be estimated from the intercept on the pressure axis. This method suffers from the large artifact associated with the introduction of a cannula into the anterior chamber and induced alterations in volume of the anterior chamber, but it is independent of ocular rigidity, corneal curvature, and calibration tables. Mean values of approximately 0.28 for human eyes are obtained by in vitro perfusion.

Measurements in vitro suffer from the various artifacts induced by postmortem changes in surviving tissue. However, alterations in blood volume, rate of secretion, and smooth muscle tone are avoided. Most important therefore is the finding that average values obtained by perfusion in vivo and in various laboratories are all in good agreement. Furthermore, fluorescein turnover and tonography also provide estimates that are all reasonably similar. Most impressive is the agreement obtained between tonography and perfusion values when the methods are applied to the same human eye, either normal of glaucomatous, in those few instances in which this has proved possible. In animal eyes comparisons of perfusion, tonography, and flow measurements also reveal values that agree well.

Perfusion by abrupt rise in pressure

The introduction of a known volume of fluid into the eye produces a sudden rise in intraocular pressure. The time course of the decrease in pressure that follows this disturbance of the equilibrium state can be utilized to estimate the outflow facility. The analysis of such pressure decay curves involves the conversion of the pressure changes to volume of aqueous leaving the eye per unit of time at the induced pressure gradient. Unfortunately pressure decay curves are subject to many of the artifacts mentioned in the discussion of tonography that follows. The results obtained agree qualitatively with other estimates of outflow facilities, but constant-pressure perfusion is to be preferred.

Tonography
Theory

Tonography affords one of the most convenient methods for the estimation of outflow facility. It is based on the old observation that massage of an eye lowers intraocular pressure. This effect is marked in normal eyes but occurs at a slower rate in glaucomatous eyes. Tonography attempts to quantitate the massage effect by the use of a tonometer to express fluid from the eye. It is carried out by placing a Schiøtz type tonometer on the eye for a prolonged period of time and recording the progressive indentation of the cornea by the plunger. Under these circumstances the pressure in the eye is raised abruptly from its pretonography level (P_0, the steady state pressure in the undisturbed eye) to a higher pressure ($P_{t_{av}}$, the average intraocular pressure during tonography), and the pressure decay curve recorded. With tonometry continued for 4 minutes, a volume of fluid (ΔV) is expressed from the eye as the intraocular pressure falls toward its steady state value. The rate in microliters per minute at which this occurs at a given pressure gradient is a measure of the outflow facility coefficient (C):

$$C = \frac{\Delta V}{4}/(P_{t_{av}} - P_0) \qquad (7)$$

It is necessary to examine the assumptions inherent in this tonography formulation of Grant more closely if one is to appreciate the significance of the values obtained and the sources of error. Unfortunately a number of tonographic investigations reported in the literature as well as a considerable part of tonography as performed clinically fail to take these potential errors into account.

Assumptions of tonography. When a Schiøtz tonometer is allowed to rest on the cornea, the immediate consequence is an indentation (V_{c_1}) of the cornea by the plunger, an increase in intraocular pressure to (P_{t_1}) because of the weight of the instrument, and a distention of the ocular coats (to V_{s_1}). The distention is the result of the corneal indentation, and the volume of distention is equal to the volume of corneal indentation. During tonography the fluid lost from the eye permits a further indentation ($\Delta V_c = V_{c_2} - V_{c_1}$) of the cornea by the plunger, a decrease in intraocular pressure (to P_{t_2}), and a contraction of the ocular coats ($\Delta V_s = V_{s_1} - V_{s_2}$). In addition, other possible changes during tonography include alterations in blood volume in the eye (V_B), episcleral venous pressure (P_V), the rate of aqueous secretion (F), and the outflow facility coefficient (C). The more general equation for all these changes may be written as follows:

Outflow facility = Outflow per minute/outflow pressure gradient

$$C_t \quad = \frac{\Delta V_s + \Delta V_c + \Delta_{VB} + F_t T}{T} /(P_{t_{av}} - P_{v_t}) \tag{8}$$

where
F_t = rate of aqueous secretion during tonography
T = time in minutes
ΔV_s = decrease in scleral distention during tonography
ΔV_c = increase in corneal indentation during tonography
ΔV_B = change in blood volume in eye during tonography
$P_{t_{av}}$ = average pressure in the eye during tonography
P_{v_t} = episcleral venous pressure with tonometer on the eye
C_t = facility of aqueous outflow in the eye with tonometer in place

If (1) there is no change in rate of aqueous secretion caused by the weight of the tonometer during tonography, that is, $F_t = F = C(P_0 - P_V)$;
(2) there is no change in blood volume in the eye during tonography ($\Delta V_B = 0$);
(3) episcleral venous pressure during tonography is the same as in the undisturbed eye ($P_{v_t} = P_V$); and
(4) facility of aqueous outflow with a tonometer on the eye is the same as that in the undisturbed eye ($C_t = C_0$);
then Equation 8 is simplified to

$$C_t = C_0 = \frac{\Delta V}{T}/(P_{t_{av}} - P_0)$$

where $\Delta V = \Delta V_c + \Delta V_s$.

Values for corneal indentation (V_c) and ocular distention (V_s) are available for all tonometric scale readings, as are values of P_t and P_0 (Tables 28-2, 28-3, 28-5, and 28-7).

Since $\Delta V = \Delta V_c + \Delta V_s = [V_{c_2} - V_{c_1}] + 1/E \log\dfrac{P_{t_1}}{P_{t_2}}$ (9)

where E = coefficient of ocular rigidity
P_t = intraocular pressure during tonometry
tables may be set up for values of V for all plunger readings where

$$V = V_c - 1/E \log P_t \tag{10}$$

Grant formulated such tables, setting $V = 0$ for scale reading 0 and assuming $E = 0.0215$. From these tables ΔV may be determined by simple subtraction (Table 28-4). Then from tables of P_t and P_0 (Tables 28-2 and 28-3) C may be computed by the use of Equation 7.

Possible errors in tonography

From these assumptions and approximations many of the sources of error in tonography become apparent. These include errors of instrumentation, variations of the individual eye, reactions of the eye to the tonometer, patient response, and operator errors.

Errors of instrumentation. Tonography is dependent on estimation of pressure and volume inferred from tonometer calibrations. Although the 1955 calibration tables appear to be reasonably accurate, they are subject to uncertainties and revision. In addition, there are inaccuracies in the calibration and standardization of the individual tonometer. Other instrumental errors in the practice of tonography include sticking of a dirty plunger, variations in line voltage, and magnetic material near the tonometer. Such instrumental variations as unusual plunger diameters and edge curves, curvature of the test block, and variations in plunger weight fortunately tend to be self-compensating in tonography insofar as outflow facility is concerned.

Variation of the individual eye. Individual eyes may vary from the assumed average value of corneal curvature. The corneal curvature may be precisely measured by a keratometer, and tables are available for applying correction factors (Table 28-6). In practice variations in corneal curvature are largely self-compensating in tonography and alter very little the values obtained.

As indicated previously, variations in ocular rigidity influence the Schiøtz tonometer reading enormously. This may produce false estimates of not only intraocular pressure but also outflow facility. Details of methods for correcting for ocular rigidity are described in the Appendix. It is important to appreciate that deviations from normal ocular rigidity rarely alter the empirical impression as to presence or absence of glaucoma and its status of control. In practice, ocular rigidity corrections are used only occasionally.

Variations in viscoelastic properties of the individual eye may provide an important source of error. The depth of the anterior chamber has been demonstrated to alter outflow facility in the perfused eye. There is no evidence that this has any influence on tonography as applied clinically.

Reaction of the eye to the tonometer. The eye may respond to the pressure rise induced by the tonometer in a number of ways.

Aqueous secretion. In the living eye the secretion of aqueous humor is a metabolic process and is subject to nervous and vascular influences. Tonography asumes that the eye is in a steady state and that no disturbances are induced in the eye except the increased rate of outflow of aqueous humor produced by the tonometer. Evidence indicates that such is not the case. Studies have demonstrated that aqueous secretion decreases as intraocular pressure increases. Such a change in aqueous formation during tonography gives an overestimation of outflow facility. This overestimation has been termed *pseudofacility,* and appears to account for about 20% of the total tonographic facility in normal eyes (about 0.06 μl/min/mm Hg). Pseudofacility is independent of trabecular outflow and therefore accounts for a larger portion of the tonographic outflow facility in glaucomatous eyes.

Blood volume. The living eye contains a large vascular bed. In tonography it is assumed that any changes induced in blood volume of the eye by the tonometer are vary rapid and that no further alterations in blood volume occur during tonography. Within the limits of error of measurements with labeled red cells, this assumption is approximately true for the cat eye. However, variable expulsion of blood from the human eye during tonography remains a distinct possibility, at least in some eyes. The problem is difficult to resolve, for even small percentage changes in total ocular blood volume could represent large fractions of the relatively small volume of fluid expressed from the globe during tonography.

Episcleral venous pressure. In the original formulation episcleral venous pressure was assumed to remain unaltered when the tonometer was applied to the eye. It has been demonstrated that episcleral venous pressure actually increases (ΔP_V) by an average of 1.25 mm Hg on application of the tonometer. This increase persists during tonography. The formula for tonography thus requires a correction factor.

$$C = \frac{\Delta V}{T} / [P_{t_{av}} - (P_0 + \Delta P_V)] \qquad (11)$$

Table 6-1. Comparison of tonography with perfusion in vivo and in vitro on human eyes

Method	Outflow facility					
	Patient 1	Patient 2	Patient 3	Patient 4	Patient 5	Patient 6
Tonography	0.27	0.22	0.20	0.25	0.27	0.28
Perfusion in vivo	0.26	0.21	0.21	0.24	0.29	0.27
Perfusion in vitro	0.29	0.24	0.23	0.26	0.35	0.33

This correction factor has been incorporated in current tables (Table 28-1). However, there is some evidence that the increase in episcleral venous pressure may be greater than this mean value in normal eyes. Ideally the magnitude of the correction factor should be computed for each eye. It is possible that this might better separate normal from glaucomatous eyes.

Constancy of outflow facility. Finally, it is assumed that the outflow facility is not altered by the application of the tonometer and that outflow facility remains constant at various presssures. There are some indications in the literature that outflow facility values are lower when obtained with heavier weights. However, when the 1955 tables are used, this is less often seen, and outflow facility is essentially the same with all weights. Furthermore, outflow obtained in the undisturbed eye by turnover measurements agrees well with that obtained during tonography. On the other hand, in the individual eye, reflex, vascular, or other changes in outflow facility induced by the tonometer cannot be ruled out, and the correctness of the 1955 tables remains open to scrutiny.

Patient response. Gross abnormalities in the tonogram are induced by the patient's squeezing, blinking, breath holding, pain, sleeping, loss of fixation, fear, distraction by noises, coughing, cardiac irregularities, changes in blood pressure, contraction of extraocular muscles, etc. (Figs. 29-22, 29-24 to 29-26).

Operator errors. Operator errors include improper retracting of the lids, fingers pressing on the globe (Fig. 29-6), inadequate cleaning of the tonometer (Fig. 29-23), poor positioning of the tonometer or tilting of the instrument, disturbing the patient, inadequate reassurance of the patient, lack of attention, improper calibration, incorrect calculations or use of the wrong weight table, use of the wrong weight, etc.

Validity of tonography

In spite of the many possible errors, careful tonography provides a reasonable estimate of the outflow facility in the living eye.

Comparison with other methods. The major evidence for the validity of tonography measurements stems from a comparison of average values with those obtained by other methods. In particular, in those instances in which it has been possible to compare perfusion in vivo and in vitro with tonography on the same human eyes, the agreement has been excellent (Table 6-1). Comparisons with outflow facility determined from turnover studies have been largely confined to animals. Here again, reasonable agreement has been established.

In general, the agreement of various methods is better when comparative measurements are made on the same eye than when absolute values are required. From the clinical point of view *it is also the comparative measurements that are of much more interest than the individual measurement.* This is as true of tonography as of other laboratory procedures.

Constant-pressure tonography. Constant-pressure tonography has been developed as a method to avoid the errors induced by variations in ocular rigidity and the pressure decay artifacts. As with constant-pressure perfusion, this is accomplished by maintaining P_t and ocular distention (ΔV_s) constant during tonography. In constant pressure tonography, all volume changes are estimated from corneal indentation (ΔV_c). The values obtained for outflow facility are reasonably similar to those obtained by conventional tonography. Unfortunately the method is still too experimental for clinical use at the present time.

●　　●　　●

In conclusion it is apparent that many of the errors inherent in tonography can be avoided, are partially self-compensating, or can be corrected by application of suitable factors. As will be seen from the discussion that follows, in spite of all potential and actual sources of error, tonography remains a useful empirical tool in clinical diagnosis and evaluation of therapy of the glaucomas.

Method of tonography (Fig. 6-1)

In practice, tonography is carried out with an electronic tonometer connected to a suitable recorder. A voltage regulator and meter are needed to assure minimal variations of line voltage. After a warm-up period of at least 30 minutes and after the 0 and 7 settings on the test block are adjusted, the tonometer is calibrated for each scale division protrusion of the plunger (0.050 mm), with a suitable micrometer gauge (Fig. 6-2). Calibration should be repeated at least daily. Before and after each use, the tonometer must be cleaned with distilled water and dried with lint-free material, for example, Kimwipes.

It is wise to perform applanation tonometry before tonography to provide data for estimates of ocular rigidity as well as to determine the weight necessary for tonography. Horizontal applanation measurements avoid the variable effects of position on intraocular pressure. They may be performed just prior to the tono-

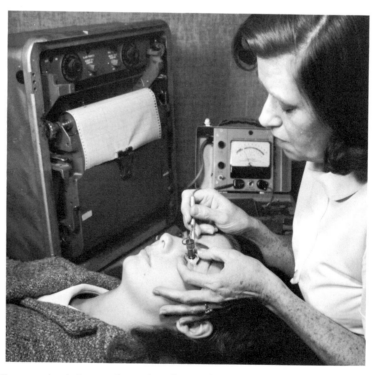

Fig. 6-1. Tonography being performed with an electronic Schiøtz tonometer connected to a Leeds & Northrup recorder.

grams without change of position of the patient. If applanation readings are under 20 mm Hg, tonography is carried out with a 5.5-gram weight; between 20 and 29 mm Hg, the 7.5-gram weight is used; at 30 mm Hg and over, the 10-gram weight is required. The applanation measurements do not appear to alter the subsequent tonogram.

Technique of tonography (Fig. 6-1). With the patient lying comfortably and fixating on a small red or white light, tonography is carried out for 4 minutes on each eye. The tonometer should be held over the eye for 20 to 30 seconds and lowered to the cornea gently and without the patient's knowledge. Caution must be exercised to avoid tilting the tonometer or pressing on the globe with the fingers used for retracting the lids. The tonography room should be isolated and free of interruptions, noises, distracting lights, and visitors. Fixation must not be interrupted, and the scale indicator should show definite pulsations.

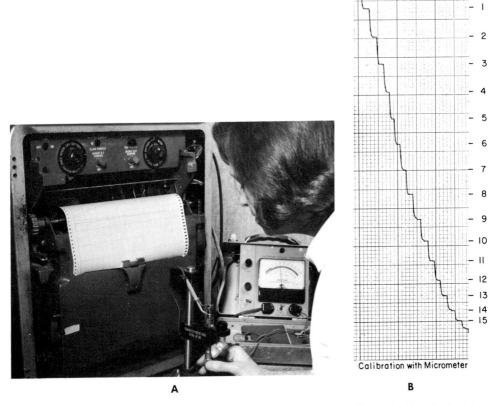

Calibration with Micrometer

A   B

Fig. 6-2. A, Calibration of tonometer with a micrometer gauge. The technician looks into a prism, which permits visualization of an enlarged image of the micrometer gauge. **B,** Example of calibration with a micrometer. The figures on the right-hand side represent scale readings.

For the water-drinking tonogram the initial tonogram is done in the fasting (over 4 hours) state. The patient is then asked to drink 1 L of water in 5 minutes. Applanation tonometry and tonography are repeated 40 minutes later.

Calculations (Fig. 6-3)

From the best smooth curve through the tonographic tracing, the initial intraocular pressure (P_0) and outflow facility (C) are estimated. It must be emphasized that, with the exception of eyes with markedly impaired outflow facilities, the tracing is *not a straight line*. The line curves because of the usual manner of approach to a steady state, because of viscoelastic properties of the eyes, and because the scales of some tonometers and many recorders are compressed at higher scale readings. The 1955 Friedenwald tables provide the values for P_t, P_0, and ΔV needed for the calculations (Tables 28-2 to 28-4 in the Appendix). $P_{t_{av}}$ can be determined by averaging P_t values (in mm Hg) for each 30 or 60 seconds, by taking the mean of the logarithm of the P_t values, and less accurately by merely averaging arithmetically the initial and final P_t values. For convenience, nomograms and tables have been derived that provide at a glance the P_0 and C values (Table 28-1). These tables include a correction for an average increase in P_V (1.25 mm Hg) during tonography. This avoids repeating the calculations for each tracing.

Table 28-1 does not give meaningful values for outflow facility if used for only the latter part of a tonographic tracing. If one insists on using the last 2 or 3 minutes of tracing, the entire calculation must be made, and an estimate of P_0 must be obtained, either by applanation tonometry or from the beginning of the tonogram.

Ocular rigidity. Corrections of the tonograms for ocular rigidity are rarely necessary. They can be accomplished by algebraic or graphic means. The graphic method is demonstrated in Figs. 28-1 and 28-2. The algebraic method consists of correcting $\Delta V_{s_{av}}$ for the rigidity of the individual eye (Table 28-7).

In a tonogram with a 5.5-gram weight, which starts at scale reading 4.5 and reaches 6.5 at 4 minutes, the effects of various ocular rigidity coefficients on values for pressure and out-

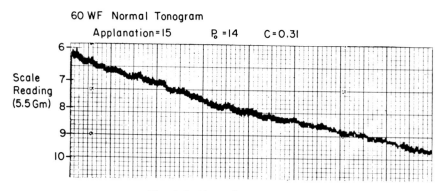

Fig. 6-3. Normal tonogram.

Table 6-2. Effects of ocular rigidity coefficient on interpretation of tonogram (initial reading, 4.5/5.5-gram weight; at 4 minutes, 6.5/5.5-gram weight)*

	A	*P_0*	*C*	*P_0/C*
Average rigidity (0.0215)	19.5	19.0	0.18	106
Low rigidity (0.0135)	23.5	23.0	0.38	61
High rigidity (0.0315)	15.5	15.0	0.11	136

*See Figs. 28-1 and 28-2 and Table 28-7.
A = applanation reading.
P_0 = intraocular pressure corrected for ocular rigidity.
C = outflow facility.

flow facility are calculated in Figs. 28-1 and 28-2 and Table 28-7 and are summarized in Table 6-2. It is seen that whereas a correction for ocular rigidity changes the P_0 and C values and the interpretation of the mechanism of glaucoma involved, it does not usually remove such a borderline tracing from the group of eyes in which glaucoma is suspected. Thus, in the case of average ocular rigidity, a C of 0.18 is a borderline value. With the correction for an assumed low ocular rigidity, C is estimated at 0.38 and P_0 as 23 mm Hg, values high enough to arouse suspicion of hypersecretion glaucoma. When the tonogram is corrected for an assumed high ocular rigidity, P_0 is as low as 15 mm Hg but C equals 0.11, and one must conclude that this is an eye with poor facility of outflow but in a hyposecretory phase.

The use of the applanation and Schiøtz tonometers provides a better estimate of ocular rigidity than Schiøtz tonometry with two weights. However, routine corrections are not advocated and rarely alter the management of the individual patient. At present it is believed to be worthwhile to recognize large deviations from normal rigidity only if they are repeatable and to understand the nature and direction of the corrections to be applied. It is also well to appreciate the self-correcting features of tonography in this regard.

Suction cup decay curves

Raising the intraocular pressure by occluding the outflow with a suction cup provides another method for following the rate at which intraocular pressure returns to its steady state. This method is in principle the same as the abrupt introduction of fluid into the eye (perfusion) or the application of a Schiøtz tonometer (tonography). The greater the obstruction to outflow (the lower the facility of outflow), the longer it will take for sufficient fluid to leave the eye to restore intraocular pressure to its original value.

In practice, the suction cup is set at –50 mm Hg pressure and is applied to the anesthetized eye for 10 to 15 minutes. The intraocular pressure is measured by applanation or Schiøtz tonometry before application of the cup, immediately after its removal, and at intervals of 1 to 3 minutes thereafter for 15 to 20 minutes or longer. To estimate the volume of fluid leaving the eye per minute per outflow pressure gradient, it is necessary to convert the measurements of changes in pressure to volume of aqueous leaving the eye. As in tonography or perfusion, this depends on pressure-volume relationships (ocular rigidity) for the individual eye.

The results reported with suction cup decay curves are usually in qualitative agreement with the tonographic findings on the same eyes. The quantitative results of suction cup decay leave much to be desired, however. They do not agree well with other clinical information about the patient or with perfusion data on the same eyes in vitro. The lack of agreement occurs in a disappointingly large number of both normal and glaucomatous eyes. All the errors inherent in non-constant pressure methods must play some role in creating the discrepancies. These include changing blood volume in the eye, variations in ocular rigidity, alterations in aqueous secretion, and various calibration problems. Most important, however, is the introduction by the suction cup of additional artifacts of large magnitude, which have definite clinical importance. These must account for the greater discrepancies found by this method than by tonography. The suction cup was designed to occlude outflow channels of the eye. It has been shown to result in a temporary reduction of outflow facility after the cup is removed. The measurement of outflow facility is thus made at a time when this factor is considerably reduced and during recovery from the trauma. In addition, the suction cup has been demonstrated to produce a variable suppression of aqueous secretion, and this is also in process of recovery during the decay curve. Since these are variable effects in the individual eye, correction factors cannot be applied.

In summary, the suction cup decay curve method suffers from the fact that the method alters the very parameters it seeks to measure. In its present state it has limited clinical usefulness. However, with the accumulation of as much clinical data as are available for tonography, certain important empirical correlations may become available.

NORMAL OUTFLOW FACILITY AND ITS VARIATIONS

The mean value for outflow facility in a large population of normal patients as measured tonographically was 0.28 ($\sigma \pm 0.05$). Thus values less than 0.18 occur in less than 2.5% of the normal population, and values below 0.13 are seen in less than 3 in 2000 normal eyes. As with intraocular pressure, there are differences in mean values for outflow facility in the various subpopulations comprising the general population. The statistical concept of "normalcy" is useful, so long as one is careful not to equate the absence of normalcy with the presence of disease.

Site of resistance

In enucleated normal eyes some 75% of the resistance to outflow is in the trabecular meshwork as demonstrated by the dissections of Grant. Calculations and perfusion of particles in the normal human eye suggest critical openings of approximately 1 μm or less. As indicated in Chapter 3, pores of this size are indicated by electron microscopy to be present in the cells of the inner wall of Schlemm's canal.

Mucopolysaccharides

In vitro, in rabbit eyes it has been demonstrated that a part of the perfusion resistance to outflow can be reduced by hyaluronidase injected into the interior chamber. In some human eyes, especially those with malignant melanomas of the choroid, a homogeneous material has been demonstrated in the trabecular meshwork, which stains with iron or Alcian blue or metachromatically with toluidine blue and can be removed by hyaluronidase. The amount of acid mucopolysaccharides present may provide another mechanism for control of outflow facility. The mucopolysaccharides may be formed locally by endothelial cells of the trabecular meshwork or may be filtered from the aqueous humor, being carried from vitreous humor or from the internal limiting membrane on the surface of the ciliary epithelium. Their clinical significance in vivo remains obscure.

Anterior chamber volume

In vitro, outflow facility varies with the volume of the anterior chamber. This effect of volume change in the enucleated human eye may well be a mechanical one on the meshwork. However, within reasonable limits, variations in the depth of the anterior chamber do not appear to be of clinical significance. Except in some of the angle-closure glaucomas, the changes in anterior chamber volume produced by the tonometer either do not alter outflow facility or compensate for other consequences of the tonometer application, for example, effects of the pressure increase on the trabecular meshwork.

Comparisons of various species also demonstrate that outflow facility varies with the volume of the anterior chamber. The large anterior chamber of the cat is associated with a facility some twenty times that of the guinea pig. Interestingly, the value of the ratio $C/(\text{volume of anterior chamber})$ is reasonably constant for all species studied.

Effects of accommodation and trabeculotomy

Outflow facility is increased by stimulation of the ciliary ganglion (in intact cats or their enucleated eyes) and during accommodation in man—probably the effect of traction by the muscles of the ciliary body on the scleral spur and trabecular meshwork. Total trabeculotomy markedly increases the outflow facility in the enucleated eye and abolishes the response to deepening the chamber or stimulating the ciliary ganglion. Partial trabeculotomy (30° of circumference) produces only a limited increase in outflow, which is somewhat increased by deepening the anterior chamber. This suggests that there is a resistance to circumferential flow in Schlemm's canal that is reduced by traction on the scleral spur and trabecular wall.

Effects of superior cervical ganglionectomy

Twenty to 24 hours after excision of the superior cervical ganglion in rabbits there is a dramatic decrease in outflow resistance (increase in outflow facility) and fall in intraocular pressure on the ganglionectomized side. Apparently this effect on outflow facility results from the release of alpha-adrenergic substances into the anterior chamber. By one week after ganglionectomy, outflow facility is subnormal because of the absence of catecholamines. At this time the outflow mechanism is exquisitely sensitive to *l*-norepinephrine, responding with large increases in outflow facility to as little as 20 mμg injected into the anterior chamber.

Changes with age

Outflow facility declines with age in both animal and human eyes. This is observed by tonography as well as by turnover studies. A part of the decrease may be accounted for by progressive decrease in the volume of the anterior chamber with age, due to the increase in lens size, etc. The decrease in outflow facility appears to be a structural change, for it persists in vitro as demonstrated by perfusion.

Endocrine factors

The variations of facility of outflow with the menstrual cycle and the large increase of facility during pregnancy suggest direct or indirect endocrine factors of control.

The effects of corticosteroids on intraocular pressure are described in more detail in Chapters 14 and 15. When corticosteroids are administered systemically, there is a tendency in some individuals for a decrease in outflow facility and an increase in intraocular pressure. The topical application of corticosteroids results in much more dramatic changes in outflow facility and intraocular pressure. Interestingly enough, the greater degrees of responsiveness are seen in patients with primary open-angle glaucoma and in their close relatives. Evidence has been accumulated that the degree of responsiveness is genetically determined. It is becoming increasingly apparent that large human populations can be divided into three reasonably discrete categories on the basis of their pressure response to topical corticosteroids. By means of family studies, it is suggested that the group which responds minimally represents a homozygous nonresponsive group (nn). Those individuals who demonstrate a dramatic pressure elevation to values in the thirties and forties after six weeks of topical betamethasone or dexamethasone closely resemble patients with primary open-angle glaucoma and are believed to be homozygous responders (gg). By such steroid testing, there is suggestive evidence that one can delineate the heterozygous responsive state (ng), and these individuals may be the carriers of primary open-angle glaucoma.

The pressure elevation induced in a susceptible person by topical corticosteroids resembles primary open-angle glaucoma. It demonstrates decreased outflow facility, increased intraocular pressure, and positive water provocative test. If pressure elevations are continued, cupping and field loss appear. The individual is usually asymptomatic and free of pain. If the induced pressure elevation is sufficiently high (sixties), corneal edema may appear. The corticosteroid pressure elevations can be reversed or modified by miotics, epinephrine, and carbonic anhydrase inhibitors in much the same fashion as in the glaucomatous eye. When topical corticosteroids are discontinued, outflow facility and intraocular pressure return slowly to normal values. Very recent field loss usually improves slowly, but long-standing field loss persists. It is not known at the present time whether spontaneous primary open-angle glaucoma will occur at a later time in eyes demonstrating a marked pressure response to topical corticosteroids.

Effects of therapy

Resistance to outflow can be altered by surgery (filtering operations) or by drugs (e.g., parasympathomimetic and anticholinesterase agents). The former is largely mechanical, but the latter may act at a cellular or enzymatic level or by muscular effects on the size and shape of the trabecular spaces. The effects of miotics on facility of outflow can be demonstrated to be independent of the pupillary action.

Effects of water drinking

The hemodilution produced by the consumption of large volumes of water results in decreases in outflow facility and elevations of intraocular pressure. In rabbits it can be demonstrated that with large enough volumes of water (by stomach tube) the normal rabbit eye will respond in this fashion. Animals with developmental glaucoma respond more dramatically to smaller volumes of water. Thus, when lesser amounts of water are used, significant changes are noted only in the glaucomatous eye. As indicated in Chapter 8, the same principle has been applied to the clinical detection of primary open-angle glaucoma. It is also of considerable interest that one can demonstrate decreases of outflow facility in perfused human and monkey eyes by the use of hypotonic perfusion fluids. The in vitro perfusion changes are associated with swelling of the trabecular endothelium, especially of the endothelium lining Schlemm's canal. A unilateral open-angle glaucomatous state closely resembling primary open-angle glaucoma has been induced by means of topical corticosteroids. Before any other changes were noted, consumption of 1 L of water was found to decrease outflow facility and raise intraocular pressure exclusively in the corticosteroid-treated eye.

Compensatory changes

In addition, there is some evidence that outflow facility may change in compensatory fashion with variations in aqueous secretion so as to maintain a relatively normal intraocular pressure (e.g., decrease in outflow facility after carotid ligation or acetazolamide administration). Such changes may be neurogenic or neurovascular. Nerve endings have been found in the trabecular meshwork, but their nature and function remain obscure. Conceivably a decrease in outflow facility when secretion is reduced may reflect nutritional or other effects on the capacity of the outflow mechanism, resulting from the decreased rate of aqueous flow.

It is clear that the mechanisms of regulation and alterations of outflow facility remain largely unknown. There are undoubtedly neurogenic and reflex controls, structural and cellular changes, and mechanical and muscular effects as well as endocrine, chemical, and enzymatic alterations. Methods are needed for more accurate determination of the mechanisms involved.

ABNORMAL OUTFLOW FACILITY

In glaucoma the outflow facility is impaired. This has been demonstrated by tonography, fluorescein-turnover studies, pressure-decay curves after suction cup, and perfusion in vivo and in vitro. In angle-closure glaucomas this impairment results from obstruction to outflow by the approximation of iris and trabecular meshwork. In the glaucomas with open angles the obstruction is probably in the trabecular meshwork itself.

In those eyes with primary open-angle glaucoma that have been studied by microdissection, the increased resistance has been found in the trabecular meshwork and is probably localized in its outermost portion bordering Schlemm's canal (juxtacanalicular meshwork or "pore" tissue). Attempts have been made to correlate the appearance of the trabecular meshwork in both normal eyes and those eyes suffering from chronic simple glaucoma with the tonographic and perfusion outflow facility measurements.

Pathology of the trabecular meshwork

In addition to the increasing collection of autopsy specimens, valuable biopsy material of the trabecular meshwork has been provided by sclerectomy, trabeculectomy, and trephine buttons removed from eyes with chronic simple glaucoma. It is most important that such studies be correlated with functional studies (perfusion and tonography) as well as with pressure damage to the optic nerve to determine which pathologic findings relate to glaucoma. In glaucomatous eyes histologic changes occur in both the trabecular sheets and the tissue adjacent to the inner wall of Schlemm's canal. In routine light microscopy there appears to be hypercellularity and thickening of the juxtacanalicular tissue. Electron microscopy of trabeculectomy specimens from such eyes demonstrates focal deposits of homogeneous osmiophilic material between the cell layers of this juxtacanalicular tissue. In advanced stages, the entire region is filled with osmiophilic plaques of this kind (Fig. 6-4). Similar deposits, but to a much lesser extent, may be seen in eyes of elderly nonglaucomatous patients. The nature of this material and how (or if) it contributes to the reduced outflow facility in glaucoma are unknown.

Changes in the trabecular sheets in advanced glaucoma may also be quite pronounced. Thickening of the basement membranes of the entire trabecular meshwork occurs, the trabecular sheets become thickening and hyalinized, and the spaces between them are narrowed. Electron microscopy confirms the increased thickness of the trabecular sheets (more than twice the normal values). This increased thickness occurs in spite of marked thinning of the central collagen core and is largely accounted for by an enormous increase in the surrounding homogeneous matrix with clumps of material of 1000 Å periodicity (Fig. 6-5).

Attempts to correlate the changes in the trabecular meshwork of human eyes with the clinical status of the patient and more specifically with the outflow facility have been most interesting. Thus, as summarized in Table 6-3, moderate and marked degrees of alterations in structure are seen much more commonly in glaucomatous eyes (24 out of 26) than in eyes believed to be normal (4 out of 56). It is also of interest, in view of recent genetic studies, that approximately

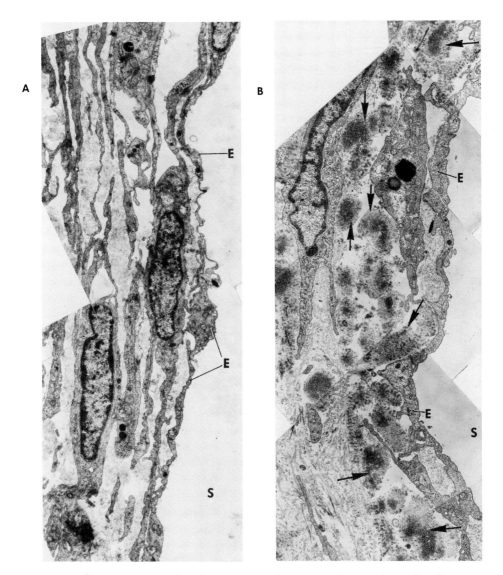

Fig. 6-4. Electron micrographs of juxtacanalicular tissue obtained by trabeculectomy in, **A,** normal and **B,** glaucomatous eyes. Note thickening of the juxtacanalicular zone in glaucoma caused by deposition of osmiophilic material (arrows) between the cell layers. *E,* Inner wall endothelium; *S,* lumen of Schlemm's canal. (**A,** ×7000; **B,** ×10,000.) (From Rohen, J. W., and Witmer, R.: Graefes Arch. Klin. Exp. Ophthal. **183:**251, 1972.)

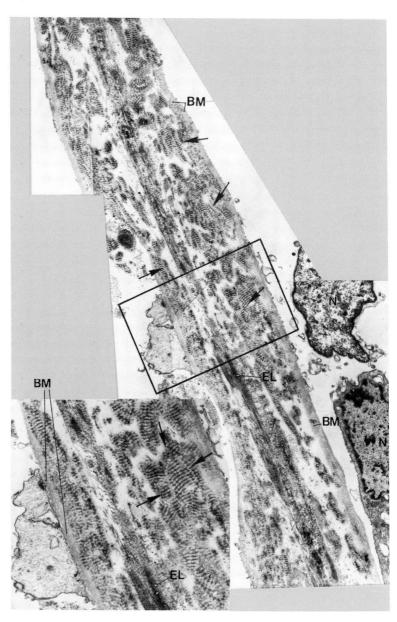

Fig. 6-5. Sagittal section through hyalinized trabecula in open-angle glaucoma. (Trabeculectomy specimen, ×7500; inset, ×15,000.) Note thickening of the basement membranes, marked widening of the trabecular sheet, and massive deposits of lattice (curly) collagen (arrows). Compare with Fig. 3-10, made at almost the same magnification. *BM,* Basement membrane; *EL,* elastic fibers; *N,* nuclei. (From Rohen, J. W., and Witmer, R.: Graefes Arch. Klin. Exp. Ophthal. **183:**251, 1972.)

Table 6-3. Histologic changes in the trabecular meshwork compared with clinical diagnosis

	Clinical diagnosis	
Trabecular pathology	Normal (number of eyes)	Open-angle glaucoma (number of eyes)
None	38	0
Minimal	14	2
Moderate	4	9
Marked	0	15
Total	56	26

Table 6-4. Comparison of tonographic or perfusion outflow facility and histologic changes in the trabecular meshwork

Trabecular pathology	Number of eyes	Outflow facility (mean)
None	20	0.28
Minimal	5	0.18
Moderate	8	0.11
Marked	10	0.05

one third of "normal" eyes demonstrated trabecular disease. Furthermore, those eyes with marked changes had C values averaging 0.05; those with moderate changes, 0.11; and those with minimal alterations, 0.18 (Table 6-4). Eyes without trabecular abnormalities had perfusion values for C that averaged 0.28.

With the use of fluorescein-labeled antihuman gamma globulin the presence of gamma globulin has been demonstrated in the trabecular meshwork of eyes with proved primary open-angle glaucoma (Fig. 6-6). In addition, the trabecular meshwork of the same eyes has demonstrated the presence of plasma cells. Although these changes are not seen in all eyes with open-angle glaucoma and occasionally can be found in some routine autopsy eyes, their more frequent occurrence in primary open-angle glaucoma is statistically highly significant (Table 6-5). Questions are thus raised as to possible roles of immunogenic mechanisms in the pathogenesis of primary open-angle glaucoma. It remains to be determined whether such mechanisms play a primary role or are merely secondary to the effects of the glaucomatous process or a reaction in the trabecular meshwork to antiglaucomatous medications. The relationship of gamma globulin and plasma cells to the material found deposited in the juxtacanalicular tissue in glaucoma is also unknown.

Unfortunately, as demonstrated in Tables 6-3 and 6-5, occasional areas of localized proliferation of endothelial cells of the inner wall of Schlemm's canal, gamma globulin, and plasma cells are seen in some apparently "normal" human eyes at autopsy. It is not known whether these eyes represent unrecognized glaucoma that has not yet produced damage to the optic nerve or perhaps a manifestation of the carrier genetic state. It is also unknown whether any of the changes

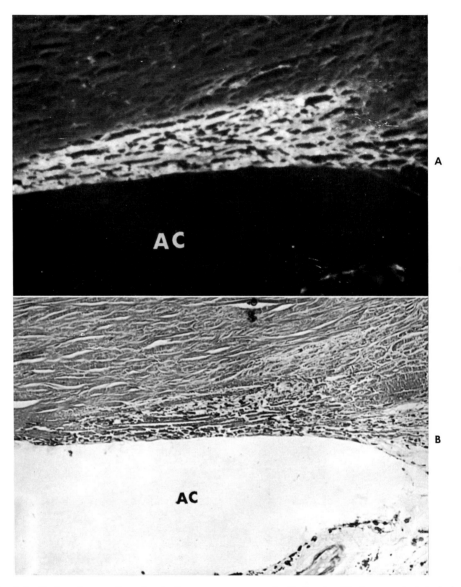

Fig. 6-6. Trabecular meshwork of glaucomatous eye. **A,** Stained with fluorescein-labeled antihuman gamma globulin. **B,** Same section stained with hematoxylin and eosin. *AC,* Anterior chamber. (From Becker, B., Keates, E. U., and Coleman, S. L.: Arch. Ophthal. **68:**643, 1962.)

Table 6-5. Gamma globulin and plasma cells in trabecular meshwork (comparison of routine autopsy eyes and trephine buttons and eyes of patients with proved primary open-angle glaucoma)

Diagnosis	Number of eyes	Number of eyes staining for gamma globulin	Number of eyes with plasma cells
Primary open-angle glaucoma			
Eyes	28	22 (79%)	23 (82%)
Buttons	52	39 (75%)	37 (71%)
Total glaucoma	80	61 (76%)	60 (75%)
Routine autopsy eyes	65	9 (14%)	13 (20%)

described are the cause or a consequence of the elevated intraocular pressure. It is hoped that further histologic and electron microscopy studies of the meshwork in eyes carefully evaluated by gonioscopy, tonography, perfusion, and response to topical corticosteroids will resolve this important problem. The opportunities afforded for a careful study and comparison of the histochemistry and ultrastructure of the chamber angles of both eyes when one eye is subjected to topical corticosteroids may help to answer many questions about the pathology and pathogenesis of primary open-angle glaucoma.

The obstruction to outflow in phacolytic and some of the various secondary glaucomas is often apparent. However, others such as siderogenic glaucoma appear to have open angles and much the same pictures in the trabecular meshwork as are seen in primary open-angle glaucoma.

UVEOSCLERAL OUTFLOW

Throughout the previous discussions attention has been directed toward the outflow of aqueous via the trabecular meshwork–Schlemm's canal system. The presence of a uveoscleral pathway for aqueous outflow has been demonstrated in the monkey but not yet studied in man. In the monkey, aqueous passes from the anterior chamber along the longitudinal muscle fibers of the ciliary body to the choroidal vessels and even through the sclera. This pathway is not altered by changes in intraocular pressure and so does not enter into the calculation of tonographic outflow facility. It does, however, account for a significant portion of outflow of aqueous from the eye (about 0.50 μl/min in the monkey). The presence of this pathway is not considered in the estimation of aqueous flow by Equation 3, p. 69. Therefore, by the use of this equation, the rate of aqueous production is underestimated, assuming the uveoscleral outflow pathway exists in the human eye.

In the monkey, pilocarpine decreases uveoscleral outflow and atropine increases it—just the reverse of the actions on aqueous flow through the trabecular meshwork. For pilocarpine to lower intraocular pressure, therefore, it must first overcome this effect on uveoscleral outflow.

CHAPTER **7**

Formation of aqueous humor

In recent years considerable information has been added to our knowledge about the formation of aqueous humor. This has been a consequence of the use of radioisotope and microchemical techniques, better mathematical analysis, and the availability of carbonic anhydrase and sodium-potassium activated adenosinetriphosphatase inhibitors.

The aqueous humor is a relatively cell-free, protein-free, transparent fluid secreted by the epithelial cells of the ciliary processes into the posterior chamber. It passes through the pupil into the anterior chamber and leaves through the trabecular meshwork to Schlemm's canal and the venous system. In the anterior chamber the aqueous humor is subject to thermal currents because of the temperature difference between the iris and the cornea. During its passage through the eye its composition is altered by diffusional exchange with the blood as well as by the metabolism of the ocular tissues. In addition, evidence suggests that its composition may be modified by active transport processes out of the eye.

ANATOMY OF THE CILIARY PROCESSES (Fig. 7-1)

Each ciliary process consists of a central core of stroma and blood vessels covered by a double layer of epithelium derived from the two layers of the embryonic optic cup. The inner layer, facing the vitreal chamber, is continuous with the nonnervous retina of the pars plana and with the nervous retina; it contains sparse melanin granules. The outer layer, containing numerous melanin granules, is the homologue of the pigment epithelium of the retina and is often referred to as the pigmented layer. Electron microscopic findings have revealed some of the complexity of the ciliary epithelium (Figs. 7-2 to 7-6).

Internal limiting membrane (Figs. 7-2 and 7-3)

In contrast to the sheetlike and faintly fibrillar basement membrane between the retina or pars plana and the vitreal chamber, the basement membrane covering the ciliary body may in areas be vastly more complex. In part, this complexity is due to the surface of the ciliary epithelium, which may vary from smooth to

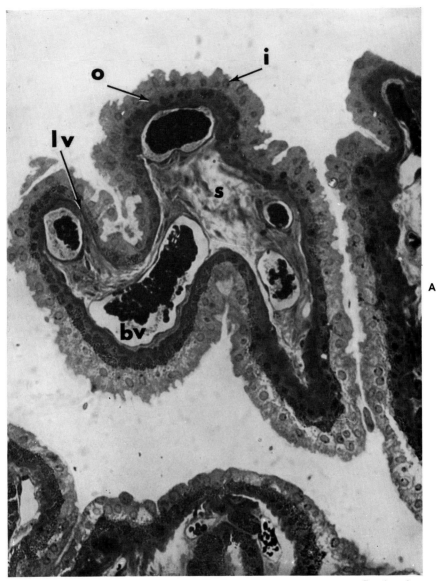

Continued.

Fig. 7-1. A, Light micrograph of a cross section of a ciliary process of the human eye, showing the inner, *i,* and outer, *o,* layers of the epithelium and the underlying lamina vitrea, *lv.* The stroma, *s,* with sectioned blood vessels, *bv,* comprises the core of the process. (×270.) **B,** Low-power electron micrograph of the human ciliary epithelium. *PC,* Posterior chamber; *ILM,* internal limiting membrane; *NPE,* nonpigmented epithelium; *PE,* pigmented epithelium; *EN,* endothelial cell; *CAP,* capillary. (**A** courtesy Dr. A. I. Cohen, St. Louis; **B** courtesy L. Feeney, San Francisco.)

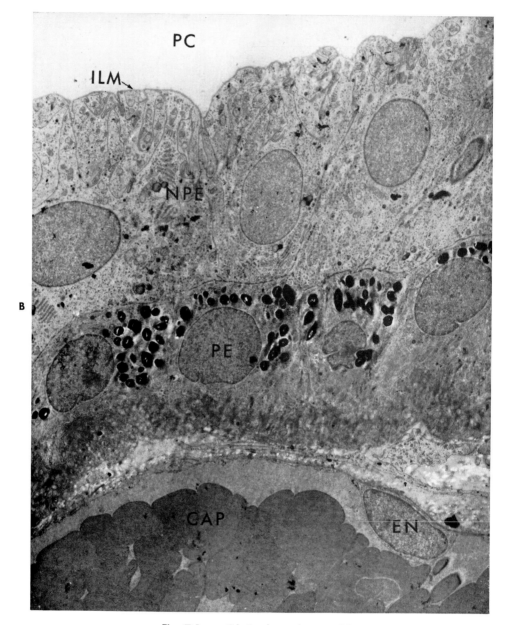

Fig. 7-1, cont'd. For legend see p. 89.

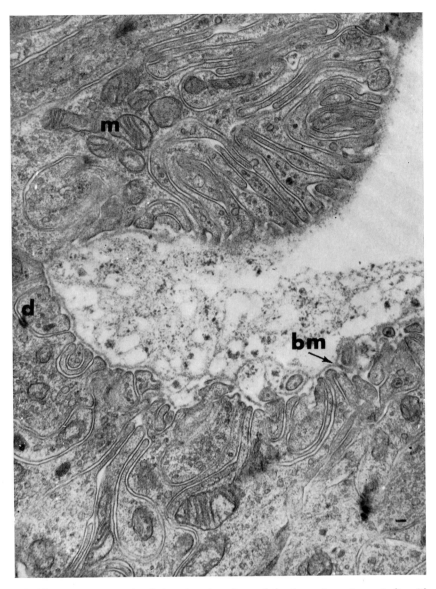

Fig. 7-2. Electron micrograph of the vitreal surface of the inner (nonpigmented) epithelial layer of human ciliary epithelium, showing the highly plicated surface, mitochondria, *m*, desmosomes, *d*, and the complex basement membrane, *bm*, or inner limiting membrane. Note the amorphous material trapped in what appears to be spongelike basement membrane and its resemblance to some cytoplasmic material. (×21,000.) (Courtesy Dr. A. I. Cohen, St. Louis.)

highly irregular, with numerous knobs and projections of the epithelial cells as well as the grosser foldings of the ciliary processes. Although uncomplicated in the former areas, in the latter the basement membrane often appears in sections to be replicated into a spongy meshwork with the spaces in the meshwork often exhibiting amorphous dense material as well as components resembling those seen in the epithelial cells and possibly extruded by or from them.

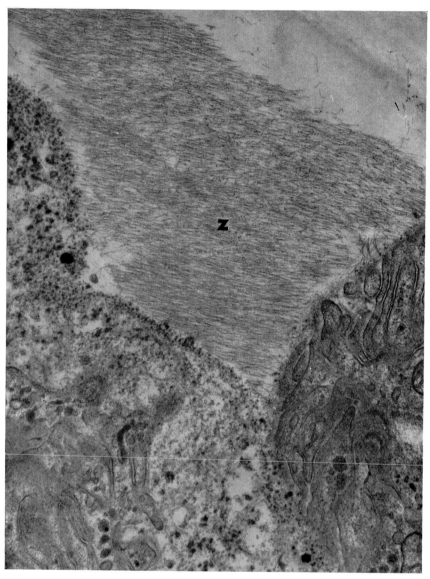

Fig. 7-3. Electron micrograph of the surface of human ciliary epithelium, showing zonule fibers, Z, apparently infiltrating the basement membrane material comprising the inner limiting membrane. (×30,000.) (Courtesy Dr. A. I. Cohen, St. Louis.)

Some components of the meshwork appear to be rich in acid mucopoly-saccharides, as demonstrated by staining with colloidal iron, Alcian blue, and toluidine blue. The acid mucopolysaccharide stains are much less intense after incubation of sections with hyaluronidase, suggesting that at least a part of the acid mucopolysaccharide is sensitive to this enzyme. The thickening of the basement membrane becomes more pronounced with age. Electron micrographs further reveal that the zonule fibers filter into the basement membrane (Fig. 7-3). In the pars plana area, bundles of fibers penetrate the inner limiting membrane and run a tangential course through the intercellular spaces of the nonpigmented epithelium.

Inner epithelial layer
(Figs. 7-2 to 7-5)

The cells of the inner epithelial layer are 10 to 15 μm in height and appear cubical or cylindrical. Adjacent cells are interdigitated elaborately by processes resembling flattened sheets and may further be united on their lateral aspects by desmosomes of the macula densa variety. The cells possess numerous mitochondria, membranous saccules studded with ribosomes, oil droplets, and some pigment granules, the latter being more numerous in cells toward the iris root. In addition, small apical vacuoles of varying diameter often appear to have a fibrous or granular content. At times these may be so numerous in the apex of a cell as to constitute the predominant cytologic feature. Cytoplasmic fibrillar material is also evident on occasion. The most prominent anatomic, and most important functional, features of these cells are the interdigitations at the apical and lateral borders plus the abundance of mitochondria in the cytoplasm and well-developed rough endoplasmic reticulum. These features are characteristic of cells engaged in active transport of salts and fluids.

Outer or pigmented epithelial layer
(Figs. 7-4 and 7-5)

The outer or pigmented layer of cells is characterized by numerous melanin granules and appears united to the inner layer by a combination of desmosomes of the macula densa type and by tight junctions or zones (zonulae occludens) where the usual intercellular gap of 200 Å is reduced to about 100 Å. In addition to possible mechanical strengthening, such tight junctions have been shown in other tissues to permit the electrotonic spread of current or the passage of small molecules or ions, thus bypassing the extracellular phase between adjoining cells. Tight junctions also have been seen to occur between the lateral aspects of cells of the outer layer and sometimes between the membrane of a fingerlike process of one of these cells and the membrane of a neighboring cell indented by the process. The cells also may exhibit patches of fibrillar cytoplasmic material of unknown character. When these cells are depigmented, acid mucopolysaccharides may be demonstrated by Alcian blue or colloidal iron staining.

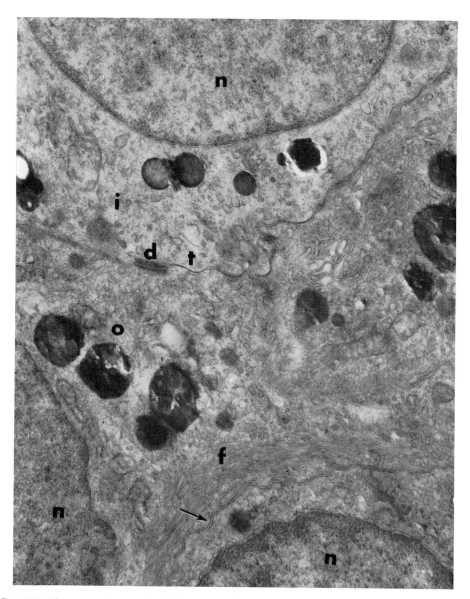

Fig. 7-4. Electron micrograph of the junction of the inner, *i*, and outer, *o*, layers of the human ciliary epithelium. Note that the membranous junction contains desmosomes, *d*, of the macula densa type as well as tight, *t*, or occluded zones. Note cytoplasmic fibrous material, *f*, cell nuclei, *n*, and pigment granules. Arrow points to a nonspecialized cell junction for purposes of comparison. (×24,400.) (Courtesy Dr. A. I. Cohen, St. Louis.)

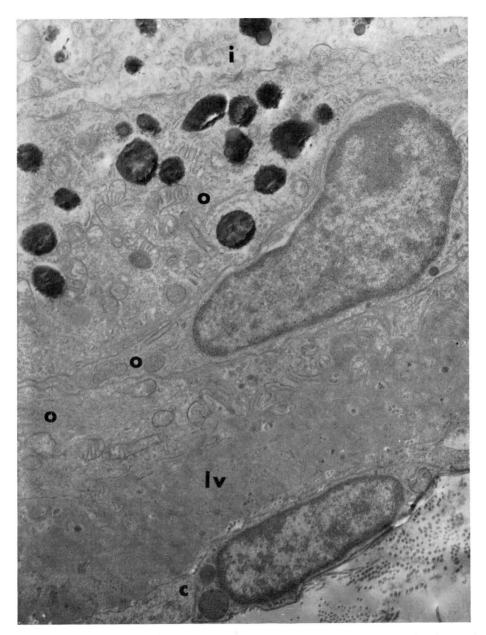

Fig. 7-5. Electron micrograph of human ciliary epithelium, showing several imbricated cells of outer or pigmented layer, *o*, and the edge of a cell of the inner layer, *i*. Below the outer cells is the lamina vitrea, *lv*, penetrated by processes of the outer cells and connective tissue fibers. Below the lamina vitrea is a connective tissue cell, *c*. (×12,800.) (Courtesy Dr. A. I. Cohen, St. Louis.)

Lamina vitrea (Fig. 7-5)

Below the outer epithelial layer is a thick basement membrane, the homologue of the lamina vitrea or Bruch's membrane of the pigment epithelium of the retina. It often contains thick collagenous bundles, other extracellular fibrils, and cell processes extending from the cells of the outer epithelial layer as well as from connective tissue cells commonly seen in the stroma of the ciliary processes. Occasionally nerve cell processes may be observed here. Sections of the undulating contours of the ciliary processes often result in oblique views in which the thickness of the lamina vitrea varies and is often exaggerated, but it is substantially thicker than the internal limiting membrane or other basement membranes of the eye. It thickens with age and becomes especially thickened in diabetics.

Stroma

The stroma consists of a gel-like volume in which are found connective tissue cells as well as extracellular fibers of at least two varieties, one a collagen with typical banding and the other of finer diameter. The capillaries of the stroma are typically thin walled and resemble the choroid capillaries of the pigment epithelium of the retina except that the ciliary body capillaries exhibit relatively fewer focal attenuations or pores. The capillaries have a basement membrane that is not interrupted over the pores (Fig. 7-6). The pores probably facilitate movement of substances into and out of the capillary lumen.

The blood supply of the ciliary processes is derived from the greater arterial circle of the iris, formed by anastomoses of two long ciliary arteries entering the eye posteriorly in the horizontal meridian and the anterior ciliary arteries entering at the muscle insertions.

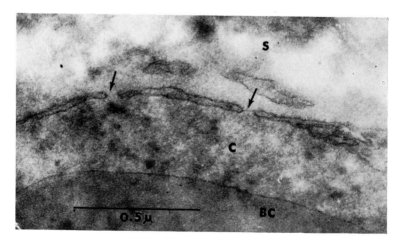

Fig. 7-6. Capillary wall with two pores (arrows). C, Capillary lumen; BC, part of a red blood corpuscle; S, ciliary stroma. Rabbit eye. (×84,000.) (From Holmberg, A.: Arch. Ophthal. **62:**949, 1959.)

CHEMICAL COMPOSITION OF AQUEOUS HUMOR

Evidence that the aqueous humor is the product of secretion includes the finding that, as formed in the posterior chamber, it differs from plasma in its concentration of several constituents. It is convenient to express aqueous humor values as a fraction of blood plasma concentration in the same animal at the same time. Most of the work along these lines has been done in the rabbit, but limited posterior chamber as well as anterior chamber data are also available on the guinea pig, monkey, and man.

In Table 7-1 are compared the relative concentrations of bicarbonate, ascorbate, chloride, protein, and hydrogen ions of aqueous humor from the posterior and the anterior chambers of rabbit eyes. It is seen that there are large excesses of bicarbonate and ascorbate and deficits of chloride, protein, and hydrogen ions, the greatest deviations from plasma values occurring in the posterior chamber. In the anterior chamber there is a tendency for equilibration with plasma values. The data for monkeys are more limited (Table 7-2). Here, too, there are greater deviations from plasma in the posterior chamber fluids than in the anterior chamber fluids. As compared with plasma concentrations, the monkey eye has an excess of hydrogen and chloride ions and a deficit of bicarbonate ions. Interestingly enough, the composition of aqueous humor in the monkey eye differs considerably from that of the rabbit and resembles more closely that of spinal fluid. The composition of human aqueous humor resembles closely that of the monkey, whereas the guinea pig aqueous humor is similar to that of the rabbit. All four species have large excesses of ascorbate and lactate in the aqueous humor, the former on the basis of secretion and the latter largely accounted for by glycolytic activity of the lens, cornea, and other ocular structures.

Table 7-1. Average steady state composition of rabbit aqueous humor*

Constituent	Posterior chamber	Anterior chamber
Chloride	0.88	0.94
Hydrogen ion	0.70	0.80
Bicarbonate	1.70	1.35
Ascorbate	57	44
Protein	0.007	0.009

*Expressed as fraction of plasma concentrations in mM/kg water.

Table 7-2. Average steady state composition of monkey aqueous humor*

Constituent	Posterior chamber	Anterior chamber
Chloride	1.25	1.11
Hydrogen ion		1.60
Bicarbonate		0.76
Ascorbate	19	15

*Expressed as fraction of plasma concentrations in mM/kg water.

Carbonic anhydrase inhibition

In all species studied, the partial suppression of secretion of aqueous humor that follows the systemic administration of carbonic anhydrase inhibitors results in alterations in the relative concentrations of these important constituents. As shown in Table 7-3, the concentrations of Cl^-, H^+, and HCO_3^- ions and proteins show less deviations from plasma values after carbonic anhydrase inhibition. On the other hand, the transport of ascorbate into the eyes of various species appears to be less inhibited than is the entry of water, resulting in substantial rises in ascorbate concentrations, especially in the posterior chamber. As might be anticipated, the decreased rate of flow that follows carbonic anhydrase inhibition results in a rise in aqueous lactate concentrations, probably as a consequence of the relative stagnation produced.

Sodium-potassium activated adenosinetriphosphatase inhibition

The injection of cardiac glycosides such as ouabain into the vitreous humor of rabbit eyes results in profound reduction in intraocular pressure. Tonography reveals no change in outflow facility and suggests a reduction of secretion to one third that of the contralateral control eye. As summarized in Table 7-4, the concentration of bicarbonate is not altered in the aqueous humor secreted into the posterior chamber, demonstrating an equal suppression of water and bicarbonate transport. The concentration of bicarbonate in the anterior chamber falls toward plasma levels exactly as predicted for a two-thirds reduction in rate of aqueous flow and the greater time provided for diffusional exchange. Similarly, although

Table 7-3. Effect of acetazolamide on the composition of anterior chamber aqueous humor*

Constituent	Man		Rabbit		Guinea pig	
	Before	After	Before	After	Before	After
Chloride	1.08	1.02	0.94	0.96	0.90	0.93
Hydrogen ion	1.53	1.30	0.70	0.89	0.73	0.83
Bicarbonate	0.83	0.94	1.35	1.11	1.42	1.19
Ascorbate	15	18	44	52	17	24
Protein	—	—	0.009	0.011	—	—

*Expressed as fraction of plasma concentrations.

Table 7-4. Effect of intravitreal ouabain (0.5 μg) on composition of rabbit aqueous humor*

Constituent	Posterior chamber		Anterior chamber	
	Control	Ouabain-treated	Control	Ouabain-treated
Bicarbonate	1.42	1.43	1.25	1.13
Ascorbate	55	90	46	52
Protein	0.007	0.008	0.009	0.016

*Expressed as fraction of plasma concentrations.

posterior chamber protein is altered very little, the anterior chamber concentration is increased because of the reduced flow rate and more time for diffusion into the anterior chamber from the plasma. As found after carbonic anhydrase inhibition, the ascorbate concentration of the fluid secreted into the posterior chamber increases dramatically, again suggesting less inhibition of ascorbate transport than of water.

Sodium

The relative concentration of sodium is much the same in the aqueous humor of all species studied. It appears to be in small excess over that of a dialysate of plasma. Experimental data also suggest a small osmotic excess over plasma in anterior chamber aqueous humor. However, it is possible that the osmotic and overall ionic excesses in the aqueous humor may be negligible. The failure to alter apparent osmotic excess in rabbit aqueous humor in spite of effective lowering of intraocular pressure by acetazolamide (Diamox) raises serious doubts as to the role of hypertonicity as a driving force for the transfer of water into the eye. Furthermore, experimental alterations of osmotic factors fail to alter aqueous flow as much as anticipated. This may mean that the measured hypertonicity merely results from water loss by evaporation through the cornea. Perhaps the apparent ionic excesses result from errors of in vivo interpretation of dialysis and osmotic data obtained in vitro.

THEORIES OF AQUEOUS SECRETION

The secretion of aqueous humor has been demonstrated to be an energetic process that is temperature dependent and requires oxygen.

Redox pump theory

Friedenwald postulated a barrier between the epithelium and stroma of the ciliary body with an electron transport system across this barrier. As represented

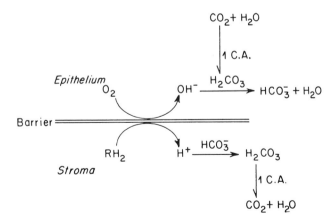

Fig. 7-7. Friedenwald's redox pump theory of aqueous secretion as applied to rabbits.

in Fig. 7-7, on the stromal side of the barrier the substrate RH_2 is oxidized, producing hydrogen ions. The electrons lost from the substrate are carried by a postulated electron transport system from the dehydrogenases through a series of oxidation-reduction reactions across the barrier to the epithelium where the cytochrome system has the capacity of using these electrons to reduce oxygen to hydroxyl ions. Such an electron pump would thus result in the production of hydroxyl ions in the ciliary epithelium. With the ever-present bicarbonate buffer, this would be measured as the appearance of bicarbonate ions in the epithelium and aqueous humor. The hydrogen ions remaining on the stromal side would also be buffered by the bicarbonate system. Both of these buffering systems would be more efficient in the presence of carbonic anhydrase. In its absence or effective inhibition, the secretory site or step most sensitive to alterations in pH would be impaired. Friedenwald found evidence for the ascorbic acid–glutathione system as well as for an epinephrine system as steps in the oxidation-reduction reactions.

This theory of secretion of aqueous humor is of considerable historical interest and served as an extremely useful stimulus for research. It offered explanations for the anomalous dye transport of the ciliary body (cationic dyes in epithelium and anionic dyes in stroma) and for the localization of cytochrome oxidase exclusively in the epithelium. It predicted the bicarbonate excess of the rabbit posterior chamber and postulated an important role for carbonic anhydrase. One practical consequence of the theory has been the use of carbonic anhydrase inhibitors to suppress aqueous formation.

Unfortunately the redox pump theory as presented by Friedenwald does not account for the secretion of aqueous humor in all species. A most important criticism of it is based on the finding that the ciliary body does not utilize stoichiometrically enough oxygen to account for the number of hydroxyl ions formed. It is possible, however, that some modification of this ingenious theory, such as the secretion of only the excess of hydroxyl ions or the recycling of electrons by carriers, may explain all the facts about secretion of aqueous humor.

Bicarbonate transport

Another speculative approach to the mechanism of secretion of aqueous humor supposes, rather than the indirect need for carbonic anhydrase to provide efficient buffering, that this enzyme plays a direct role in the transport process. On this basis one may postulate the active transport of bicarbonate into the rabbit eye and of hydrogen ions into the human eye, both of these made available from carbon dioxide and water in the presence of carbonic anhydrase. The mechanisms by which these ions could be carried into the aqueous humor remain unknown, but one may consider carriers or ion exchange systems.

Histochemical studies have demonstrated the presence of concentrations of carbonic anhydrase along the apical borders and lateral interdigitations of the nonpigmented epithelium of the rabbit ciliary body and at the basal parts of the pigmented epithelium. The enzyme is not present in the fetal ciliary body, but appears with increasing concentration during the first few weeks of life. This correlates well with the onset of aqueous secretion in the rabbit. The histochemical reaction is blocked, partially or totally, by the addition of varying amounts of the carbonic anhydrase inhibitor acetazolamide to the medium.

Sodium-potassium activated adenosinetriphosphatase and active cation transport

The enzyme sodium-potassium adenosinetriphosphatase has been studied extensively and found in cell membranes of many transport sites. Bonting has found an equivalence between cation flux and sodium-potassium adenosinetriphosphatase activity over a 25,000-fold range of cation flux rates in such different tissues as the human erythrocyte and the herring gull salt gland. In the eye two important transport sites, the ciliary epithelium and the lens epithelium, have been shown to have high sodium-potassium adenosinetriphosphatase activity. Both the enzyme and the cation transport system at both sites are similarly located, require sodium and potassium, and are inhibited by cardiac glycosides such as ouabain. In the ciliary epithelium the magnitude of the suppression of aqueous secretion parallels the degree of inhibition of the enzyme. Bonting postulates the enzyme to be on the side of the ciliary epithelium facing the aqueous humor. This would account for the easier ouabain inhibition on that side and would suggest sodium transport from cell to posterior chamber. In this hypothesis, water enters passively with the salt, and the enzyme carbonic anhydrase probably plays an indirect role such as maintaining cellular pH. Histochemical evidence has been presented that demonstrates the presumptive sites of adenosinetriphophatase on the apical and lateral interdigitations of the cell membranes of the nonpigmented epithelium of rabbit ciliary body. Activity was also noted in the boundary between the pigmented and nonpigmented epithelia. The localization of adenosinetriphosphatase is in the same regions shown to contain carbonic anhydrase. Both enzymes appear to be present in epithelial cells of tissues known to transport electrolytes.

Pinocytosis

The electron microscopic finding of vesicles in the ciliary epithelium has raised the question as to whether membrane flow and pinocytosis ("cell-drinking") may play an important role in the formation of the intraocular fluids. The increase in the number of vesicles after administration of acetazolamide or systemic hypothermia led Holmberg to postulate that the vesicles might transport aqueous humor to the posterior chamber. However, other evidence suggests that the vesicles may be derived from the breakdown of the surface infoldings of the ciliary epithelium and represent a fixation artifact. They are seen only in tissue fixed with osmium tetroxide and are not noted in gluteraldehyde-fixed specimens. At any rate, pinocytosis as a mechanism of transport is intriguing. However, it does not offer an explanation as to the mechanism of production of aqueous humor but merely places the primary secretory product at the less accessible intracellular level.

Other transport systems into the eye

There are at least four other transport systems into the ocular fluids. These include ascorbate, neutral amino acids, basic amino acids, and acidic amino acids. Such transport systems appear to be separate and discrete, with individual carriers, as demonstrated by studies designed to attempt to saturate or compete for the carriers. In each instance the Michaelis-Menten type of kinetics has been demonstrated (Fig. 7-8).*

*An excellent review of this material is to be found in Kinsey, V. E., and Reddy, D. V. N.: Chemistry and dynamics of aqueous humor. In Prince, J. H., editor: The rabbit in eye research, Springfield, Ill., 1964, Charles C Thomas, Publisher.

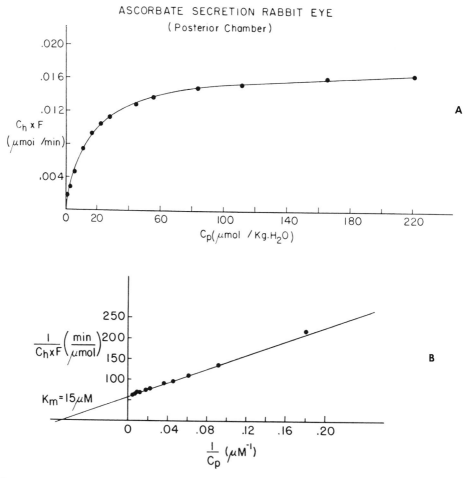

Fig. 7-8. **A,** Rate of ascorbate transport (μmol/min) at various concentrations of ascorbate (μmol/kg plasma water). **B,** Lineweaver-Burke plot of the data presented in **A.** The straight line obtained demonstrates the Michaelis-Menten type of kinetics, with half-saturation concentration (K_m) μmol.

Transport out of the eye

The recent finding of effective anion transport systems out of the eye further increases the complexity of aqueous secretion. One secretory system appears to be almost identical with the organic anion transport mechanism of the renal tubules of many species. It results in the renal excretion of such large anions as para-aminohippurate (PAH), phenolsulfonphthalein (PSP), Diodrast, penicillin, glucuronides, and sulfates. The transport of some of these anions out of the eye contributes to their exclusion from the vitreous humor and posterior chamber aqueous humor and may well alter the composition of the aqueous humor. Transport of these organic anions out of the eye can be saturated, demonstrates Michaelis-Menten kinetics, and is inhibited by probenecid or systemic hypothermia, much as in the renal tubule. Such inhibition appears to be associated with the appearance of large vesicles and distortion of the pigmented epithelium in the rabbit eye. This association suggests the pigmented layer as a possible site for this transport process.

Iodide is also secreted out of the eye by a transport system related to that in the thyroid and salivary glands. It also demonstrates characteristic saturation kinetics with iodide and competitive inhibition by perchlorate. It is not altered by probenecid and appears to be independent of the Diodrast system.

There is also evidence that amino acids may be actively transported out of the posterior segment of the rabbit eye, thus accounting for their low steady-state concentrations in the vitreous.

Other factors in aqueous flow

In the previous paragraphs attention has centered on transport of electrolytes and fluid across the ciliary epithelium into the posterior chamber. The rate of transport of these substances depends not only on the integrity of the secretory mechanisms involved but also on the availability of electrolytes and tissue fluid within the connective tissue stroma of the ciliary processes. This, in turn, is dependent on blood pressure in the ciliary body and permeability through the capillary walls. When intraocular pressure is elevated, blood flow into the ciliary processes is reduced, and aqueous formation decreases. Elevation of intraocular pressure during tonography induces this situation, producing the phenomenon of "pseudofacility." Similarly, reduction in blood pressure and blood flow by carotid ligation results in decreased aqueous production (p. 110).

RATE OF AQUEOUS FLOW

The rate of secretion of aqueous humor may be measured by a number of methods. Unfortunately each of these methods is subject to a large number of errors. The errors stem from analytical methods, inadequacies of theory, biologic errors, etc. It has therefore been of considerable interest to compare different methods, each with its own sources of errors, in the same animal species. The availability of carbonic anhydrase inhibitors and their ability to decrease the rate of aqueous secretion have been of enormous heuristic value in studies of aqueous humor formation. For the first time it was possible to alter the flow parameter and to measure the effects of this alteration. It has been demonstrated that cardiac glycosides and systemic hypothermia to 20° C both decrease markedly the rate of aqueous production in rabbit eyes. These have provided independent methods for altering aqueous humor dynamics and have permitted the application of the various methods of measurement.

The methods for measuring aqueous flow may be subdivided into chemical and physical methods. Chemical methods include the turnover of test substances, the determination of steady-state chemistries, and the fluorescein appearance time. The physical methods depend on the estimation of aqueous flow from facility of outflow and intraocular pressure, facility of outflow being determined by either tonography or perfusion.

Chemical methods
Turnover of test substances

The most precise chemical method is the study of turnover of test substances in the posterior and anterior chamber fluids. This method is largely confined to animal eyes except for the use of fluorescein turnover in human eyes. The method that is applied is laborious, and a number of approximations have to be made in interpreting the results. Nevertheless, a number of laboratories have accumulated data which indicate that roughly 3 to 4 μl/min are secreted into and leave the rabbit eye. After the administration of various effective carbonic anhydrase inhibitors, there is a decrease of approximately 50% in the rate of aqueous flow. Lowering the body temperature to 20° C results in some 80% to 90% decrease in the rate of formation of aqueous humor.

The para-aminohippurate technique of Bárány and Kinsey is a most ingenious method for estimating the rate of flow, which involves only anterior chamber and plasma concentration data. PAH is excluded from the posterior chamber and vitreous body and is rapidly excreted by the kidneys. After its intravenous infusion, PAH enters the anterior chamber by diffusion to a steady state approximately one-sixth that of plasma. On cessation of intravenous injection the plasma is rapidly cleared, and the decline in aqueous humor concentration gives an estimation of the flow rate. Unfortunately the data are limited to the two concentrations available by anterior chamber puncture of the two eyes at different time intervals, and it is required that both eyes have similar rates of flow at a particular time.

The finding that iodide is secreted out of the eye behind the iris but diffuses into the anterior chamber from the plasma permits the use of this anion for turnover studies in the anterior chamber. The concentration of iodide in the rabbit anterior chamber aqueous humor rises exponentially to a steady state of 30% to 50% of the plasma concentration. The rate constant of this exponential is a direct measure of k_0, the fraction of iodide in the anterior chamber that leaves per minute by diffusion and flow. Previously administered nonlabeled iodide may be

Table 7-5. Iodide measurement of rate of aqueous flow

Treatment	Number of rabbits	Treated eye/nontreated eye (mean ± σ)
Carotid ligation	15	0.83 ± 0.087
Pilocarpine, 2%	20	1.16 ± 0.095
Atropine, 2%	20	0.79 ± 0.090

used to determine the steady-state ratio of concentration in the anterior chamber (C_a) to that in the plasma (C_p) by chemical means. From the same anterior chamber tap, the values at other time intervals are measured with radioisotopes, permitting a derived estimate of k_{fa}, the flow rate for the individual eye:

$$k_{fa} = \frac{C_p - C_a}{C_p} k_0$$

The applications of this method to animals subjected to hypothermia or carbonic anhydrase inhibition provide results in excellent agreement with other methods of measurement. The method may also be used to compare treated and untreated eyes of the same animal at the same time. This permits an evaluation of unilateral procedures such as carotid ligation or topical application of pilocarpine or atropine (Table 7-5).

Fluorescein appearance and steady state

The more approximate chemical measurements of alterations in the steady-state chemistries in the posterior and anterior chambers and fluorescein appearance time permit determinations on single animals rather than on large series required for conventional turnover studies. These simpler methods of measurement do not provide absolute estimations of aqueous flow and require that no alterations are induced in the diffusion of the particular ion. Furthermore, the steady-state method depends on both eyes behaving identically and having the same rate of flow initially. With attention to their limitations, these approximate methods may be used for relative measurements, however. In the case of carbonic anhydrase inhibitors, for instance, the results are in excellent agreement with the turnover studies—that is, some 50% inhibition of flow. The effects of intravitreal ouabain on steady-state concentrations in the posterior and anterior chambers also provide estimates of reduction of flow in good agreement with tonographic findings (to approximately one-third that of the control eye). Hypothermia, however, alters the diffusion coefficients of various ions, and the simpler methods cannot be applied.

Photogrammetric estimation

A photographic estimation of aqueous flow through the pupil, described by Holm, provides another method for measurement of aqueous production. Fluorescein staining of the anterior chamber is induced by iontophoresis, with the pupil miotic. Aqueous passing into the anterior chamber appears at the pupillary border as a progressively enlarging, nonstaining vesicle. Rapid-succession photographs of optical sections of the anterior chamber demonstrate the vesicle and permit estimation of its volume. Two series of photographs are made about 15 seconds apart, and the difference in vesicle size per unit of time gives an estimate of aqueous flow. Possible errors in the method arise from the necessity for miosis, the possible effects on aqueous production of iontophoresis and strong illumination during the rapid-sequence photography, and the accuracy of the vesicle volume calculations. Rapid changes in aqueous production rate and factors altering development of the vesicle at the pupillary border are also important. In spite of the potential errors, the method is interesting and is applicable to human eyes. Flow rate estimates are in agreement with those obtained by other methods. In addition, carbonic anhydrase inhibition produces a reduction in flow of approximately the same degree as determined with turnover studies and tonography.

Physical methods

Most physical methods of measurement involve the concept of outflow facility. The rate of aqueous flow, F, is assumed to be proportional to the outflow pressure gradient $(P_0 - P_V)$, where P_0 is the intraocular pressure and P_V is the episcleral venous pressure. The proportionality constant, C, is defined as the facility of aqueous outflow:

$$F = C(P_0 - P_V) \tag{3}$$

Perfusion

As indicated previously, when the eye of the living animal or the enucleated eye is perfused at a pressure P_I greater than P_0, perfusion fluid enters the eye at rate I. When the rate of inflow, I, is plotted against perfusion pressure, P_I, not only is an estimate of the outflow facility, C, obtained from the slope of the straight line, but also the intraocular pressure, P_0, may be determined from the intercept. The rate of flow may then be calculated from Equation 3 or from the ordinate at a pressure equal to the episcleral venous pressure.

The results obtained in a large series of rabbits give average pressures of 19 to 20 mm Hg with outflow facilities of 0.35. If it is assumed that $P_V = 9$ mm Hg, these values are compatible with a secretory rate of 3.5 to 4.0 $\mu l/min$.

Tonography

Tonography provides a more practical method for measurement of outflow facility and intraocular pressure in the living eye. With this technique estimates for the normal rabbit are a P_0 of 20 mm Hg and an outflow facility of 0.33. This again suggests a rate of aqueous flow between 3.5 and 4.0 $\mu l/min$. It has been possible to compare tonography and perfusion on the same eye of the same animal. The fact that under these circumstances the agreement is very good suggests that errors either compensate for one another or are of insufficient magnitude to alter the data. The tonographic method has the advantage that it may be applied repeatedly to the same eye. Under these circumstances many of the errors inherent in the technique, the calibration, and the characteristics of the eye tend to cancel out, producing reasonable estimates of alterations in the rate of aqueous formation. The effects of carbonic anhydrase inhibitors have been evaluated by this method by performing tonography before and after the administration of the agent. The results again demonstrate a decrease of aqueous flow of approximately 50% to 60% in rabbit eyes. By injecting ouabain into the vitreous of one eye, one is able to compare injected and control eyes. Four to five days after injection the ouabain-treated eye demonstrates flow values reduced to approximately one-third those of its contralateral control. Similar studies during systemic hypothermia demonstrate an exponential decrease in aqueous secretion and in intraocular pressure with a decrease in temperature. At 20° C, tonography indicates a suppression of secretion of approximately 80% to 90%, which is in excellent agreement with turnover studies. It is most reassuring that the diverse approaches to the problem of estimating alterations in secretory rate provide such consistent data. The agreement of such independent methods of measurement, each with its own assumptions and errors, strongly suggests the basic validity of the methods.

Tonography is one of the methods that can be applied to human eyes. Here the rate of secretion appears to be somewhat less than that of the rabbit, roughly 1.5 to 2.0 μl/min. On occasion the outflow facility values obtained by tonography may be compared with perfusion values in vivo and in vitro. In the few instances in which this has been possible, the agreement was excellent. Furthermore, by the comparison of tonographic tracings before and after the administration of carbonic anhydrase inhibitors, some 45% to 50% suppression of aqueous flow has been demonstrated in human eyes. This reduction in flow may also be estimated by fluorescein appearance time, and one may even compare the alteration in fluorescein appearance time with the changes in the tonogram for the same eye. Estimates obtained in this fashion are in reasonable agreement.

Suction cup

The suction cup method attempts to measure the rate of aqueous secretion by obstructing outflow channels with a vacuum of 50 mm Hg below atmospheric pressure. Under these circumstances intraocular pressure rises by an amount that depends on the distensibility of ocular coats, the rate of secretion of aqueous humor under the conditions of the test (suction and elevated intraocular pressure), the degree to which outflow pathways are occluded (whether all aqueous humor retained in perilimbal tissues results in expected rise in intraocular pressure), and possible alterations in blood volume in the eye. The method is much improved by repeated applanation tonometer readings during the occlusion by a suction ring. Normal ocular rigidity is often assumed, or Schiøtz measurements may be carried out as well as applanation to determine the ocular rigidity of the individual eye.

Although there is evidence that the rate of secretion may be decreased progressively as intraocular pressure is elevated by the suction cup, this may be merely incomplete occlusion of outflow channels, with progressively increasing leak. At any rate, relative values can be obtained that provide estimates of alterations in flow. By this method it can be demonstrated that carbonic anhydrase inhibitors suppress the formation of aqueous humor in human eyes some 40% to 60%. It has also been demonstrated that diurnal variations in intraocular pressure are a consequence of alterations in secretory activity, partly compensated by changes in outflow facility in the normal eye and uncompensated (and thus of greater magnitude) in glaucomatous patients. Also confirmed by the suction cup method is the reduction in rate of flow with age. When the test is carried out for 15 minutes at a vacuum of 50 mm Hg, the mean values for inflow vary from approximately 0.8 to 1.0 μl/min, relatively low values. However, 5-minute compression values average 1.1 to 1.5 μl/min, and these probably still represent an underestimation of the secretory rate. As indicated in the preceding chapter, the rate of return of intraocular pressure to original values after removal of the suction cup produces a crude estimate of outflow facility. More detailed studies of the effects of the suction cup itself on intraocular pressure, on deformation and rigidity of the globe, on aqueous secretion, and on possible expression of fluid from the eye are needed.

ALTERATIONS IN FLOW
Spontaneous alteration

The rate of aqueous flow in human eyes varies spontaneously in a diurnal fashion. This largely accounts for the diurnal fluctuations in intraocular pressure. The variations correlate with diurnal changes in plasma corticosteroid levels, both being higher by day than by night. In certain individuals the pressure variations appear of much larger magnitude than they are in others. This may result from less compensatory change in outflow facility or from a reduced and fixed outflow facility as in glaucoma. However, some few people are even able to raise their intraocular pressure to abnormal levels intermittently, largely by hypersecreting. Little is known about the details of metabolic, hormonal, vascular, neurogenic, and psychogenic factors that alter the rate of aqueous secretion. Alterations in rate of aqueous flow are probably only one of the means by which centrally innervated influences may alter intraocular pressure.

Age

There is convincing evidence that the rate of aqueous flow decreases with advancing age, with a particularly sharp decline after the age of 60 years. Thus, in spite of the decrease in outflow facility found in human and animal eyes with advancing age, intraocular pressure is maintained at about the same level by a progressive decline in aqueous secretion. It is not clear at present whether the decrease in secretory activity and outflow facility are independent of each other or whether there is a relationship between the two. It is of considerable interest that many younger members of the families of patients with glaucoma are found to have impaired outflow facility but hyposecrete aqueous humor, maintaining normal intraocular pressures for considerable periods of time. Here again, it is not known whether there is a causative relationship between the two factors. The problem becomes even more difficult to evaluate when it is appreciated that the reduction of aqueous secretion by such means as the administration of acetazolamide does not always result in a fall in intraocular pressure. Some normal eyes maintain pressure in spite of the decrease in aqueous secretion and do so by decreasing their outflow facility. In this instance it would appear as if the decreased outflow facility were a response to the lower aqueous secretion rather than a causative factor. One may even speculate that a reduction in aqueous secretion with age or in the relatives of patients with glaucoma may decrease the nutritional supply of the trabecular meshwork and result in temporary or permanent alterations in trabecular function.

Glaucoma with hyposecretion

An intermittently decreased rate of aqueous secretion is a common finding in glaucomatous eyes. This serves to lower intraocular pressure in spite of the impaired outflow facility and may account for the long interval of delay in damage to the optic nerve and loss of visual field. The mechanism of hyposecretion in glaucomatous eyes remains unknown. The understanding of this protective device is of key importance, especially in the families of patients with glaucoma. The finding of similar hyposecretion in hereditary glaucoma of rabbits offers an experimental approach to this intriguing mechanism. Unfortunately intermittent hyposecretion often makes it most difficult to diagnose glaucoma before damage to the optic nerve has taken place, since intraocular pressure may be normal at the time of examination.

Hyposecretion is more common in advanced glaucoma and may account for many instances of so-called low-tension glaucoma with cupping of the optic disc and visual field loss. In such long-standing glaucoma, histologic findings of an atrophic fibrotic ciliary body with hyalinized shrunken processes are compatible with the hyposecretion observed.

Drugs

A number of pharmacologic agents alter the secretion of aqueous humor and have become of clinical importance in glaucoma therapy.

Carbonic anhydrase inhibitors (Chapter 19). The rate of aqueous flow may be altered by any of a large number of carbonic anhydrase inhibitors. At maximum dosage almost all these agents result in some 50% decrease in the rate of aqueous flow. Secretion of aqueous humor is not further reduced by increasing the dose by tenfold above this level. This built-in safeguard in the use of carbonic anhydrase inhibitors may account for the lack of toxicity to the eye.

Epinephrine. The topical application of high concentrations of epinephrine (e.g., 2% epinephrine bitartrate or hydrochloride) results in suppression of aqueous secretion by approximately 30% to 35%. This effect is additive to that produced by carbonic anhydrase inhibitors. The therapeutic possibilities of these two agents are discussed in Chapter 19.

Cardiac glycosides. Cardiac glycosides have been demonstrated to inhibit the sodium-potassium adenosinetriphosphatase of the ciliary epithelium and to reduce the rate of formation of aqueous humor in experimental animals. Unfortunately, at dosage levels that prove practical, digoxin has proved to be of very limited value in the therapy of glaucoma, and the dangers of inducing cardiac toxicity are considerable.

Other agents. A number of sedatives and anesthetic agents may also decrease the rate of aqueous formation. There is some evidence that stimulation of the ciliary ganglion (in cats) or administration of some of the parasympathomimetic or anticholinesterase drugs may produce increases in aqueous humor production (Table 7-5).

Surgery

The secretion of aqueous humor can also be modified by surgical procedures.

Carotid ligation. Carotid ligation in rabbits results in a 20% decrease in aqueous flow on the homolateral side. The decrease in flow is largely compensated by a decrease in outflow facility, so that pressure is little altered. A temporary decrease in aqueous secretion is also noted in the human eye after carotid ligation, and more permanent decreases may follow carotid occlusion.

Eye surgery. Many surgical procedures on the eye are followed by a period of hyposecretion. This is often associated with separation of the choroid, but cause-and-effect relationships have not been established. Hyposecretion may persist for days or weeks after a cataract operation or for months or years after cyclodialysis or cyclodiathermy. The hyposecretion that follows surgical procedures may lower intraocular pressure in the presence of impaired outflow facility and make difficult the recognition of glaucoma or its precarious state of control.

Inflammatory diseases of the eye. In uveitis, particularly when there is involvement of the ciliary body, a profound hyposecretion is apparent. This may be a manifestation of an increased permeability between blood and aqueous humor, making the secretory pump leak. Hypotony may occur after an attack of acute angle-closure glaucoma, trauma, radiation, or retinal detachment or with active uveitis in spite of possibly obstructed outflow channels. In the recovery period, if the ciliary body recovers before the trabecular meshwork is functional, intraocular pressure may be elevated.

CHAPTER **8**

Clinical applications

It is clear that there are a large number of possible errors and many limitations in the methods of measurement of intraocular pressure and outflow facility. Although some of these may be corrected or avoided, conclusions should not be drawn hastily from single determinations. However, in spite of errors and theoretical difficulties in interpretation, repeated consistent values obtained by tonometry and tonography provide useful information about the status of the eye. As with other laboratory procedures, when taken in conjunction with the history and clinical findings, the data obtained have proved of considerable value to the clinician in both diagnosis and management of the glaucomas.

DIAGNOSIS OF OPEN-ANGLE GLAUCOMA

Classic findings

As compared to the normal eye (Fig. 6-3), the eye with open-angle glaucoma has classically an elevated intraocular pressure and decreased outflow facility (Fig. 8-1). Thus 80% of patients with proved open-angle glaucoma have intraocular pressures over 21 mm Hg at the time of diagnosis (Table 8-1). Furthermore, the likelihood of visual damage is directly related to the height of the pressure and

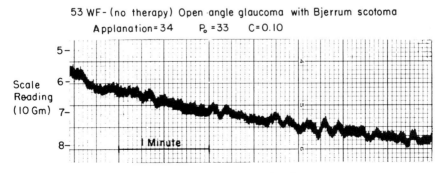

Fig. 8-1. Tonogram—open-angle glaucoma.

age of the patient (Table 8-2). Glaucoma is clearly associated with elevation of intraocular pressure. In the absence of ocular damage and functional loss, the diagnosis of glaucoma can be suggested only by tonometric and tonographic findings. Therefore *every* patient old enough to cooperate should be subjected to tonometry unless there are specific contraindications (such as corneal ulcer). Only in this way can patients with ocular hypertension be discovered and followed closely to determine when therapy might be necessary. All patients with a pressure of 21 mm Hg or more should be subjected to further study.

As indicated previously, an intraocular pressure greater than 21 mm Hg (two standard deviations from the mean) would be expected to occur in less than 2.5% of the normal population if pressures were distributed equally above and below the mean. Intraocular pressures are not evenly distributed, however, and pressures over 21 mm Hg are seen more frequently than statistically anticipated in the non-

Table 8-1. Prevalence of tonometric and tonographic findings in normal eyes and patients with untreated glaucoma

	Prevalence	
Finding	*Normal eyes*	*Untreated glaucoma*
Applanation pressure > 21	4.7-6.5%	80%
C < 0.16	8%	83%
P_0/C > 100 after water	16%	94%

Table 8-2. Frequency of field defects with elevated pressure*

Applanation pressure (mm Hg)	*Age (yr)*	*Number of eyes*	*Number of field defects*
20-25	30-39	117	0
	40-49	275	9
	50-59	321	35
	60-69	101	11
Total		814	55 (6.8%)
26-30	30-39	5	1
	40-49	91	6
	50-59	163	22
	60-69	32	7
Total		291	36 (12.4%)
> 30	30-39	0	0
	40-49	8	3
	50-59	29	8
	60-69	16	4
Total		53	15 (28.3%)

*From Armaly, M. F.: Invest. Ophthal. **11**:75, 1972.

glaucomatous population (Table 8-1). It is for this reason that an elevated intra-ocular pressure cannot be considered synonymous with a diagnosis of glaucoma. The problem is further complicated in that 20% of patients with proved glaucoma have pressures within normal limits at the time of any one measurement. Some of these represent instances of "low-tension glaucoma," in which visual damage is caused by ischemic optic nerve changes unrelated to increased intraocular pres-sure. Others may represent patients with decreased ocular rigidity (if Schiøtz tonometry is used) or transient hyposecretion. Tonography may help in identify-ing these patients by demonstrating impaired outflow facility with normal Schiøtz pressure readings.

Impaired outflow facility with normal Schiøtz tension readings

There are at least two mechanisms of clinical importance that result in flat tonographic tracings without apparent pressure elevations. One of these is a de-creased ocular rigidity, and the second, a decreased rate of aqueous formation.

Decreased ocular rigidity (Figs. 29-7 to 29-9). Decreased ocular rigidity occurs especially in myopic eyes, in thyrotropic exophthalmos, and after consumption of a liter of water. In such eyes the true status may be detected by applanation to-nometry, by tonography, or preferably by a combination of the two.

Hyposecretion (Fig. 29-3). The second mechanism resulting in a flat tonographic tracing in the absence of pressure elevations is a decreased rate of secretion of aqueous humor. Hyposecretion may normalize intraocular pressure in spite of impaired outflow facility. This mechanism may delay damage to the optic nerve and affords a physiologic counterpart to the clinical use of secretory suppressants. Unfortunately the spontaneous diurnal, or even more prolonged, periods of de-pression of secretion are frequently not permanent. Eyes with impaired outflow mechanisms often sustain pressure elevations at times other than physicians' office hours. Thus field loss may occur in spite of apparently normal office or survey tonometric measurements. In fact, without tonography the diagnosis in these pa-tients is often not suspected until damage to the optic nerve has occurred.

Water-drinking provocative test and P_0/C ratio (Fig. 29-3)

In the glaucomatous patients described in Table 8-1, 83% were found to have an outflow facility, C, less than 0.16. It has been found empirically that 40 to 45 minutes after the consumption of a liter of water, the patient having fasted for the previous 4 or more hours, a rise in intraocular pressure and a decline in outflow facility occur in many glaucomatous eyes. When only 1 L of water is used, the normal eye rarely reacts in this manner (Chapter 6). To maximize the rec-ognition of glaucomatous eyes, one may therefore use the P_0/C ratio. A P_0/C ratio greater than 100 after water drinking occurred in 94% of eyes with proved untreated glaucoma and in less than 2.5% of *selected* normal eyes, and P_0/C values greater than 138 were seen in 73% of the glaucomatous eyes and in only 0.15% of the *selected* normal eyes.

When this information first became available, it appeared that the ratio P_0/C applied to tonography after the ingestion of water would provide a convenient method for the recognition of early glaucoma. Although this may be true, it is erroneous to assume that this parameter represents the basis for initiation of anti-glaucomatous therapy in patients without other abnormalities. It is true that in *selected* normals, a P_0/C ratio over 100 after water drinking is seen very infrequently. Normals in this instance were young volunteers with no ocular abnormalities and no family history of glaucoma. As noted previously, intraocular pressure increases slightly with age, and outflow facility decreases with age. Both of these factors increase the likelihood of a high P_0/C ratio in older individuals. Since the general population consists of many subpopulations, including those of all ages, the results of the water drinking test in the general population differ from the findings in the selected normals. More recent statistics indicate that a P_0/C ratio greater than 100 after water drinking is found in about 16% of the general, nonglaucomatous population. This is still considerably less frequent than in glaucomatous eyes, where 94% have this finding. Since the prevalence of glaucoma is small, however, the water-drinking provocative test fails to accurately separate the glaucoma and normal populations. Although most patients with glaucoma have an abnormal water-drinking provocative test, most patients with an abnormal test do not have glaucoma. One cannot say that because a $P_0/C > 100$ is found in glaucoma, the finding of a $P_0/C > 100$ means the individual has glaucoma. This finding in eyes without cupping or field loss should classify the patient as a glaucoma suspect who needs prolonged reappraisal. In a relatively small series of 26 such patients (40 eyes) studied for 5 years (Table 8-3), 6 eyes (15%) developed field loss (Bjerrum's scotomas). However, a number of the eyes showed progression of their outflow impairment (to less than 0.13 in one half of the eyes) and elevated intraocular pressures (to over 24 mm Hg in more than one third of the series).

Glaucoma with $P_0/C < 100$. Some few patients who subsequently develop proved glaucoma demonstrate P_0/C values within normal limits on one or more occasions. Some of these cases go through repeated periods of abnormal tonometric and tonographic findings interspersed with remissions to normal values.

Table 8-3. Five-year follow-up on 40 "normal" eyes with initial $P_0/C > 100$ after drinking water

Finding	Incidence
$P_0 > 21$	24 (60%)
$P_0 > 24$	15 (38%)
$P_0 \geq 30$	6 (15%)
$C < 0.18$	30 (75%)
$C < 0.13$	20 (50%)
P_0 rise, 8+ mm after drinking water	4 (10%)
Field loss	6 (15%)

Possible causes for fluctuation in the water-drinking provocative test may relate to inadequate water absorption and hemodilution, errors in tonographic technique, or the *intermittent nature of glaucoma in its early stages*. The fact that outflow facility can show spontaneous improvement in some instances provides hope that the biochemical factors responsible for such improvement may someday be discovered and applied to the therapy and prevention of glaucoma.

Corticosteroid response

Topical corticosteroids produce decreases of outflow facility and elevations of intraocular pressure. As suggested in Chapter 6, the response appears to be genetically determined. Almost all eyes with primary open-angle glaucoma respond with dramatic elevations of intraocular pressure. In groups of glaucoma suspects selected because of $P_0/C > 100$ after water drinking, some 25% to 30% respond as dramatically as do the glaucomatous eyes (gg); the remaining 70% to 75% resemble the heterozygous responders (ng). Even in selected normal populations (no family history, normal discs and fields, and negative water-drinking provocative test), almost one third of individuals respond with pressures over 20 mm Hg, resembling the heterozygous state (ng), and a few (approximately 4%) respond as dramatically as the homozygous responders (gg). It must be reemphasized that the same cautions must be used here as with the water tonogram and other provocative tests. "Positive" testing results mean that the individual resembles persons in the glaucoma or carrier states but not that he has the disease. Only time and close observation can establish the diagnosis. The provocative test can only call certain suspects to the attention of the ophthalmologist so that they may be followed more closely and earlier discovery can be made of those who develop glaucoma.

Interestingly enough, in studies of the offspring of patients with proved primary open-angle glaucoma, some 20% respond to topical corticosteroids as homozygous marked responders (gg), and almost all of the remaining 80% respond as do the heterozygous responders (ng). Among the homozygous responders, 93% demonstrated a positive water-drinking provocative test, whereas only 41% of the heterozygous responders had a $P_0/C > 100$ after water drinking. Thus the group that behaved like glaucoma patients in their response to topical corticosteroids also resembled glaucoma patients in their response to water drinking.

Family studies

When diagnostic methods are applied to the immediate families of patients with proved open-angle glaucoma (siblings, parents, and children) in which the prevalence of glaucoma is high, it is found that even the relatives who do not demonstrate pressure elevation or field loss have a very high prevalence (20% of 220 eyes studied) of significantly decreased outflow facility (less than 0.18) and almost one third have a P_0/C over 100 after drinking water. As many as 85% to 90% of the offspring of patients with primary open-angle glaucoma respond to topical corticosteroids with significant pressure elevations, and 20% or more of these offspring present responses of such magnitude as to resemble their glaucomatous parents.

Elevation of intraocular pressure and outflow facility impairment after six weeks of dexamethasone may occur when there is no other manifestation of an abnormality in the eye. At this time, without steroids the water-drinking provocative tonogram may be normal. With repeated water-drinking tonograms more than one half of such responders to steroids demonstrate $P_0/C > 100$ after water drinking on one or more occasions. It may be intermittent or persistent, and many never go beyond this stage. It may subsequently be followed by impaired outflow facility before drinking water. Later intermittent elevations of intraocular pressure may be recognized (with variations in secretory state). All these findings may revert to normal and then recur.

Most relatives of glaucoma patients remain in the suspect stage for many years or for their lifetime and never sustain any damage to their optic nerves. As time goes on, the outflow impairment in some individuals becomes sufficiently marked and inflexible as to produce more persistent elevations of intraocular pressure. At a still later time those patients destined to develop glaucoma begin to demonstrate field loss and cupping. It has been possible in the relatives of some patients with glaucoma to follow this sequence from perfectly normal pressures and outflow facilities to the onset of field loss (Fig. 8-2). In such patients fol-

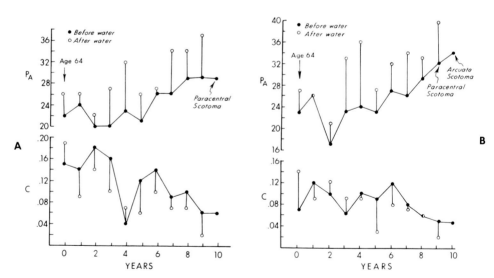

Fig. 8-2. Intraocular pressure (above) and outflow facility (below) of right eye, **A,** and left eye, **B,** with changes produced by water drinking, in a patient during the ten years preceding the development of field loss. Note that progressive outflow impairment occurred prior to marked rise in pressure and field loss. (From Kolker, A. E.: Proceedings of Jerusalem Seminar on the Prevention of Blindness, New York, 1972, Academic Press, Inc.)

lowed for ten years before the development of field loss, the pattern of progressive impairment in outflow facility followed by increase in intraocular pressure was apparent. Progressive changes with time, rather than the status when first examined, appear to be the most significant.

Elevated Schiøtz tension readings with steep tonographic tracings

In the vast majority of patients with an elevated intraocular pressure in the presence of open angles, tonography merely confirms the diagnosis and demonstrates the impaired outflow facility. There are a very few patients who have an elevated Schiøtz estimate of intraocular pressure but with steep tonographic tracings. The points to consider in the differential diagnosis of such patients are the following.

1. *Is the patient capable of angle closure?* (Fig. 29-5.) Some patients with early angle-closure glaucoma are brought out of the attack by the tonometer displacing fluid behind the cornea, thus opening the angle and producing a very steep curve in spite of elevated initial pressure. Similar opening of a closed angle may be demonstrated by use of the Zeiss gonioscopic prism with pressure. Unless recognized as such, the diagnosis of angle-closure may be missed.

2. *Is this an instance of abnormally high ocular rigidity?* An elevated ocular rigidity will produce a false high pressure estimate by Schiøtz readings if only one weight is used and can produce a sizable overestimation of the outflow facility. Applanation tonometry before tonography is the best method for ruling this possibility in or out. Ocular rigidity may also be evaluated, but less adequately, by Schiøtz tonometry with two different weights.

3. *Is there an artifact in the tracing?* (Fig. 29-6.) An inexperienced operator may inadvertently press on the globe during tonography. This will produce an abnormally high reading and a steeper than normal curve. Similar effects can be produced by use of too light a weight, so that scale readings less than 4.00 are recorded (effect of too large a footplate hole, p. 63), by squeezing, by spontaneous or induced changes in the steady state of the eye (e.g., decrease in secretion), and by excitement and blood pressure changes. These factors are best ruled out by repeated measurements and experience.

4. *Does this particular patient have chronic simple glaucoma but respond to the application of the tonometer by inhibiting aqueous secretion (pseudofacility)?* (p. 72.) This is an important possible interpretation of this type of tracing and may be ruled out only by repeated measurements. These patients are sometimes distinguished only by their response to miotic therapy.

5. *Does the eye in question have an elevated episcleral venous pressure?* This results in millimeter for millimeter rise in intraocular pressure and may occur without alteration in outflow facility, thus simulating hypersecretion. These eyes are easy to recognize, however, by the marked engorgement of the episcleral veins, and the diagnosis can be confirmed by measurement of the P_V.

6. *Is true hypersecretion present?* (Fig. 29-4.) If all the foregoing considera-

tions can be ruled out, then and only then can one interpret elevated pressure and high outflow facility as manifestations of hypersecretion (Chapter 15). Even under these circumstances another possible explanation exists. Uveoscleral pathways for aqueous outflow have been demonstrated to account for about 25% of the aqueous leaving the monkey eye (p. 87). Since this pathway does not enter into the calculation of tonographic outflow facility, selective obliteration of this aqueous exit route could produce the findings of elevated pressure and high outflow facility. It has not been demonstrated that such localized pathologic changes occur, or even if this pathway is present in the human eye.

Diurnal fluctuations

Diurnal variations in intraocular pressure are largely dependent on alterations in secretory activity. Since eyes with impaired and less flexible outflow facility sustain greater pressure fluctuations with variation in secretory rate than do eyes with more adequate and easily varied outflow facility, the deviations in intraocular pressure are magnified in glaucoma. Measurements around the clock have proved of considerable value in the early diagnosis of the glaucomas. Furthermore, normalization of outflow facility by miotics tends to minimize diurnal variations in intraocular pressure in glaucomatous eyes. Since in many patients the peaks of intraocular pressure occur before or after office hours, diurnal measurements permit a more adequate appraisal of status of control as well as a more rational basis for time and frequency of administration of therapy. Thus pressure determinations around the clock supplement tonography in both the early diagnosis and more adequate management of the glaucomas.

Conclusion

It is apparent that tonography is not essential for the diagnosis of classic primary open-angle glaucoma. It is, however, a simple laboratory test that measures one of several important parameters involved in glaucoma. Periodic estimation of this parameter provides a convenient and useful means to detect the glaucoma suspect and follow the progression of the disease. As such, it is a valuable adjunct to other methods in the diagnosis of this condition.

DIAGNOSIS OF ANGLE-CLOSURE GLAUCOMA
Tonography

The diagnosis of angle-closure glaucoma may be suggested by the history but rests primarily on the gonioscopic appearance of the angle. If the angle is closed and the pressure is elevated, there is no question about diagnosis. In some instances, however, the angle appears closed in some or all areas without significant pressure elevations but with impaired outflow facility. Such patients are apparently capable of hyposecreting and thus avoid pressure elevations. This occurs more frequently following pupillary dilation.

Provocative tests (Figs. 29-1 and 29-2)

The provocative tests for angle-closure glaucoma include dark room mydriasis for 60 to 90 minutes or the use of mydriatics such as 5% eucatropine (Euphthalmine). Mydriatics should be confined to one eye at a time. They should be followed by prompt routine administration of miotics until the pupil is constricted. As compared with pressure measurements alone, a larger number of eyes capable of occluding can be recognized by a significant reduction (25% to 30%) in outflow facility in association with gonioscopic evidence of occlusion. In several independent studies, although less than one half of the eyes with a proved capacity for angle-closure glaucoma could be detected by an 8 mm. rise in intraocular pressure, some 80% to 85% of the same eyes demonstrated a significant flattening of the tonographic tracing. It is to be noted that negative provocative tests do not rule out the possibility of subsequent episodes of angle-closure glaucoma. Therefore all patients with gonioscopic evidence of narrow angles should be followed closely and warned of the symptoms of angle-closure glaucoma. Only repeated provocative testing may reveal their capacity for angle-closure glaucoma. It is apparent that a significant decrease in outflow facility after a mydriatic provocative test is strongly indicative of angle-closure glaucoma. However, some patients with early open-angle glaucoma demonstrate a similar decrease in outflow facility after parasympatholytic agents, especially if homatropine or cyclopentolate (Cyclogyl) is used. Although this occurs much less often with eucatropine, it is absolutely essential to examine patients with a gonioscope after the mydriatic tonography provocative test. Only if the angle appears occluded at the time of the flattening of the tracing can one establish a diagnosis of a capacity for angle-closure glaucoma.

MEDICAL THERAPY FOR OPEN-ANGLE GLAUCOMA
Miotics (Fig. 29-20)

Miotics improve outflow facility and thus lower intraocular pressure. Tonometry permits evaluation of the pressure level obtained under such therapy. However, because of variations in secretory behavior, the patient's intraocular pressure may be elevated at times when he is not seen in the physician's office. In fact, several studies have indicated that this is the rule rather than the exception. The best preventive measure against pressure elevations is the normalization of outflow facility by miotics. Tonography therefore is of help in the evaluation of miotic therapy.

Prognosis. In a series of patients followed for a period of over three years on miotic therapy, the initial tonographic response to miotics could be related to the prognosis for continued pressure control. Of 250 eyes with chronic open-angle glaucoma, those eyes that could be brought to pressures of 24 mm Hg or less with miotic therapy were found to have a 50% chance of continued control at this level over a three-year period. If pressure could be reduced to levels of 21 mm Hg or less, the chances of continued successful control for three years rose to approximately 2 out of 3. Outflow facility values of 0.13 or more with miotic therapy alone also assured continued control in approximately 70% of eyes. Values of 0.18 or more increased the chances of success to better than 5 out of 6. A P_0/C ratio of 100 or less was associated with continued control in 90% of the eyes.

In an independently studied series of 185 eyes similarly followed with miotic therapy for one-and-one-half to nine years, field was lost in 31% of eyes with pressure of 21 or less, but in 48% of those eyes with pressure over 21 mm Hg. However, in this series, field was lost in 82% of eyes with outflow facilities below 0.18 but in only 11% of those maintained at facility values of 0.18 or higher.

In a third series of patients with proved open-angle glaucoma controlled by miotics, the therapy was deliberately reduced to the point at which the pressures were maintained at 17 to 25 mm Hg at all office visits. Outflow facilities were permitted to attain any value. This resulted in a high incidence of progression of field loss. Thus, in the series of 72 eyes observed in this fashion for periods of one to six years, 32% lost field. Of the eyes with outflow facilities of less than 0.18, 45% suffered field loss, whereas only 4% sustained such damage with facility values of 0.18 and above. Most important, these two selected facility populations did not differ at all in mean intraocular pressure (20.7 mm Hg). Such data from three separate laboratories provide abundant evidence for the importance of maintaining a normal outflow facility by miotic therapy.

Inadequacy of glaucoma control as measured by tonometry or tonography indicates the need for more intensive medical (miotic or secretory suppressant) therapy. However, it must be emphasized that an abnormal tonogram, even with the patient on maximum tolerated medical therapy, does not constitute a criterion for operative intervention unless there is evidence of progressive field loss or increased cupping.

Carbonic anhydrase inhibitors (Fig. 29-18)

Carbonic anhydrase inhibitors lower intraocular pressure by suppressing secretion and do not alter outflow facility in glaucomatous eyes. In patients whose outflow facility cannot be improved by any of the miotic agents available, the addition of carbonic anhydrase inhibitors permits lowering of intraocular pressure and maintaining it at a lower level throughout the day. In these patients tonography merely confirms tonometry in revealing the reduction of intraocular pressure. It also provides a method for following the progression of the outflow impairment. Particularly in the secondary glaucomas, tonography may demonstrate spontaneous improvement in outflow facility of sufficient magnitude to suggest the cessation of carbonic anhydrase inhibitor therapy. This is of particular importance because the systemic side effects of carbonic anhydrase inhibitors are to be avoided if at all possible. If a patient who requires carbonic anhydrase inhibitors demonstrates an improvement in outflow facility, efforts should be made to stop systemic therapy until such time as it is again needed. Interestingly enough, the same applies to some patients with open-angle glaucoma; that is, they go through phases of spontaneous improvement in their outflow facility on the same miotic therapy, and for a period of time they may do without carbonic anhydrase inhibitors.

Epinephrine (Fig. 29-19)

Topical epinephrine hydrochloride or bitartrate (2%) also suppresses the secretion of aqueous humor. Its effects appear to be additive to those of Diamox. The information derived from tonometry and tonography in epinephrine therapy is similar to that described above for carbonic anhydrase inhibitors. Most patients respond to epinephrine with improved outflow facility in additon to the decrease in aqueous secretion. Some eyes demonstrate dramatic increases in outflow facility soon after epinephrine therapy is begun, but others show improved outflow facility only after prolonged administration. The mechanism of the improvement remains unknown but is still being actively investigated (Chapter 18).

SURGERY FOR OPEN-ANGLE GLAUCOMA

It is our firm conviction that open-angle (simple) glaucoma should be controlled medically if at all possible. The only indications for surgery in the open-angle glaucomas are the progressive loss of visual field and cupping of the optic disc while maximum medical therapy is used and tolerated. Tonometry and tonography may confirm the inadequate medical control and suggest more intensive therapy, but these tests do not indicate the decision as to surgical intervention. In fact, even in patients referred for surgery because of progression of field loss, if the medical therapy can be altered to improve tonometric and tonographic status of control, additional periods of medical care under close supervision may be indicated. It has been our experience that under these circumstances few operations are necessary in the open-angle glaucomas. Furthermore, the vast majority of patients can be carried through their lifetime by medical therapy without significant loss of function and without the hazards, complications, and sequelas of surgical procedures.

Filtering procedures (Figs. 29-20 and 29-21)

Successful filtering operations improve outflow facility and thus lower intraocular pressure. The scarring down of a filtering bleb may be detected by a decrease in tonographic outflow facility before it can be recognized clinically or tonometrically. A progressive decrease in outflow facility is usually the first sign predicting the failure of the filtering bleb. Most glaucoma surgery is followed by a variable period of hyposecretion. During this interval tonometry is of little help in evaluating the results of the surgical procedure. In the case of cyclodialysis and cyclodiathermy, the hyposecretion may persist for prolonged periods of time.

Ocular rigidity

An important effect of surgery is the frequent apparent decrease in ocular rigidity postoperatively. The decrease in rigidity occurs after various types of surgery on the eye and results in underestimation of intraocular pressure by Schiøtz tonometry with one weight. The underestimates provide false assurance to the ophthalmologist as to the success of his procedure. Applanation tonometry reveals the true status. Tonography in these eyes also causes concern because, in spite of the apparent normalization of intraocular pressure, the tracing remains flat. This is particularly true after cyclodiathermy.

MEDICAL THERAPY FOR ANGLE-CLOSURE GLAUCOMA

The angle-closure glaucomas are surgical problems. Medical therapy of such eyes is to be considered a preoperative measure. The rare exceptions may be old and disabled patients who perhaps cannot tolerate surgical procedures or patients who refuse surgery. The latter group appears to be most frequent in the hands of ophthalmologists not completely convinced of the merits of surgery in early angle-closure glaucoma.

Most patients with angle-closure glaucoma can be brought out of the acute attack and their pressures normalized with miotics, carbonic anhydrase inhibitors, and/or osmotic therapy. Under these circumstances, tonography permits evaluation of the status of the outflow channels. Although gonioscopy may reveal the anatomic changes in the angle, it is not possible by gonioscopy alone to evaluate the functional status of the trabecular meshwork. Patients are seen in whom the angle appears to be still largely occluded but in whom the normalization of outflow facility demonstrates a functioning trabecular meshwork. It has been demonstrated that this is much more common than was supposed, and many eyes have been controlled with peripheral iridectomy, avoiding the hazards of the filtering procedure. On the other hand, in those eyes with pressures lowered by carbonic anhydrase inhibitors and hyperosmotic agents the outflow facility may remain impaired in spite of hypotony. Tonography permits the important distinction between these two groups of eyes. The one with normalization of outflow facility will do extremely well with a peripheral iridectomy, whereas the eye with impaired outflow facility may require postoperative medical therapy or a filtering procedure. It is clear that tonography and gonioscopy complement each other in these cases.

SURGERY FOR ANGLE-CLOSURE GLAUCOMA

As noted previously, tonography plays a role in the decision as to the type of surgery to be done for some patients with angle-closure glaucoma. It permits evaluation of the status of the trabecular meshwork and a more rational decision as to whether peripheral iridectomy will normalize the eye. Thus, in a series of operations on 182 eyes of 110 patients with angle-closure glaucoma, the results of surgery could be compared with the preoperative tonogram (Table 8-4). The failure rate following iridectomy was negligibly small in eyes with outflow facility greater than 0.13 but rose to 62% of eyes with outflow facility less than 0.13. On the other hand, a filtering procedure was approximately equally successful regardless of preoperative outflow facility. Fortunately, filtering operations proved as suc-

Table 8-4. Failure rate of initial surgery for angle-closure glaucoma and preoperative outflow facility

Preoperative outflow facility	Initial surgery performed			
	Iridectomy		Iridencleisis	
	Number of eyes	Failures	Number of eyes	Failures
≥ 0.18	60	0 (0%)	21	4 (19%)
0.13 – 0.17	19	1 (5%)	23	5 (22%)
< 0.13	21	13 (62%)	38	9 (24%)
Total	100	14 (14%)	82	18 (22%)

cessful after an iridectomy failure as they were when performed as initial procedures. In a series of 35 iridencleisis operations on eyes with previous iridectomies there were 9 eyes (26%) that failed to be controlled. This is quite comparable to the average failure rate (22%) of iridencleisis as a primary procedure. Therefore, in cooperative and understanding patients, the simpler and safer iridectomy should be done. This permits the use of strong miotics and epinephrine preparations that may normalize or improve remarkably the outflow facility in eyes that were thought to need filtering procedures. Filtering procedures are reserved for iridectomy failures or for those eyes with hopelessly impaired outflow facility and completely occluded angles.

CONGENITAL AND SECONDARY GLAUCOMAS

The tonographic findings in the congenital and secondary glaucomas follow in general those of the primary glaucomas. The elevation of intraocular pressure is almost always a consequence of obstructed outflow. Tonography gives no indications as to the cause of the obstruction, and this information must be derived from gonioscopic, slit-lamp, and other methods of examination. In the handling of the angle-closure group, tonography permits an evaluation of the function of the trabecular meshwork when the visible obstruction by the iris has been relieved (medically or surgically). The need for further therapy may then be anticipated.

In the secondary glaucomas with open angles and in congenital glaucomas, especially when pressure has been lowered by secretory suppression, it is often difficult to evaluate the status of the outflow channels by pressure measurements alone or by gonioscopy. In fact, an inflammatory process itself may so decrease secretion that pressure may not be elevated in spite of marked damage to the trabecular meshwork. Here tonography provides important information as to the patency of the outflow channels and may afford the first means of suggesting a diagnosis of glaucoma or of alerting the ophthalmologist to its future occurrence. Furthermore, it is an excellent means for following the progression of the outflow disorder and for evaluating the need for continuation of secretory suppressants. Poor outflow facility after an inflammatory process has subsided may also suggest the need for miotic therapy. Successful goniotomy in congenital glaucoma has been demonstrated to improve outflow facility and thus normalize intraocular pressure even when the period of postoperative hyposecretion is over.

OCULAR RIGIDITY AND GLAUCOMA DIAGNOSIS AND THERAPY
Definition

As defined by Friedenwald (p. 62), the coefficient of ocular rigidity is the factor E that relates changes in intraocular volume to alterations in pressure:

$$E = \frac{\log P_2 - \log P_1}{V_2 - V_1}$$

When measurements of intraocular pressure are made by applanation tonometry, the changes in pressure induced by the procedure are so slight that ocular rigidity variations have little effect on the determination. However, in Schiøtz tonometry and tonography the variations in ocular rigidity can lead to serious error. When the Schiøtz tonometer is applied to the eye, the intraocular pressure is raised by some 15 to 25 mm Hg. Since calibration tables assume an average value for E, deviations from this value in individual eyes lead to false estimates of the true intraocular pressure. Ocular rigidity may be approximated by Schiøtz tonometry using two different weights but is best measured by an applanation and Schiøtz reading.

Measurement (Table 28-7 and Figs. 28-1 and 28-2)

A simple check on the possibility of deviations of ocular rigidity from the normal in the individual eye is the measurement with two different weights or with applanation and one weight. Since patients vary in the magnitude of pressure elevation induced by changing from sitting to reclining positions, horizontal applanation measurements are preferable. If the values obtained from the ordinary calibration tables for "average" eyes agree, ocular rigidity is normal; if they differ, then the scale readings should be plotted on the nomogram, and further study is indicated. It is readily appreciated that if the scale reading with the heavier weight gives the lower pressure reading, the ocular rigidity coefficient, E, is less than the mean value and the true intraocular pressure, P_0, is higher than that indicated in the tables. If the heavier weight suggests a higher pressure reading, ocular rigidity is higher than normal, and the true intraocular pressure is lower than indicated.

Decreased ocular rigidity (Figs. 29-7 to 29-9)

A lower than average ocular rigidity coefficient such as is found in some cases of myopia or thyrotropic exophthalmos results in an underestimation of intraocular pressure by Schiøtz tonometry if only one weight is used. Such an underestimation of pressure may lead to failure to recognize glaucoma or to the false assumption that it is adequately controlled. Some operative procedures lower ocular rigidity, and in certain glaucomatous eyes the administration of stronger miotics also results in lowering of the ocular rigidity coefficient and similar false assurances as to glaucoma control. Applanation measurements indicate the true intraocular pressure and resolve the problem.

In tonography an ocular rigidity coefficient lower than the assumed normal results in a false flat tracing in addition to a low estimate of intraocular pressure. If no corrections are made, such findings simulate glaucoma with hyposecretion (controlled pressure but inadequate outflow facility). Fortunately, on an empirical basis these tonographic findings alone suggest the importance of close follow-up and further study whether or not attention has been called to the decreased ocular rigidity. This again demonstrates the rare need clinically for applying rigidity corrections to the tonogram.

Increased ocular rigidity

An ocular rigidity coefficient higher than the assumed average will lead to erroneously high estimates of intraocular pressure by Schiøtz tonometry and may result in a misdiagnosis of glaucoma or may incorrectly suggest poor control. The uncorrected tonographic tracings on such eyes are steep, thus simulating hypersecretion glaucoma. As indicated previously, the differential diagnosis between elevated ocular rigidity and hypersecretion glaucoma can be made only after estimation of rigidity of the given eye.

It must be emphasized again that corrections for ocular rigidity rarely rule out a suspicion of glaucoma. Random errors in tonometric readings can lead to serious errors in estimation of E and P_0. Patients with borderline tensions should not be dismissed on the basis of high estimates of ocular rigidity without due caution, repeated measurements, and considerable follow-up.

SUMMARY

In summary, it is apparent that tonography, when performed carefully and suitably corrected for the individual eye, provides information of considerable value for the early diagnosis of glaucoma as well as for the study of the progress of the disease and its status of control. It must be reemphasized that this laboratory test can supplement and corroborate other findings, but it is not a substitute for other tests and for good clinical judgment.

Problems for consideration

Intraocular pressure. Of all the parameters of aqueous dynamics, intraocular pressure is the one most accurately determined by present methods. Applanation tonometry provides the best estimate of intraocular pressure, and values agree well with those obtained by direct cannulation of the eye. The instrument, however, is expensive and a slit lamp is required for its use. Development of the Draeger and Perkins applanation tonometers appears to meet the requirements for hand-held, portable instruments that are accurate. Expense still remains a problem.

The Schiøtz tonometer is subject to considerably greater error than the applanation tonometer. Ultimate replacement of this method of measuring intraocular pressure by applanation tonometry is envisioned.

Outflow facility. The development of more accurate, clinically applicable methods of estimation of outflow facility is of prime importance in the future study of glaucoma. All the methods presently utilized introduce considerable error and assumptions, since all require disturbance of steady-state dynamics. Nevertheless, tonography is practical, and the values of outflow facility obtained have been demonstrated to be clinically valuable in the management of glaucoma. Fundamental studies are needed, however, to understand and correct the errors and artifacts of the method. Corrections must be made for viscoelastic expansion of the ocular coats, expulsion of blood from the eye when the tonometer is applied and re-entry of blood during the procedure, alterations in aqueous production during tonography, and posterior deformation of the globe from the weight applied. The last is also dependent on the firmness of the orbital tissues and the suspension apparatus of the eye. Possible changes in outflow facility induced by the procedure itself must also be considered. Constant-pressure tonography avoids some of these fundamental problems but is not yet a practical clinical test.

Aqueous production. Accurate and rapid determination of the rate of aqueous flow presents many difficulties, some of which have been described. A measure of inflow rate independent of assumptions pertaining to outflow facility would be of great value in the understanding of aqueous physiology. Extension of the studies of Holm might provide such a method.

EPIDEMIOLOGIC STUDIES

Epidemiologic studies aimed at improving our understanding of the beginning and natural history of primary open-angle glaucoma are needed. The hypothesis that eyes which will develop glaucoma in the future belong to a distinct population that can be detected early by abnormalities of aqueous dynamics requires testing. Prospective studies aimed at long-term follow-up of individuals with no glaucoma but with different intraocular pressures and outflow facilities will be invaluable in determining whether such measures can predict later glaucoma and thus indicate the beginning of the clinical disease. The meaning of "ocular hypertension" without visual field loss or optic nerve damage must be elucidated. The complex frequency distribution of intraocular pressure and the biologic factors responsible for it need exploration so that more meaningful statistical conclusions can be formulated.

PHYSIOLOGIC INVESTIGATIONS

Factors responsible for fluctuation in aqueous secretion, outflow facility, and intraocular pressure are important but poorly understood. Diurnal variations of these parameters exist, but the regulatory mechanisms are unknown.

Electron microscopic studies indicate that aqueous secretion is probably closely related to the interdigitations between epithelial cells. Anatomically, the nonpigmented epithelial cells are much more complex than the pigmented cell layer. Anatomic studies after modifications of transport systems may clarify the role of the pigmented epithelium.

Several systems transporting substances into and out of the eye are involved in the aqueous secretory process. Other systems almost certainly remain to be discovered. The exact functions of these systems, nutritional or otherwise, are unknown, but their elucidation may hold the key to the understanding of glaucoma as well as other ocular diseases. The possibility exists that alterations in enzyme systems, genetic or induced, may greatly influence aqueous formation or outflow. In view of the prominent role played by carbonic anhydrase in aqueous secretion, it would be interesting to determine qualitative and quantitative alterations in this enzyme in patients with and without glaucoma.

Several investigators have demonstrated the presence of vacuoles in the endothelial cells of the inner wall of Schlemm's canal. These vacuoles connect the trabecular spaces with the lumen of Schlemm's canal and can be seen as pores on scanning electron micrographs of the inner canal wall. It is not known whether these vacuoles represent the normal channels for aqueous outflow, whether they exist in vivo, or if they represent rapidly occurring fixation artifacts. Elucidation of these questions is necessary for the understanding of the physiology of aqueous outflow in the human eye.

Most studies have indicated that the major site of obstruction to aqueous outflow is in the trabeculum bordering Schlemm's canal (juxtacanalicular tissue). The fact that glaucoma patients were successfully treated by removing the *outer* wall of Schlemm's canal suggests that, in some cases at least, the obstruction may be peripheral to Schlemm's canal. It has not been demonstrated, however, that this procedure can be performed without damage to the *inner* wall of Schlemm's canal or that the improved glaucoma status is not due to alterations of the trabecular meshwork. Careful studies are necessary to clarify these observations.

The nature of changes in the trabecular meshwork in patients with glaucoma is poorly understood. Age changes must be carefully differentiated from those due to disease. Electron microscopic studies of the trabecular meshwork after pharmacologic alteration of outflow facility are needed. These will be particularly valuable in eyes treated with topical steroids before death. The finding of plasma cells and gamma globulin near the inner wall of Schlemm's canal in eyes with open-angle glaucoma requires explanation regarding their role in trabecular function and disease.

References—Section III

Armaly, M. F.: On the distribution of applanation pressure. I. Statistical features and the effect of age, sex, and family history of glaucoma, Arch. Ophthal. **73:**11, 1965.

Armaly, M. F.: Interpretation of tonometry and ophthalmoscopy, Invest. Ophthal. **11:** 75, 1972.

Bárány, E. H.: Pseudofacility and uveo-scleral outflow routes. In Leydhecker, W., editor: Glaucoma; Tutzing Symposium, Basel, 1967, S. Karger.

Bárány, E. H., and Scotchbrook, S.: Influence of testicular hyaluronidase on the resistance to flow through the angle of the anterior chamber, Acta Physiol. Scand. **30:**240, 1954.

Becker, B.: Carbonic anhydrase and the formation of aqueous humor, Amer. J. Ophthal. **47:**342, 1959.

Becker, B., and Friedenwald, J. S.: Clinical aqueous outflow, Arch. Ophthal. **50:**557, 1953.

Bengtsson, B.: Some factors affecting the distribution of intraocular pressures in a population, Acta Ophthal. **50:**33, 1972.

Bill, A.: Further studies on the influence of the intraocular pressure on aqueous humor dynamics in cynomolgus monkeys, Invest. Ophthal. **6:**364, 1967.

Bill, A., and Bárány, E. H.: Gross facility, facility of conventional routes, and pseudofacility of aqueous humor outflow in the cynomolgus monkey, Arch, Ophthal. **75:**665, 1966.

Bonting, S. L.: Na-K activated ATPase and active cation transport. In DeGraeff, J., and Leijnse, B., editors: Water and electrolyte metabolism. II, Amsterdam, 1964, Elsevier Publishing Co.

Clark, W. B., editor: Symposium on glaucoma, St. Louis, 1959, The C. V. Mosby Co.

Corboy, J. M., and Borchardt, K. A.: Mechanical sterilization of the applanation tonometer. I. Bacterial study, Amer. J. Ophthal. **71:**889, 1971.

Corboy, J. M., Goucher, C. R., and Parnes, C. A.: Mechanical sterilization of the applanation tonometer. II. Viral study, Amer. J. Ophthal. **71:**891, 1971.

Davson, H.: The eye. Vol. 1. Vegetative physiology and biochemistry, London, 1969, Academic Press, Inc.

Draeger, J.: Principle and clinical application of a portable applanation tonometer, Invest. Ophthal. **6:**132, 1967.

Forbes, M., Pico, G., and Grolman, B.: A non-contact applanation tonometer, description and clinical evaluation, Arch. Ophthal. **91:**134, 1974.

Friedenwald, J. S.: The formation of the intraocular fluid, Amer. J. Ophthal. **32:**9, 1949.

Friedenwald, J. S., and Becker, B.: Aqueous humor dynamics, Arch. Ophthal. **54:**799, 1955.

Friedenwald, J. S., and others: Standardization of tonometers, decennial report of the American Academy of Ophthalmology and Otolaryngology, Rochester, Minn., 1954, The Academy.

Goldmann, H.: Abflussdruck, Minutenvolumen und Widerstand der Kammerwasserstromung des Menschen, Docum. Ophthal. **5-6:**278, 1951.

Grant, W. M.: Tonographic method for measuring the facility and rate of aqueous flow in human eyes, Arch. Ophthal. **44:**204, 1950.

Grant, W. M.: Clinical measurements of aqueous outflow, Arch. Ophthal. **46:**113, 1951.

Holm, O.: A photogrammetric method of estimation of pupillary aqueous flow in the living human eye, Acta Ophthal. **46:**254, 1968.

Holmberg, A.: Ultrastructure of the ciliary epithelium, Arch. Ophthal. **62:**935, 1959.

Kinsey, V. E., and Reddy, D. V. N.: Chemistry and dynamics of aqueous humor. In Prince, J. H., editor: The rabbit in eye research, Springfield, Ill., 1964, Charles C Thomas, Publisher.

Kronfeld, P. C.: The new calibration scale for Schiøtz tonometers, Amer. J. Ophthal. **45:**308, 1958.

Kronfeld, P. C., and others: Tonography symposium, Trans. Amer. Acad. Ophthal. Otolaryng. **65:**133, 1961.

Kupfer, C.: Clinical significance of pseudofacility, Amer. J. Ophthal. **75:**193, 1973.

Kupfer, C., and Sanderson, P.: Determination of pseudofacility in the eye of man, Arch. Ophthal. **80:**194, 1968.

Linnér, E.: Episcleral venous pressure during tonography, Acta XVII Concilium Ophthalmologicum (1954) **3:**1532, 1955.

Moses, R. A., and Becker, B.: Clinical tonography: the scleral rigidity correction, Amer. J. Ophthal. **45:**196, 1958.

Newell, F. W., editor: Glaucoma; Transactions of the First, Second, Third, Fourth, and Fifth Conferences, New York, 1956-1960, Josiah Macy, Jr. Foundation.

Raviola, G.: The fine structure of the ciliary zonule and ciliary epithelium, Invest. Ophthal. **10:**851, 1971.

Rohen, J. W., and Witmer, R.: Electron microscopic studies on the trabecular meshwork in glaucoma simplex, Graefes Arch. Klin. Exp. Ophthal. **183:**251, 1972.

Van Buskirk, E. M., and Grant, W. M.: Lens depression and aqueous outflow in enucleated primate eyes, Amer. J. Ophthal. **76:**632, 1973.

Weekers, R., editor: Glaucoma symposium, Docum. Ophthal. **13:**1959.

Zimmerman, L. E., and others: Symposium: Contribution of electron microscopy to the understanding of the production and outflow of aqueous humor, Trans. Amer. Acad. Ophthal. Otolaryng. **70:**737, 1966.

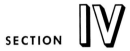

OPHTHALMOSCOPY AND PERIMETRY

Ophthalmoscopy provides an objective method of viewing the actual site of damage to the optic nerve produced by increased intraocular pressure. Perimetry permits a subjective evaluation of the extent of that damage. In addition to being of great diagnostic value, they are the final criteria of success or failure of glaucoma therapy.

9
Optic discs

EQUIPMENT

Accurate ophthalmoscopy is of particular importance in glaucoma to evaluate the health of the optic nerve. The examiner must often look through tiny miotic pupils. It is therefore important to have a good ophthalmoscope with a small aperture and a sufficiently powerful light to illuminate the interior of the eye through the small pupil. The Keeler, the Propper, and the Welch-Allyn with halogen bulb have been particularly useful.

Although direct ophthalmoscopy is usually used in the United States, indirect ophthalmoscopy has occasional distinct advantages. This is particularly true in high myopia or when the media are hazy. Often a definite diagnosis can be made by its use that would be impossible by the direct method.

An even more effective ophthalmoscopic method is the slit lamp with a Hruby lens or a fundus contact lens such as the Goldmann or Zeiss goniolens. Since the slit beam can pass to one side of any opacities in the media, visibility is not obstructed by reflected light, as with the other methods. Furthermore, the slit beam is of great value in determining the extent of excavations of the optic disc, particularly when they are shallow. Certainly the slit-lamp evaluation of the optic disc is quite accurate and should be applied when field defects are inconsistent with disc examination by other forms of ophthalmoscopy. Any question of the configuration of the optic disc should be resolved by slit-lamp examination.

The smooth-domed Koeppe lens provides a clear ophthalmoscopic view of the fundus and is especially useful for infant examination. During the first 2 months of age, the Richardson-Shaffer infant diagnostic lens is inserted more easily than the 16 mm Koeppe lens. In any patient the smooth-domed lens has several advantages. It can hold an unanesthetized infant's lids open for easy examination. Irregular, uncontrolled eye movements are reduced by holding the lens more firmly against the eye. When there are minor irregularities on the corneal surface, the lens provides a smooth surface to view the posterior pole. The optics of the lens minimizes the effect of a small pupil.

ANATOMY OF THE OPTIC DISC

The axons of the retinal ganglion cells join as a common cable at the optic disc. As they turn back to form the optic nerve, a central funnel-shaped depression, called the physiologic excavation, is left in the middle of the optic disc. If the posterior scleral foramen is small, the axons are crowded together, and the physiologic excavation is small or absent. If a large posterior scleral foramen is present, the physiologic excavation may occupy more than half the disc. When glaucomatous cupping of a disc occurs, the width and depth of that cup will depend at first on the configuration of the disc before it was damaged. The size of the cup is inherited. Therefore families of patients have a tendency toward cupping of the same degree. This fact may provide help in the interpretation of a large cup in a glaucoma suspect. Most reports, old and recent, show a slight increase in cupping with age. It should be noted, however, that some statistical analyses have refuted this.

The floor of the physiologic cup or the glaucomatous cup is formed by the lamina cribrosa, which is the white, sievelike connective tissue stretched across the posterior scleral foramen (Fig. 9-1). The larger the cup, the more easily this lamina can be seen. The gray dots in its surface mark the openings through which the axons pass into the optic nerve itself. The lamina cribrosa lies 0.7 mm behind the retinal surface in hyperopic eyes and half that distance in myopic eyes.

Normally the retinal elements, the pigmented epithelium, and the choroid terminate abruptly at the nerve head. Anatomic variations in this termination, such as the scleral crescent in myopia, may alter the appearance of the disc and its surroundings. The optic canal itself has varying degrees of obliquity, which alter the disc appearance. The slope of the walls of the cup is partially dependent on the obliquity of the scleral canal. In myopia the canal has an exaggerated obliquity directed temporally. Because of these changes and the fact that the position of the cribriform plate prevents the formation of any deep cup, it is easy to miss glaucomatous excavation in the myopic eye. In this situation it is particularly valuable to examine the disc with the slit-lamp beam and either a Hruby lens or a flat-surfaced contact lens.

BLOOD SUPPLY OF THE OPTIC NERVE AND DISC
(Plates 2 and 3)

It seems increasingly probable that the nerve destruction which results from glaucoma is based on vascular insufficiency to the nerve. The relationship between intraocular pressure and systemic blood pressure, or more specifically, ophthalmic artery pressure, may be of extreme importance. Attempts are underway to correlate the pressure gradient between these systems with visual loss. Relative systemic hypotension or carotid stenosis contributes to development of nerve damage even in eyes with relatively normal intraocular pressures. Furthermore, similar rapid changes in fields have occurred in hypertensive patients with glaucoma when their

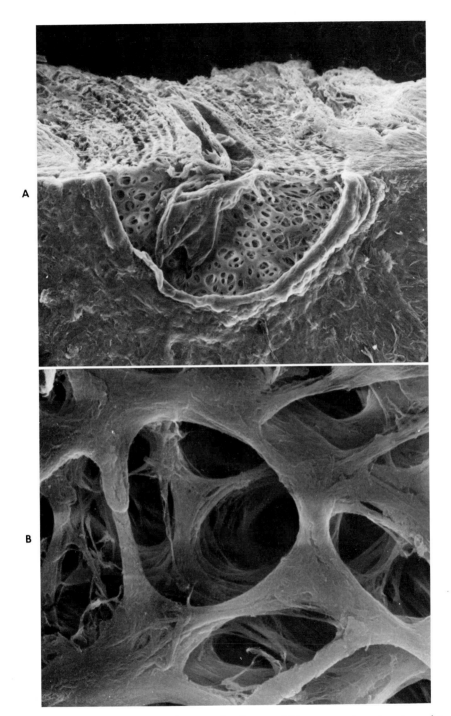

Fig. 9-1. A, Nonglaucomatous right eye of a 5-year-old boy seen at postmortem, showing the anterior surface and cross-sectional view of the lamina cribrosa. Scanning electron micrograph at 20 kv and 0 tilt. (×36.) **B,** Enlarged view of the anterior surface of the lamina cribrosa seen in **A,** showing the pores and array of the plates. (×480.) (Courtesy Dr. J. M. Emery, Houston, Texas.)

blood pressure has been abruptly lowered by antihypertensive medications. In addition, Drance found that many low-tension glaucoma subjects had histories of an episode of acute systemic hypotension due to trauma or bleeding ulcers. Patients should be questioned specifically about such episodes. Blood pressure measurements and ophthalmodynamometry are useful methods for evaluation of the glaucoma patient.

The reason for this vulnerability at the optic disc is probably the peculiarity of its blood supply. The optic nerve is nourished by tiny arterial twigs coming from the pial vessels and the central retinal artery. The short posterior ciliary arteries

---

Plate 2

A, Three-dimensional color drawing of the intraocular and part of the orbital optic nerve. Where the retina terminates at the optic disc edge, the Muller cells, *1a*, are in continuity with the astrocytes, forming the *internal limiting membrane of Elschnig, 1b.* In some specimens Elschnig's membrane is thickened in the central portion of the disc to form the *central meniscus of Kuhnt, 2.* At the posterior termination of the choroid on the temporal side, the border tissue of Elschnig, *3*, lies between the astrocytes surrounding the optic nerve canal, *4*, and the stroma of the choroid. On the nasal side, the choroidal stroma is directly adjacent to the astrocytes surrounding the nerve. This collection of astrocytes, *4*, surrounding the canal is known as the *border tissue of Jacoby.* This is continuous with a similar glial lining called the intermediary tissue of Kuhnt, *5*, at the termination of the retina. The nerve fibers of the retina are segregated into approximately 1000 bundles, or fascicles, by astrocytes, *6*. On reaching the lamina cribrosa (upper dotted line), the nerve fascicles, *7*, and their surrounding astrocytes are separated from each other by connective tissue (drawn in blue). This connective tissue is the cribriform plate, which is an extension of scleral collagen and elastic fibers through the nerve. The external choroid also sends some connective tissue to the anterior part of the lamina. At the external part of the lamina cribrosa (lower dotted line), the nerve fibers become myelinated, and columns of oligodendrocytes (black and white cells) and a few astrocytes (red-colored cells) are present within the nerve fascicles. The astrocytes surrounding the fascicles form a thinner layer here than in the laminar and prelaminar portion. The bundles continue to be separated by connective tissue all the way to the chiasm, *Sep.* This connective tissue is derived from the pia mater and is known as the septal tissue. A mantle of astrocytes, *Gl.M,* continuous anteriorly with the border tissue of Jacoby, surrounds the nerve along its orbital course. The dura, *Du,* arachnoid, *Ar,* and pia mater, *Pia,* are shown. The central retinal vessels are surrounded by a perivascular connective tissue throughout their course in the nerve; this connective tissue blends with the connective tissue of the cribriform plate in the lamina cribrosa; it is called the central supporting connective tissue strand here.

B, Diagrammatic representation of blood supply of optic nerve head and optic nerve. *A,* Arachnoid; *C,* choroid; *CAR,* central retinal artery; *CRV,* central retinal vein; *D,* dura; *OD,* optic disc; *ON,* optic nerve; *PCA,* posterior ciliary arteries; *R,* retina; *S,* sclera; *SAS,* subarachnoid space; *LC,* lamina cribrosa; *PR,* prelaminar region; *Col. Br.,* collateral branches.

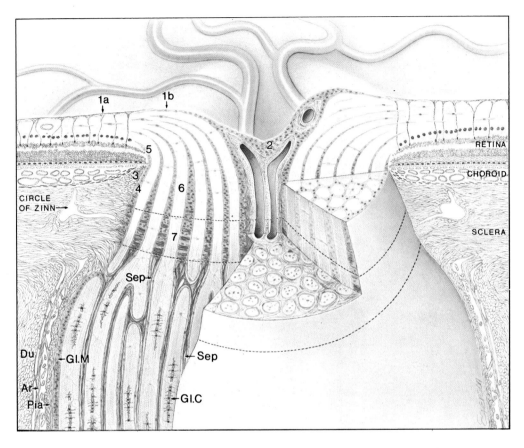

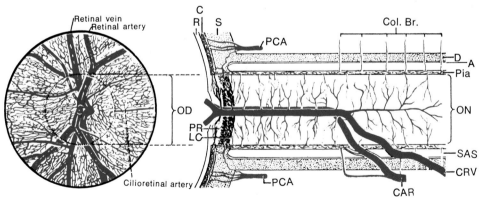

Plate 2. For legend see opposite page.

Plate 3

A to **C,** Mexican infant, 3 years old, with highly pigmented fundus. **A,** Disc at normal tension of 15 mm Hg applanation. **B,** With 35 grams added pressure (Bailliart), picture shows pallor when diastolic pulse appears. **C,** At pressure of 80 grams, systolic arrest appears, producing extremely pale disc.

D to **F,** Infantile glaucomatous patient, 6 months old. **D,** Cupped disc seen through slightly hazy cornea; intraocular pressure 36 mm Hg. **E,** Pressure of 20 grams (Bailliart) produced pulse. **F,** Pressure of 35 grams (Bailliart) produced systolic arrest, with severe pallor of disc and posterior pole.

G to **I,** A 20-year-old woman with severe open-angle glaucoma; tensions ranged from 22 to 45 mm Hg over a six-month period. **G,** Moderate-sized cup (0.4 disc diameter). **H,** Marked enlargement of cup in five months (0.7 disc diameter), with no field defect to smallest targets. **I,** Same disc three months after successful filtering surgery: retinal vessels no longer displaced nasally, disc again a pink color, no cupping visible. Vision: 20/20; tension: 10 mm Hg by applanation.

(From Shaffer, R. N., and Hetherington, J., Jr.: Trans. Amer. Acad. Ophthal. Otolaryng. **73:**929, 1969.)

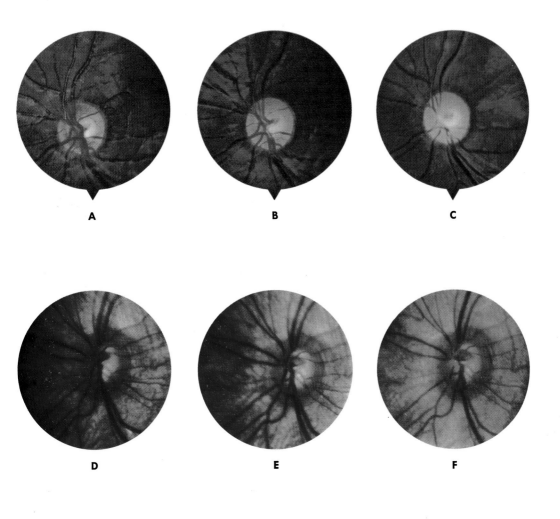

A

B

C

D

E

F

G

H

I

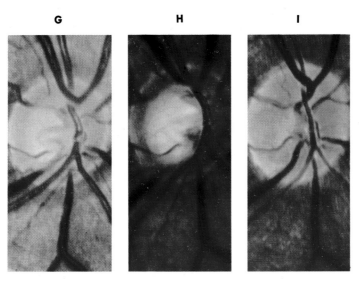

Plate 3. For legend see opposite page.

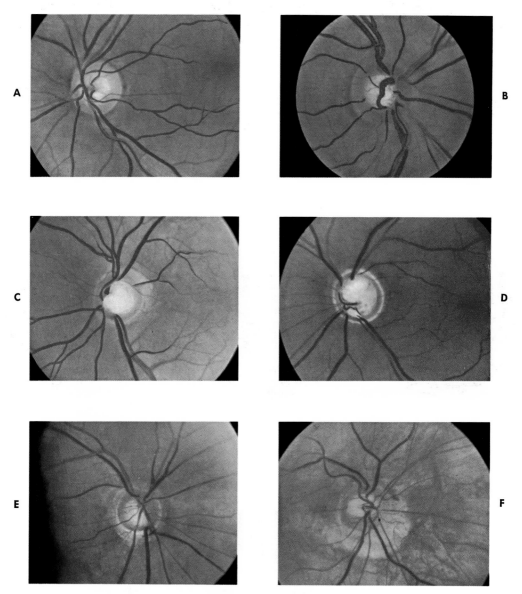

Plate 4

A, Optic disc with slight physiologic cupping, C/D 0.4.

B, Optic disc with moderate cupping, C/D 0.5.

C, Optic disc with moderate cupping, C/D 0.8.

D, Optic disc with severe cupping, C/D 0.9. History given in legend for Fig. 10-11.

E, Cupping of lower portion of the optic disc, C/D 0.5-0.6. History given in legend for Fig. 11-1.

F, Slightly cupped myopic disc with peripapillary atrophy. History given in legend for Fig. 11-5. Contact lens ophthalmoscopy demonstrates cupping that extends to the periphery of the disc.

supply the major portion of the optic disc and, of course, the choroid. These small converging vessels sometimes form a ring around the nerve head called the circle of Zinn and Haller. More often, only a portion of this circular vessel is present. A few recurrent vessels from the central retinal artery supply the superficial peripheral part of the disc. The disc circulation is a low-pressure vascular system. As described above, an increase in intraocular pressure or a decrease in intraneural arterial pressure can permit shunting of blood away from the disc. This may lead to degeneration of the glial supporting tissue and the neurons, resulting in disc cupping and nerve fiber bundle field defects. Why these defects follow such a characteristic pattern is still unknown.

Ophthalmodynamometry of infant discs provides good evidence that the damage to the optic disc by increased intraocular pressure is due to a shunting of the blood away from the disc. When an infant eye is subjected to increased pressure, this shunting mechanism is vividly shown. At relatively low intraocular pressure, pallor of the whole posterior pole of the eye begins as blood is forced out of either or both the choroid and peripapillary retinal network. At pressures of 15 to 30 grams, the diastolic pulse appears. The disc and peripapillary area become more pale until the circulation is stopped, usually at a pressure of 45 to 55 grams (Plate 3, *A* and *B*). This is in contrast to the adult disc, in which the diastolic pulse is usually seen between 60 and 80 mm Hg and systolic arrest between 100 and 120 mm Hg.

The blood pressure of infants is known to be considerably lower than that of adults. In the first few months of life, blood pressure will average 85 mm Hg systolic and 40 mm Hg diastolic; these gradually increase to 90 to 100 mm Hg systolic and 50 to 60 mm Hg diastolic by the time the infant is 1 year of age. This means that the effective pulse pressure going into an infant eye is less than in the adult, as is shown by ophthalmodynamometry. Similar increases in intraocular pressures might be expected to shunt blood more efficiently from the infant disc than from the adult one with its higher pulse pressure. It therefore seems logical to believe that the degree of ischemia is one reason for cupping of the infant disc to occur rapidly, whereas an adult disc at the same pressure may show no cupping for many years.

Fluorescein angiography in glaucoma (Figs. 9-2 to 9-4)

Early investigations with India ink and neoprene injections in monkeys show a decreased flow to the distal portion of the optic nerve when the intraocular pressure is elevated. Filling of vessels in the peripapillary area is also diminished, whereas the central retinal vessel remain less affected. The areas mainly involved are those supplied by the short posterior ciliary arteries. Fluorescein injections in animals have shown similar vascular abnormalities with artificially elevated pressures and with reductions in blood pressure.

Preliminary investigations have demonstrated marked vascular changes in some glaucoma patients with uncontrolled pressures both before and during in-

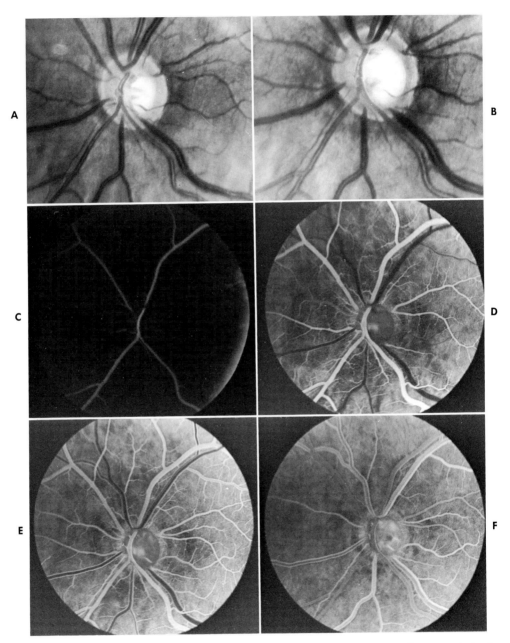

Fig. 9-2. A and **B,** Fundus photographs showing increasing disc cupping during period of uncontrolled intraocular pressure (upper thirties). No field defect demonstrable. **C** to **F,** Fluorescein angiographic series showing abnormal pattern with initial filling of central retinal artery and delayed choroidal filling during this period of uncontrolled pressure.

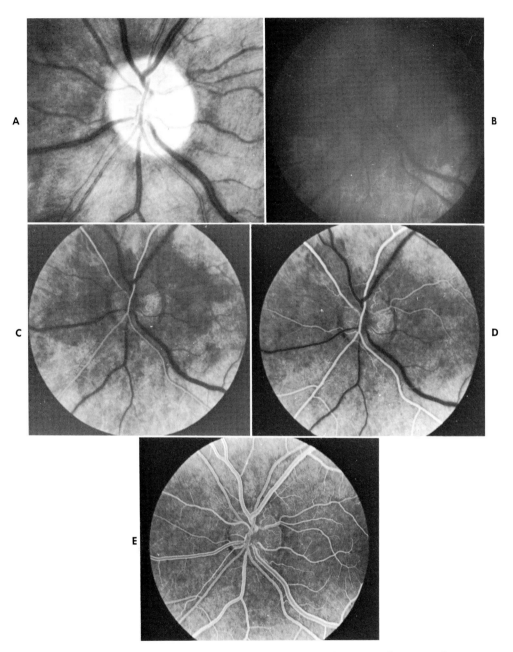

Fig. 9-3. A, Fundus photograph of same eye as Fig. 9-2 after surgical control of pressure, showing marked reduction of cupping in young patient. **B** to **E,** Postoperative angiographic series reveals a normal filling pattern, the choroid fluorescing earlier than the central retinal artery.

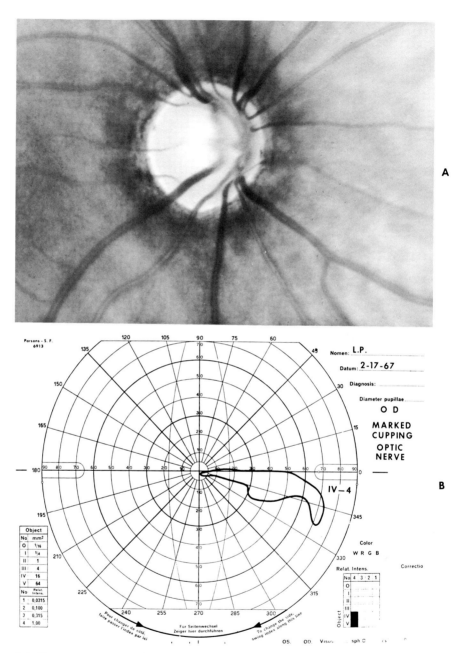

Fig. 9-4. Two years prior to the angiography seen in Figs. 9-2 and 9-3, the opposite eye had advanced glaucomatous cupping (0.9 disc diameter), **A**, and field loss, **B**.

creased cupping. Fluorescein-filling in both the central retinal vessel and choroidal circulation are delayed. In addition, this stage shows a reversal of the usual filling pattern (Fig. 9-2). Normally the choroidal circulation is apparent before the central retinal artery fluoresces. An abnormal increase in intraocular pressure produces a change in which the central vessels fluoresce prior to the choroidal flush. The vascular changes may occur before a field defect becomes evident. When the pressure is normalized and cupping disappears, a normal fluorescein pattern returns (Fig. 9-3). In man a diminution in vascular filling of capillaries on the atrophic disc in late stages of glaucoma has been described.

Fluorescein angiography not only clearly supports the vascular theories of previous studies with animals but also provides a possible test for determining the tolerance of the optic nerve to a specific level of intraocular pressure. Unfortunately similar changes can often be seen in normotensive eyes, so the test is not as yet specific.

Radial peripapillary capillaries (Fig. 9-5)

Michaelson and Henkind performed detailed studies of vessels in the superficial nerve fiber layer of the retina. Long capillaries follow nerve fiber bundles in an arcuate pattern. There is some speculation that various glaucoma field defects may originate from ischemia secondary to pressure directly on these vulnerable superficial small vessels. Supporting this theory are laboratory studies showing underfilling of these small capillaries in cats with artificially increased ocular pressure and the clinical finding of isolated scotomas in the arcuate area in eyes with early glaucoma. Selective atrophy of radial peripapillary capillaries has been shown in postmortem eyes of patients with chronic glaucoma.

Axoplasmic flow

There has been recent interest in the physiologic process of axoplasmic transport and its possible involvement in the pathogenic mechanisms of glaucomatous nerve damage. Axonal transport or flow is a physiologic property of all nerve fibers, including those of the visual system, and consists of the movement of intracellular materials up and down the length of the axon. Proteins and other substances synthesized in the retinal ganglion cells are transported in the axons of the optic nerve. The system permits movement of materials required for maintenance of the structural integrity of the axon plus substances needed at the synaptic terminals in the lateral geniculate body. Flow rates for different materials vary from a few millimeters to several centimeters per day. It is of interest that axoplasmic transport can be blocked by mechanical constriction of the axon from external pressure (e.g., by a ligature) or by localized ischemia. The demonstration by Anderson and associates and others that elevated intraocular pressure causes a blockage of axonal transport in the optic disc at the lamina cribrosa has permitted speculation that this process might be involved in the development of optic nerve damage in glaucoma. It is not clear whether the lamina cribrosa mechanically compresses the

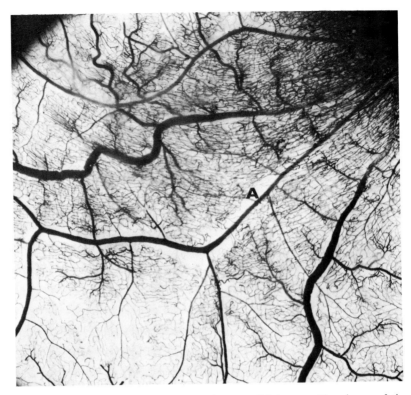

Fig. 9-5. Radial peripapillary capillaries in the superficial nerve fiber layer of the retina in man (India ink preparation). A, Inferotemporal artery. (From Henkind, P.: Invest. Ophthal. **6:**103, 1967.)

nerve fibers when intraocular pressure is elevated or if the blocked transport is a consequence of disc ischemia produced by the high pressure. Both protein synthesis within the nerve cell body and protein transport along the axon can be affected by elevation of IOP. Whether chronic alteration of either of these processes eventually leads to neuronal degeneration or functional loss is not yet known.

OPTIC DISC CHANGES IN GLAUCOMA (Figs. 9-6 to 9-12 and Plate 4, A to D)

Whether caused by vascular insufficiency, intraocular pressure excess, or a combination of both, the visible damage to the optic nerve occurs at the optic disc. In the region of the lamina cribrosa there is destruction of nerve fibers and glial tissue, which results in an increased size of the physiologic cup. The initial changes forming the cup are most likely due to loss of extracellular and intracellular fluids. Loss of astroglial tissue is followed by degeneration and atrophy of nerve fibers. In the adult, bowing of the cribriform fascia is a late change (Fig. 9-12), but it is an early change in the infant (Fig. 17-12).

The very deep, wide cups seen in advanced glaucoma are caused both by tissue destruction in the disc and by the extension of that process into the neural and

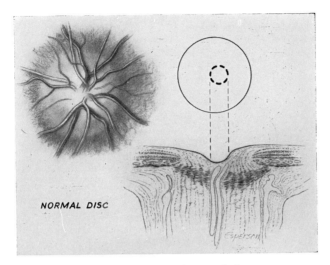

Fig. 9-6. Diagram of normal disc.

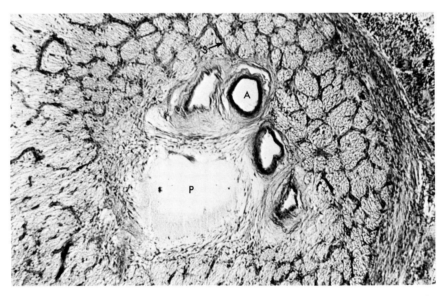

Fig. 9-7. Photomicrograph of cross section of normal human optic disc, showing physiologic cup, *P*, blood-filled channels in optic disc, *S*, and central retinal artery, *A*. (PAS stain; ×56.) (From Henkind, P., and Levitzky, M.: Amer. J. Ophthal. **68:**979-986, 1969.)

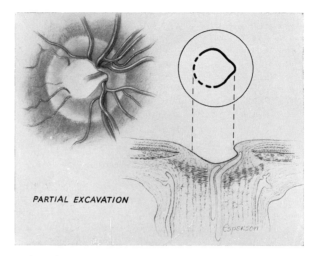

Fig. 9-8. Diagram of moderately cupped disc. Dotted line indicates a sloping edge; and solid line, an undetermined edge of the cup.

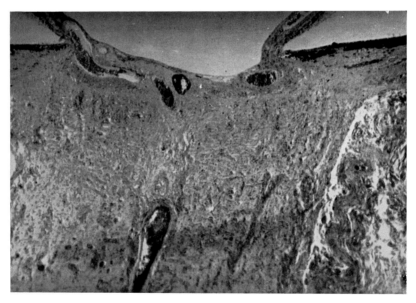

Fig. 9-9. Photomicrograph showing optic disc with no cupping. (Courtesy Dr. F. C. Cordes, San Francisco.)

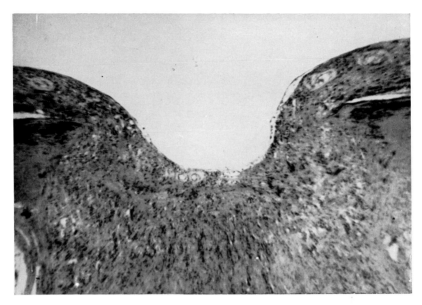

Fig. 9-10. Photomicrograph showing moderate cupping. (Courtesy Dr. F. C. Cordes, San Francisco.)

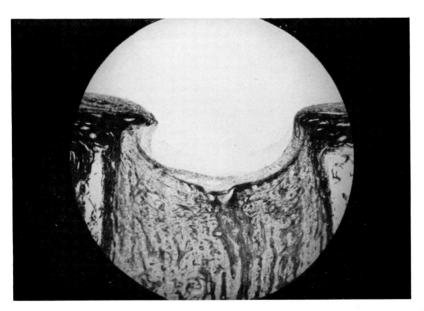

Fig. 9-11. Photomicrograph showing moderately severe cupping with undermining of the edges of the cup. (Courtesy Dr. F. C. Cordes, San Francisco.)

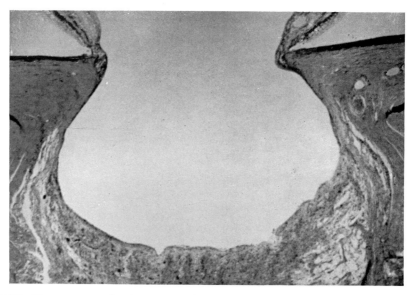

Fig. 9-12. Photomicrograph showing total excavation with undermining, the so-called bean pot excavation. (Courtesy Dr. F. C. Cordes, San Francisco.)

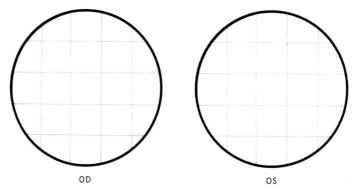

OD   OS

Fig. 9-13. Grid shown here can be stamped onto a chart. Each space represents two tenths of the diameter in the horizontal and vertical direction and acts as a guide for greater accuracy in diagramming.

glial elements behind the cribriform plate. The lamina cribrosa is then able to bow backward, increasing the depth of the cup (Figs. 9-9 to 9-12).

It is clear that early glaucomatous cupping may disappear after the intraocular pressure is lowered. Although the frequency of this occurrence is unknown, it is probably seen more often in young patients (Plate 3, *C*). This normalization of the glaucomatous cupping should not be confused with disc edema associated with hypotony. These visible cupping changes can occur without field defects.

To evaluate the disc, the examiner should be aware of the pattern in which cupping progresses. Glaucomatous cupping in many patients forms by symmetrical enlargement of the physiologic central cup. It is common, however, to detect cupping that extends toward the disc margin in a confined area, usually in the inferior temporal or superior temporal quadrant.

Early cupping may develop to form a marginal step if pressure causes a recession of the surface peripheral to the central physiologic cupped area. This is referred to as saucerization. A field defect usually corresponds to the involved area of the disc.

Normally the retinal vessels come perpendicularly through the cribriform plate into the eye, climb up the large mass of axon cylinders that occupy the nasal half of the disc, and then turn onto the surface of the retina. They either run more diagonally across the floor of the deepened cup or, in advanced cases, vanish under the nasal lip of the cup, reappearing at the edge of the excavation (Plate 4, E).

It is often possible to predict the quality of the field loss by the appearance of the disc. If the excavation is extreme in the lower portion, there will be a corresponding Bjerrum's scotoma in the upper field. A markedly cupped, atrophic disc with only a thin layer of nerve fibers about the periphery is an ominous finding. The contrary finding of a disc with little cupping and much healthy looking nerve tissue is prognostically more favorable.

Nasal displacement of the retinal vessels is no longer considered characteristic of glaucomatous cupping. The degree of vessel displacement is related to the width and depth of the cup, whether the cup is normal or excavated.

In a busy practice, careful examination of the disc can indicate areas worth greater scrutiny on field testing. It is important to remember that glaucomatous disc cupping may appear without a field defect.

Disc changes in infants

Disc cupping in infants may differ from that in adults. Contrary to information in the literature, glaucomatous cupping does occur early in the young and may be quite marked. According to Richardson and Shaffer, C/D ratios larger than 0.3 were found in 2.7% of normal infants (26 of 936 eyes) and in 61% of glaucoma infants (52 of 85 eyes); the incidence of optic cup asymmetry was 0.6% in normal infants (3 of 468 eyes) and 89% in unilateral glaucoma infants (24 out of 27 eyes). Glaucomatous cupping in infants will often diminish rapidly with pressure control. Changes in cupping provide an excellent parameter for diagnosis and follow-up of infantile glaucoma.

Clinical evaluation

If the cup is initially small, a moderate increase in its size may not attract the attention of the ophthalmologist, whereas a large cup is likely to arouse suspicion as to whether it is physiologic or glaucomatous. Therefore it becomes important for the

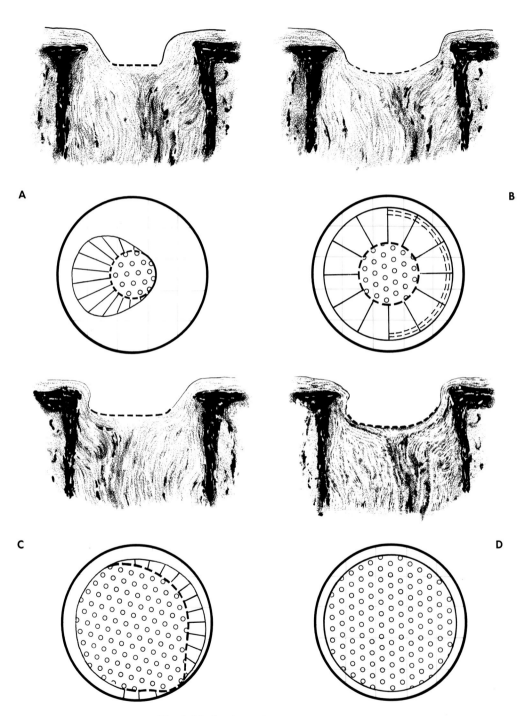

Fig. 9-14. For legend see opposite page.

ophthalmologist to make careful diagrams of discs so that changes in their contour can be evaluated in later years. Ideally, all discs examined should be photographed, preferably in stereo, or diagrammed according to the method suggested in Fig. 9-14. Any eye under suspicion of glaucoma must certainly be photographed or diagrammed. It is also helpful to include a measurement to one decimal place, indicating the size of the cup in relation to the total disc diameter, abbreviated as C/D ratio. Disc cupping greater than 0.7 disc-diameter is present in less than 1% of a normal population. A difference between eyes of 0.2 disc-diameter or greater is found in less than 1% of a normal population. These findings during ophthalmoscopy should alert a physician to further examination.

Cupping is estimated by noting the area of change in color and contour. Statistical analyses show that most experienced examiners determine the cup/disc ratio according to color differences. If a change in contour occurs, this landmark is recorded. A gradual slope ascending toward the periphery of the disc is often mistakenly disregarded. Future damage can be determined more accurately if all possible parameters are diagrammed. Focusing attention on the cup rim helps determine the location or extent of damage. A rosy-colored, vascular, wide rim of nerve tissue is probably healthy, whereas an irregularly narrowed or pale rim often indicates prior damage. Approximately 85% of field defects can be predicted on the basis of a single disc examination without any other evidence available.

Fig. 9-14. A, This optic disc has a 0.3 disc-diameter cup which is moderately deep, exposing the lamina cribrosa, shown by the small circles. The nerve fibers begin at the inner dotted circle and rise toward the retinal surface near the periphery of the disc as shown by the straight radial lines. On the other side there is a steep slope as shown by the solid line. **B,** This diagram depicts a 0.4 disc-diameter cup with an upward slope to the retinal level near the edge of the disc. At one side, the slope steepens abruptly as shown by the short concentric lines. The lamina cribrosa is exposed as shown by the circles. **C,** Contour of a typical glaucomatous cup is diagrammed. The color contrast shows a cup of 0.7 (horizontal) × 0.9 (vertical) disc-diameter with an extension to the lower temporal rim, exposing large areas of the lamina cribrosa. The loss of nerve tissue to the edge of the disc is almost invariably associated with an arcuate field defect. One half of the cup is steep-walled as shown by the solid line. The other half of the cup has a slope that reaches the retinal level near the periphery of the disc. **D,** This represents a severely cupped disc with steep edges to the cup, which measures over 0.8 disc-diameter. The lamina cribrosa is exposed. Since the nerve fibers at the disc margin may be intact, one could not predict the presence of a field defect. A patient with such a disc should have careful perimetric studies and must remain under observation. Asymmetry of cupping is a most important indication of glaucomatous damage and is often easily seen in bilateral disc diagrams. (From Shaffer, R. N., Ridgway, W. L., Brown, R., and Kramer, S. G.: The use of diagrams to record changes in glaucomatous discs, Amer. J. Ophthal. **80:**460, 1975.)

CHAPTER 10

Peripheral and central fields

Although many different instruments may be used to test the visual fields, not one is as important as a skilled perimetrist who knows what to look for in a field and who is ingenious enough to obtain reliability in a subjective type of examination. In studying the patient with glaucoma, one must map both the peripheral field and the central 30° of the field to avoid missing any important defect. The peripheral field is less valuable in following the course of a patient with glaucoma because a greater percentage of defects occur in the central field.

EQUIPMENT

Goldmann perimeter

The half-sphere perimeter is theoretically ideal. Such an instrument is the beautifully designed Goldmann perimeter (Fig. 10-1). This instrument is equipped for accurate standardization of test conditions for both peripheral and central fields, a characteristic that permits reproducibility of defects among different examiners and clinics. In addition, it provides excellent sensitivity, well-defined end points, and no visual clues other than the test object itself. The large choice of target sizes and intensities permits rapid plotting of isopters. Fixation is monitored through the centrally placed telescope. A reticule in the telescope is convenient for accurate pupillary measurements.

Tangent screen

The tangent screen is still used in many offices to examine the central 30° of the visual field. Careful tangent-screen perimetry will uncover most of the glaucoma-type defects. The advantage of the tangent screen over other perimeters is the expanded central area of testing. The screen should have a black matte finish and be illuminated uniformly to 7 footcandles.

Tübinger perimeter (Fig. 10-2)

The Tübinger perimeter has added to our knowledge of early field defects and has provided perhaps the most sensitive instrument for clinical use. The light in-

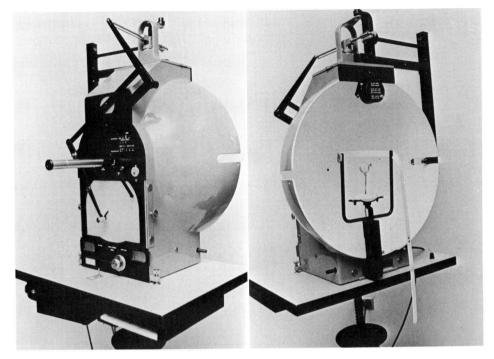

Fig. 10-1. Goldmann perimeter for visual field examination.

A

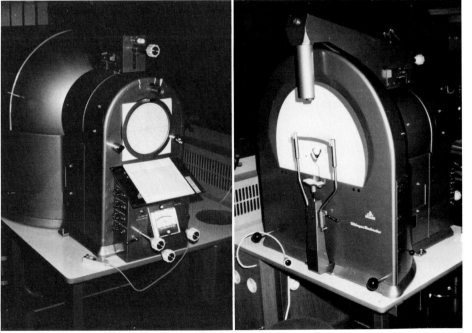

B

Fig. 10-2. Tübinger perimeter for static visual field examination.

tensity of the test target can be reduced from a maximum of 1000 apostilbs to a minimum of 0.00001 apostilb in 80 equidistant steps. Either the peripheral or central field can be tested in detail by both kinetic and static perimetry. This instrument is especially designed for static perimetry, allowing the examiner to easily plot visual response along any meridian of the visual field. Testing visual acuity at the point of fixation is a standard part of the Tübinger examination. The Tübinger is best utilized in a large clinical research setting. The cost of the instrument and the length of time required for a field examination limit its value in general ophthalmologic practice.

Other equipment

Flicker fusion, color fields, campimetry, skiascotometry, and angioscotometry all have their champions. In general, they do not add materially to the clinical information available by standard methods.

Also available are the automated visual field perimeters. Although these have some value as screening devices, they have not been found as reliable or complete as standard visual testing equipment. The Auto-Plot tangent screen, however, is a fairly reliable instrument giving good clinical results. Still, it is not as flexible as the traditional tangent screen or Goldmann perimeter.

METHOD OF EXAMINATION

The technique of field examination is well described in books on perimetry. There are a few important points that should be stressed because these are of vital importance in glaucoma.

Goldmann perimeter

Adjustment

The primary adjustment should be made daily by positioning the objective light at maximum intensity (V-4-e) toward the luxometer placed at one side of the bowl. Bulb changes or other appropriate adjustments are necessary if the intensity measures less than 1430 luxes (1000 apostilbs). Adjustment of target and bowl illumination should be checked each time before the instrument is used. This is done by matching the bowl illumination to the V-1-e target. Room illumination should be minimal, and the patient should be as comfortable as possible to reduce fatigue. The position of the headrest can be adjusted to center the eye under observation through the telescope. To avoid head movement, the patient should have available a buzzer or other simple hand signal. With the vast majority of patients the head strap need never be used.

Refraction and add

In the plotting of central fields with the Goldmann perimeter, it is necessary to utilize the patient's best refraction plus a near correction based on the age of the patient, as outlined in the instructions that accompany the instrument. If field defects are discovered, they should be rechecked with plus and minus spheres of 0.50 D in addition to the preceding correction. With the Goldmann perimeter, artifactual field defects appear to be produced in some eyes by differences in the refraction between the fovea and certain areas of the retina.

Technique (Fig. 10-3)

Methods of performing sensitive, reliable Goldmann perimetry are still under investigation. Aulhorn and Harms have contributed concepts that provide a new approach to techniques in glaucoma field analysis. The test object of greatest useful sensitivity is the smallest size and intensity detectable at the temporal horizontal meridian in the 25° isopter, 15° above and 15° below this point. This threshold target is used to define the limits of the central isopter and blind spot by kinetic perimetry. Particular attention is given to the nasal and temporal meridian for a step. Careful investigation of the 5°, 10°, and 15° isopters is necessary to reveal isolated scotomas characteristic of early glaucoma. These three central isopters are examined by static and, if necessary, by kinetic perimetry (from nonseeing to seeing). Any paracentral field defects found with the threshold target should be

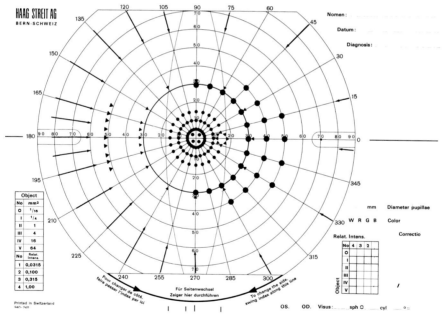

Fig. 10-3. Goldmann visual field chart illustrating both static (arrows) and kinetic (dots) points of examination. Note that 72 points are tested statically with a threshold target in the central field. This is considered a reliable search for early glaucomatous field defects. The I-4-e target is used to check for nasal step in the peripheral field. Some advocate testing of the peripheral temporal field for a step as indicated. A quick retinal scan is performed with target III-4-e.

checked at least twice, since artifacts are possible in any subjective test. The depth of field defects and any areas of consistent, hesitant response (especially in the Bjerrum area) should be noted. The I-2-e is the established standard test object for the central field and should be used when defects occur with weaker threshold targets.

Tangent screen

On the tangent screen the target should be exposed to the patient only when the examiner wishes it to be seen. The standard wands with a white bead on the end are unsatisfactory. To test the reliability of the patient, it should be possible to conceal the white targets from the patient whenever the examiner wishes. This can be done by using side-mounted wands, luminescent targets, or retractable targets.

Patient's fixation

If a refractive error of over 1.00 D is present, the patient should wear corrective lenses. The patient must look steadily at the fixation target, which should be large enough to be seen easily. With normal vision a 1 to 5 mm size is adequate. The patient's eye should be watched by the examiner. Attention, understanding, and fixation can be checked constantly by concealing and then exposing the target in areas of known sight or of known scotoma. Beware of the patient using bifocals for the examination. These may produce misunderstood artifacts.

Size of target

The field should be mapped with the smallest test object that the patient is able to see outside the blind spot and still produce a reliable and repeatable field. In early glaucoma this is usually either a 1 or 2 mm white bead at 1 or 2 meters. The plotting of the tangent screen field should follow the format suggested for the central fields on the Goldmann perimeter.

Rechecks of field

For comparable fields, the same size object at the same distance with the same illumination and by the same examiner are all important. If fields are examined by a technician, the physician should occasionally recheck these fields, since he is more conscious of the errors inherent in any subjective test.

Tübinger perimeter (Figs. 10-4, B, and 10-5)

During the last few years the principle of static, or profile, perimetry has been applied to the study of glaucomatous field changes. In this method a stationary test object is offered at a fixed position. The luminence of the test object is at first below the sensitivity threshold (i.e., the object is not visible) and is gradually increased until the patient can just perceive the target. The Tübinger is admirably designed for this method of perimetry.

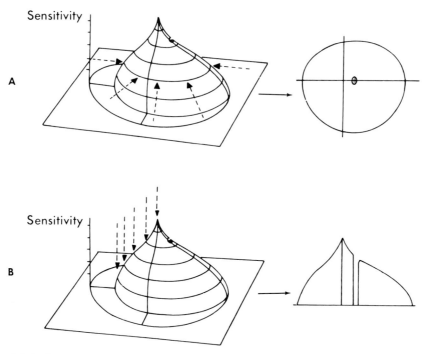

Fig. 10-4. A, Isopter (kinetic) perimetry. The test object of fixed intensity is moved along several meridians toward fixation. The points where the object is first perceived are plotted in a circle. **B,** Static perimetry. A stationary test object is increased in intensity from below threshold until perceived by the patient. Threshold values yield a graphic profile section. (Modified from Aulhorn, E., and Harms, H.: In Leydhecker, W.: Glaucoma, Tutzing Symposium, Basel, 1967, S. Karger.)

Generally four meridians within the central field are chosen for investigation. The threshold sensitivity at fixation and at each degree along the meridians is determined. In this way a "profile section" can be plotted through known defects or, in their absence, the standard test meridians: 45°, 225°, 135°, 315°. Fig. 10-5 illustrates the resulting graph. Occasionally the investigation is carried out along an isopter (circular static perimetry).

In static perimetry the findings are not influenced by the speed of moving the test object or the reaction time of the patient, since the test object is not moved during the period between patient perception and response. As a result, small, isolated scotomas characteristic of early glaucoma are more readily discovered by static perimetry. This method of field examination is much too time-consuming for routine perimetry but may prove to be of great value in following glaucoma suspects for the earliest signs of visual damage. The importance of examination of the paracentral regions of the field, best accomplished by static perimetry, has been emphasized in this chapter. Occasionally the pattern of a glaucomatous defect can be isolated from other visual reducing factors such as cataracts or inflammation.

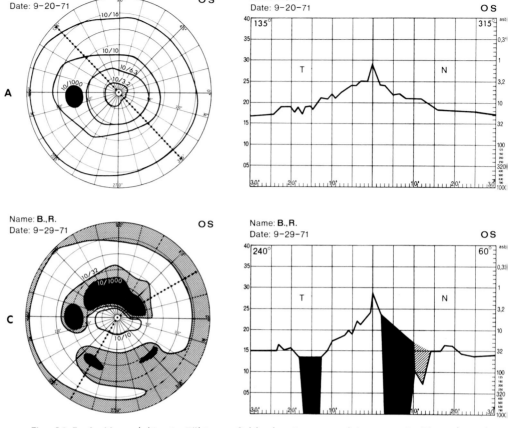

Fig. 10-5. A, Normal kinetic Tübinger field, showing central isopters. **B,** Normal static Tübinger field, showing responses along the 135 to 315 meridians in the central field. **C,** Glaucoma field of a 56-year-old patient with pressures ranging from 15 to 28 mm Hg in both eyes while on medications. Disc cupping and field damage progressed, and surgery was required. **D,** Static perimetry along the 60 and 240 meridians confirms the defect shown by kinetic perimetry.

Also, a discrepancy between the appearance of the disc and visual fields obtained with less sensitive instruments can be resolved with the Tübinger.

GLAUCOMATOUS CHANGES IN THE VISUAL FIELDS
Anatomy of field defects

One to several rods but only one cone activate each ganglion cell of the retina. The axon of this ganglion cell runs in an arcuate course from its point of origin to the optic disc and then through the nerve to the lateral geniculate body. All the axons entering the upper half of the disc originate in ganglion cells in the upper half of the retina, whereas those entering the lower half of the disc originate in the lower hemisphere of the retina. There is no cross communication above and below

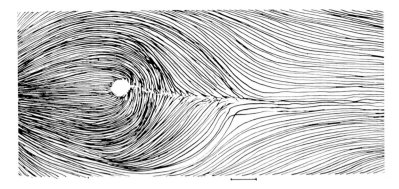

Fig. 10-6. Drawing of the region of temporal raphe, reconstructed from low-power photographs. (Scale indicates 1.0 mm.) (From Vrabec, F.: Amer. J. Ophthal. **62:**926, 1966.)

the 180° retinal meridian. This line of separation in the temporal retina is called the horizontal raphe. The arching course of the fibers is shown in Fig. 10-6.

When a field defect appears in an eye with increased intraocular pressure, it is probably caused by damage to a group of axon cylinders in the area of the optic disc. The effect is similar to cutting an electric cable supplying power to a section of a city, in that lights beyond the break would be out but adjacent areas would be normally lighted. Because the axons arch from their ganglion cell origin around the macula, an arcuate blackout of an area of field is produced. The axons from the macular area also arch slightly before entering the temporal edge of the disc. Fortunately they are usually the fibers most resistant to pressure damage, and this is the reason that good central visual acuity is commonly retained until late in the glaucomatous process.

Isolated scotomas that occur in the paracentral areas are probably partial nerve fiber bundle defects originating at the disc. Henkind, in studies of retinal blood supply, emphasizes the possible importance of radial peripapillary capillaries in the pathogenesis of the field defect. Direct pressure on these capillaries in the retina may produce damage.

It has been shown by Goldmann, Harrington, and Drance that there is an increased sensitivity to functional loss in Bjerrum's area of the central field in most eyes. The beginning of the specific arcuate defects of glaucoma can be demonstrated by increasing the tension in most normal eyes with external pressure. This sensitivity to pressure is more marked in eyes with glaucoma. It seems to be correlated in part with systemic blood pressure and with intraocular pressure. Some patients with glaucoma who have high blood pressure and stable fields develop rapid field deterioration when the systemic blood pressure is drastically reduced.

Angle-closure glaucoma

The rapid rise of intraocular pressure to a point near the systolic pressure of the retinal artery results in ischemia of the retina with generalized irregular depression of all isopters of the visual field. In addition, corneal edema further diminishes the light entering the eye from the test objects. Perimetry is largely of academic value in the acute glaucomas.

In chronic angle-closure glaucoma the changes in tension mimic those of chronic open-angle glaucoma, and therefore field defects are similar.

Open-angle glaucoma

The effect of prolonged pressure on the optic disc results in the following typical defects in the perimetric field: generalized peripheral constriction, isolated scotomas in the 5° to 15° isopters, nasal depression and nasal step, temporal step, elongation of the blind spot, and nerve fiber bundle defects.

Generalized peripheral constriction

Studies show that generalized peripheral constriction is the most common glaucoma field defect. However, because other factors such as aging, miosis, and hazy media cause the same contraction, it has little diagnostic value. If there is progressive constriction, its etiology should be identified.

Isolated paracentral scotomas (Fig. 10-7)

Careful perimetry with small test objects and reduced illumination on either the tangent screen or the Goldmann perimeter will often show small islands of relative or absolute scotoma within the Bjerrum's area. These sometimes disappear with accurate refraction but more often represent definite defects in the visual field characteristic of early glaucoma. They do not connect with the blind spot. In the series of Aulhorn and Harms, such isolated defects in the Bjerrum's area without connection to the blind spot were found in 20% of the glaucoma fields. Typically these defects enlarge and later connect with the blind spot to form the classic arcuate scotoma. It should be noted that these isolated scotomas may also be found in the paracentral region only a few degrees from fixation. This is especially true on the nasal side of fixation. Testing for defects only in a circle at the 15° eccentricity from the center will miss many of these (almost a fourth in the above series).

Nasal depression and nasal step

Depression of the nasal peripheral portion of the field may represent an early glaucoma defect. Nasal depression alone, as with generalized constriction, is not very helpful clinically in establishing the presence of a glaucoma defect. However, when the depression extends to the horizontal raphe and forms a step, a defect is evident. A nasal step can appear without evidence of a central field defect (Fig. 10-8).

Temporal step (Fig. 10-9)

Occasionally a step will occur temporal to the blind spot. Drance, on finding this defect in chronic simple glaucoma, suggested that the glaucoma field examina-

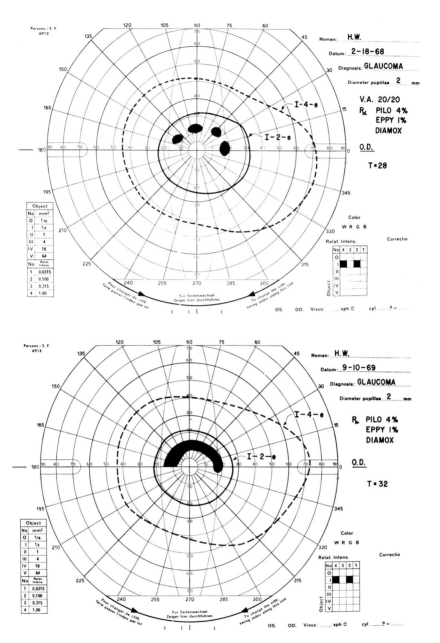

Fig. 10-7. Example of paracentral scotomas found in a patient with elevated intraocular pressure and progressive disc cupping. Note later formation of arcuate scotoma.

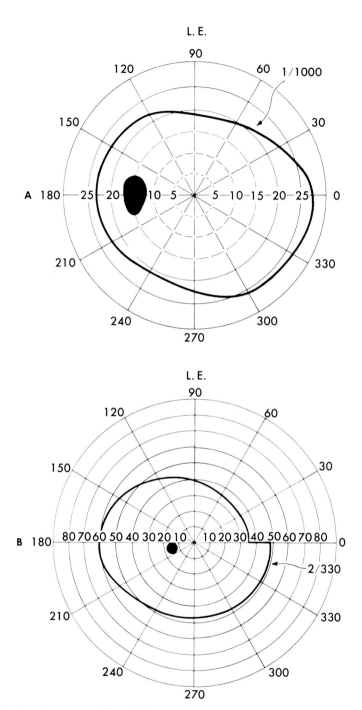

Fig. 10-8. Case history: Fields of left eye of a 58-year-old man with open angles and elevated pressure in both eyes. **A,** Examination showed deep glaucomatous cupping of the right disc and a suspiciously abnormal left disc with a normal central field on tangent screen. **B,** Peripheral field revealed a nasal step.

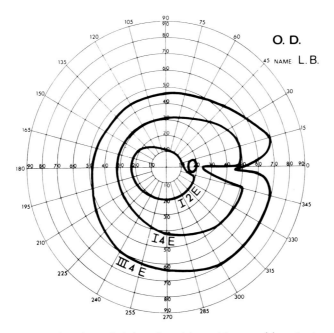

Fig. 10-9. Temporal wedge-shaped defect found in a 62-year-old patient with an eight-year history of open-angle glaucoma. Tensions measured 30 mm Hg in the right eye and 26 mm Hg in the left. The horizontal C/D was 0.8, and the cup extended to the superior temporal disc margin.

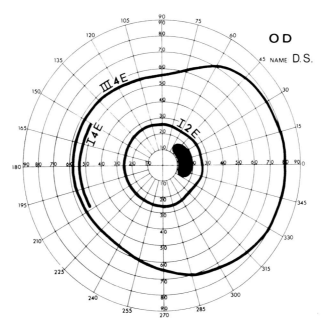

Fig. 10-10. Generalized enlargement of the blind spot is not a glaucoma defect. A small percentage of early glaucoma defects develop progressively from the blind spot in an arcuate direction.

tion include a careful search of this area. Temporal field defects are sometimes found without other visual field changes.

Enlargement of blind spot (Fig. 10-10)

Enlargement of the blind spot does not have any specificity unless enlargement occurs in an arcuate direction. Enlargement of the blind spot is an uncommon early finding in glaucoma.

Nerve fiber bundle defects

All the typical glaucoma field defects can be interpreted as variants of the nerve fiber bundle defect. The typical complete nerve fiber bundle defect is the arcuate or Bjerrum's scotoma (Figs. 10-5, C, and 10-7), representing a cut in the conduction pathway of a group of axon cylinders at the optic disc. This produces a scimitar-shaped area of blackout, arching from the blind spot around the macula in the 10° to 20° circle but often reaching to within 5° nasally. The scotoma follows the nerve fiber pattern to the horizontal meridian in the nasal field, where it ends in a sharply demarcated horizontal line or nasal step. A nasal step may also be produced by a double arcuate scotoma if the two defects are not of identical size at their junction point on the nasal horizontal meridian (Fig. 10-11). The Bjerrum's scotoma may occur either above or below fixation, but the upper is more frequent.

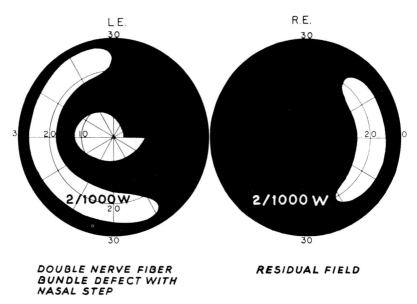

L.E.

R.E.

2/1000 W

2/1000 W

DOUBLE NERVE FIBER
BUNDLE DEFECT WITH
NASAL STEP

RESIDUAL FIELD

Fig. 10-11. Case history: Fields of a 60-year-old man with advanced open-angle glaucoma. Ophthalmoscopically, the discs are markedly cupped (Grade 4). The disc of the left eye is shown in Plate 4, D.

Baring of the blind spot (Fig. 10-12). Although baring of the blind spot may be present in glaucoma, it is not characteristic. Most investigators believe that any subject, normal included, will demonstrate baring to an appropriate test object.

Terminal field. Fortunately, the macular fibers are often most resistant to glaucomatous damage. Vision of 20/20 may be retained when only a few degrees of central field remain. There is often a tiny horizontal step just nasal to fixation. The loss of this final central island may be very sudden. Often a small crescent of vision remains in the temporal periphery, which may persist after all other areas of vision are gone (Fig. 10-11).

ARTIFACTS IN THE VISUAL FIELDS

The need for standardization of visual field methods would seem obvious. Yet many decisions in the treatment of glaucoma are based on variations noted in successive visual fields, which may have no relation at all to progression of the visual field defect. The examiner must then be on guard to watch for such artifacts.

Environmental artifacts

1. *Calibration*—illumination of screen and test object must be uniform. Reduction in illumination or in contrast will magnify a field defect.

2. *The use of small and larger objects* is necessary in the quantitative evalua-

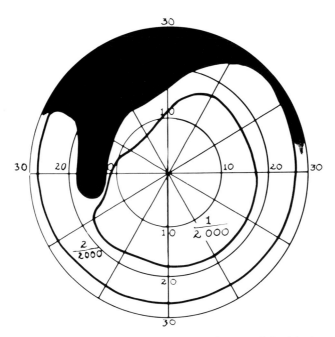

Fig. 10-12. Tangent screen visual field depicting true baring of the blind spot. This is not necessarily considered a glaucoma defect.

tion of a field defect, but the defect found with one size of target must not be compared with a field taken with a different-sized object or at a different distance. It is also important that the object be large enough to assure reliability in the patient's response.

3. The *distance* of the patient from the screen must remain standard to avoid discrepancies if a tangent screen is used.

4. The *attention of the patient* must be held at all times. If the patient is unreliable, this must be noted on the field chart so that undue emphasis will not be placed on an unreliable chart.

5. The *technique of the examiner* should be as nearly standard as possible, and the patient should be kept alert but not tense. It is impossible to compare tangent screen fields reliably when they have been done by two different examiners.

Pupillary size

1. The field may be decreased if a *miotic* has been instilled shortly before the test. Dilating the miotic pupil may give an amazing increase in the field particularly if lens opacities are present. With hazy media, luminescent targets such as the Lumiwand tend to give larger fields than do white beads of similar size. Because of changes in pupillary size and refraction whenever medication is changed, a new base-line field of vision should be established. Pupil size should be noted.

2. Drooping of the *upper lid* over the pupil will reduce the pupillary aperture, with the same effect on a field defect as decreasing the size of the target.

Glasses, eyebrows, and nose

Frames of glasses, segments of multifocal lenses, overhanging brows, and a large nose can cause abnormalities in the field and must be avoided by lifting the brows and changing the head position.

Changes in media

Cataracts tend to give a general depression of the fields, with an exaggeration of existing scotomas. The edge of the scotomatous defect will be sloping, with a much decreased field to small objects and a larger field with large objects. Any decrease in the clarity of the media will cause similar interferences (Fig. 10-13).

Uncorrected refractive errors

It has been found that artifactual scotomas are sometimes produced and existing defects are exaggerated by relatively small refractive errors. It is therefore important that central fields be done with corrective lenses that will completely correct any refractive error. An addition of 1.00 D to the distance correction for tangent screen examinations at 1 meter and an appropriate lens determined by age for the Goldmann perimeter will increase accuracy in presbyopic patients.

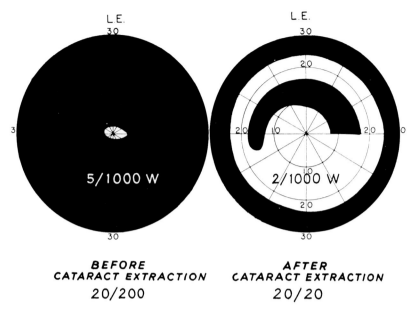

Fig. 10-13. Case history: Fields of a 72-year-old glaucoma patient taken before and after cataract operation. The other eye was enucleated for pain caused by neovascular glaucoma secondary to an occlusion of the central retinal vein.

Concomitant ocular defects

1. *Macular or myopic changes* or generalized retinal degenerative diseases such as retinitis pigmentosa may result in misinterpretation.

2. *Inflammatory lesions*—choroiditis, neuritis, and uveitis can alter the fields both by actual nerve damage and by increasing vitreous haze. Juxtapapillary choroiditis will often give a true arcuate scotoma.

3. *Vascular lesions and central nervous system tumors*—occlusions in the central vein or artery or their branches, cerebrovascular accidents, various retinopathies, and ocular, chiasmatic, and cerebral tumors can all produce marked field defects that can be confusing, especially if superimposed on a glaucomatous field defect.

4. *Drusen of the disc and a congenital coloboma of the optic disc* can produce varied field defects. The presence of an arcuate scotoma with a very full optic nerve and no cup should make one suspicious of drusen.

5. *Retinal detachment* is not an uncommon complication in glaucoma. It is often missed until advanced, since peripheral fields are not taken as routinely as they should be and examination of the retina is difficult through miotic pupils.

6. *Myelinated nerve fibers* cause relative scotomas. The corresponding area of myelination can be readily seen with ophthalmoscopy.

Psychologic artifacts

Any subjective examination is open to errors produced by the patient, which may not be recognized by an unwary clinician, such as the following:

1. Misunderstanding of the test by the patient
2. Tiring patient by prolonged testing
3. Malingering or hysteria
4. Inattention
5. Mental vagaries

CHAPTER 11

Clinical interpretation of disc and field changes

DIAGNOSTIC IMPORTANCE

The clinical examinations for glaucomatous excavation of the optic disc and the corresponding nerve fiber bundle field defects are by far the most significant part of any study of glaucoma. This fact is sometimes overlooked in the clinician's preoccupation with intraocular pressure. Actually, an increased pressure would be of no importance if one could be sure that no damage to the nerve would eventually result from it.

It has been generally accepted that by the time disc and field changes have become obvious, the patient no longer has early glaucoma, and therapy should begin before damage has occurred. There is little doubt that glaucoma is best suspected by an intelligent correlation of the findings of ophthalmoscopy, gonioscopy, tonometry, and tonography. With the development of more precise methods of visual field evaluation, there has been a greater tendency to withhold medication until the first signs of visual field or optic disc damage occurs. This presupposes that proper therapy will arrest the disease process at the stage when it is instituted. It also places great reliance on perimetry and obligates the ophthalmologist to repeated, frequent careful study of the optic disc and the visual function in glaucoma suspects. Except in cases of moderate to extreme ocular hypertension, most glaucoma suspects with normal fields and discs can be followed without medication for years without their developing field loss or cupping. It should be emphasized that this procedure can be undertaken only when reliable and frequent evaluation of the optic discs and careful visual field studies are possible. When this ideal situation cannot be obtained, one must rely on statistical correlates and clinical judgment in deciding when to institute glaucoma therapy.

Comparative disc and field findings (Fig. 11-1 and Plate 4, E)

Defects in the visual fields are usually accompanied by corresponding cupping of the optic discs. Perimetric examination of an eye with a normal upper disc, but

167

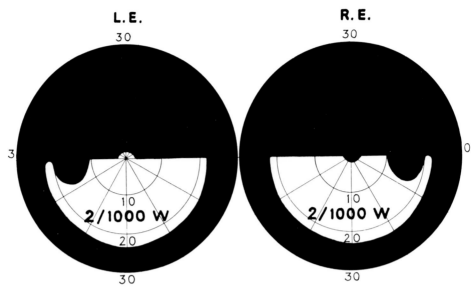

Fig. 11-1. Case history: Fields of a 57-year-old woman with low blood pressure. The intraocular pressure was never found to be above 30 mm Hg. The facility of outflow was 0.12 in each eye. The upper field loss corresponded to marked cupping of the lower disc as shown in Plate 4, E.

cupped lower disc, would be expected to reveal an upper arcuate defect. Whenever a disc is evaluated, this type of prediction should be attempted because it sharpens the examiner's eye and his diagnostic acumen.

Occasionally field findings are not only unreliable but also actually misleading. The disc examination provides an objective check on the reliability of the subjective field study. If the disc has a normal pink appearance to the nerve fibers and no cupping, the physician should be most skeptical if a marked field defect is found. Similarly, a severely cupped disc requires a thorough search for a field defect, including examination with smaller test objects and testing at increased distances from the tangent screen, the use of threshold targets with the Goldmann perimeter, and occasionally Tübinger static perimetry when available. An optic cup that extends over seven tenths of the total disc diameter should be considered pathologic until proved otherwise. In most eyes the optic cups will be similar on both sides. A discrepancy between the two is significant and should make one suspicious.

Cupping without field defect (Fig. 11-2)

The frequency with which glaucomatous disc cupping occurs without visual loss is unknown at present. Progression of cupping, however, without field defect in patients with elevated pressures is well documented and is probably due to loss of tissue fluids and glial tissue rather than of nerve fibers. Studies showing greater

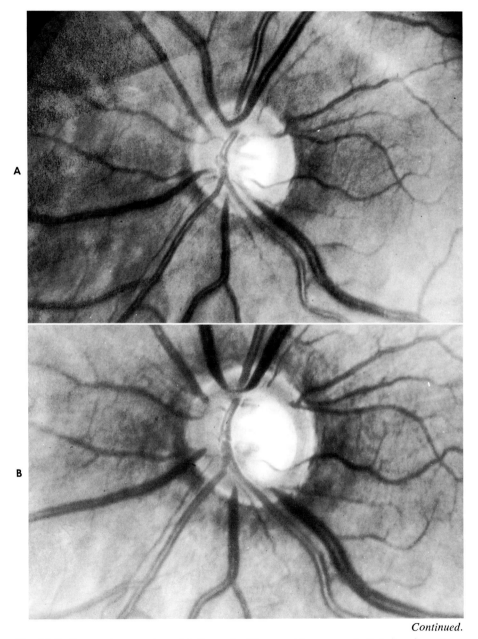

Continued.

Fig. 11-2. Progressive cupping of left eye in 18-year-old woman. **A,** 0.4 disc-diameter progressed to, **B,** 0.7 disc-diameter at pressures of 38 to 46 mm Hg. **C,** No field defect was found in the patient by static Tübinger or, as shown here, by Goldmann perimetry.

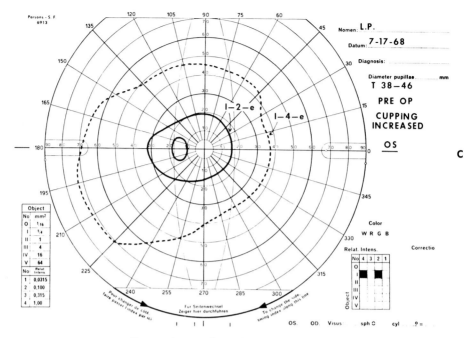

Fig. 11-2, cont'd. For legend see p. 169.

disc cupping in steroid-responsive gg eyes and in glaucoma eyes with field defects in the opposite eye support the concept that cupping precedes the field defect. The knowledge that increased cupping precedes a field defect is further supported by the fact that asymmetrical cupping in an ocular hypertensive, in the absence of field defects in either eye, is usually greater in the eye with the higher pressure. That such progression may occur before the development of glaucomatous field defects stresses the need for careful observation of the optic discs. Well-documented progression of cupping associated with elevated intraocular pressure may be an indication for further medical therapy and, if necessary, surgery.

Hemorrhages of the disc associated with field defects (Fig. 11-3)

In patients with elevated intraocular pressures, Drance found linear hemorrhages located superficially on the neuroretinal rim of the disc. Disc hemorrhages were occasionally followed by extension of disc cupping in the hemorrhagic area. In some patients the development of a specific, fresh, absolute nerve fiber bundle field defect was associated with these hemorrhages. They tend to occur more frequently in cases of low-tension glaucoma, suggesting a poor vascular status in these patients.

Red-free filter ophthalmoscopy of nerve fiber bundle defects (Fig. 11-4)

Interest in red-free examination of the retinal nerve fiber layer was revived by Hoyt. Although most descriptions of use apply to central nervous system lesions, there are encouraging reports of its value in glaucoma. Direct ophthalmos-

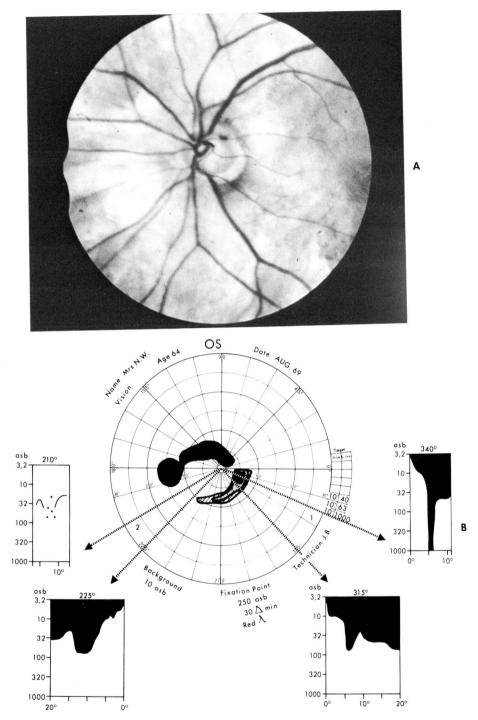

Fig. 11-3. Case history: **A,** A 64-year-old female patient in apparently good health, with chronic simple glaucoma but whose intraocular pressures were within normal limits on therapy. She developed a hemorrhage on the left disc, **B,** associated with a fresh inferior absolute arcuate scotoma. The superior absolute arcuate scotoma occurred four years earlier, associated with a hemorrhage on the lower part of the disc. (Courtesy Dr. S. M. Drance, Vancouver, B. C.)

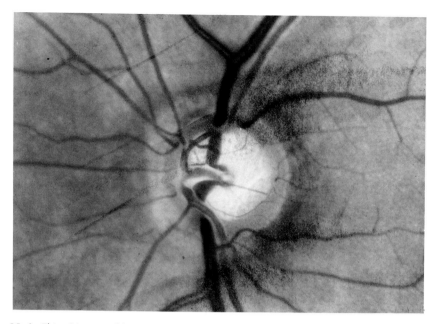

Fig. 11-4. This 54-year-old patient was followed closely for eleven years because of a family history of open-angle glaucoma. Pressures gradually increased into the low twenties, and the disc cups began to enlarge from 0.5 to 0.8 disc-diameter in both eyes. A field defect was not detectable until three years after obvious enlargement in cupping. When the red-free examination was photographed, an inferior arcuate field defect was present. (Courtesy William F. Hoyt, University of California School of Medicine, San Francisco.)

copy, preferably with a green No. 65 filter, is used to scrutinize the nerve fiber layer, especially temporal to the disc in the superior and inferior arcuate area. Atrophy of neurons shows as a loss of the uniform striated pattern at the nerve fiber layer. These striations give the retina a grayish cast, but when they are absent, the deeper red of the choroid is allowed to predominate.

Glaucoma defects appear early as grooves (slits), wide wedges, or a diffuse loss. Retinal vessels become more prominent, and there is a loss of vascularity in the superficial peripapillary layer. Excellent visibility through a dilated pupil, clear media, and a cooperative patient are necessary. Changes described are subtle, and experience is required to master the technique. The method is not foolproof and, when used, should be correlated with other findings.

Myopic disc and field in glaucoma (Fig. 11-5 and Plate 4, F)

Myopic eyes represent a special problem in the diagnosis of glaucoma. Many myopic eyes have gone blind from primary or secondary glaucoma without the ophthalmologist's being aware of the diagnosis. The reasons for this difficulty are threefold. First, as Goldmann has pointed out, the distance between the level of the lamina cribrosa and the level of the retina is much less than in normal or hyperopic eyes. The average value of this distance in the normal eye is about 0.7 mm,

L.E.   R.E.

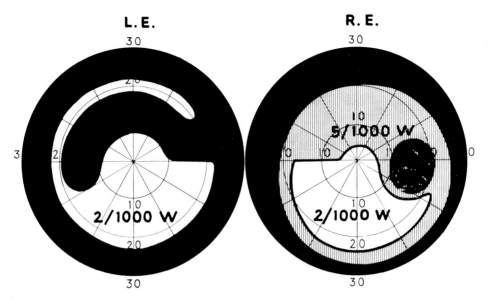

Fig. 11-5. Case history: Fields of this 62-year-old woman show loss of the upper field with a 2/1000 white target. The intraocular pressure was thought to be 21 mm Hg in the right eye and 19 mm Hg in the left eye by Schiøtz tonometry but was found to be 28 mm Hg in the right eye and 24 mm Hg in the left eye by applanation tonometry. The patient had −7.00 D of myopia with decreased ocular rigidity. The disc of the right eye is pictured in Plate 4, F.

whereas that of the myopic eye is between 0.2 and 0.5 mm. Therefore a completely cupped disc in a myopic eye will have only half the depth of the usual glaucomatous cup. Furthermore, its character is marked by the usual myopic conus, tilting of the disc, and circumpapillary atrophy. Second, the ocular rigidity is usually lower than that of normal eyes; therefore Schiøtz tensions, using the ordinary conversion tables, are lower than the actual intraocular pressure as described in Chapter 8. This particular error is avoided by the use of applanation tonometry. Third, an enlargement of the blind spot may be thought to be due to the myopic conus and choroidal atrophy. Staphylomas of the posterior pole or peripheral fundus may produce irregular refractive errors that affect visual field examination. This is especially critical with current methods of perimetry using reduced-intensity targets. Appropriate lenses are used to correct for refractive scotomas. The astute clinician must be doubly on guard for glaucoma in his myopic patients. This is especially true because glaucoma occurs more frequently in myopes.

PROGNOSTIC IMPORTANCE OF PROGRESSING DEFECTS IN DISCS AND FIELDS

In open-angle glaucoma or in angle-closure glaucoma without pupillary block, increased cupping of the optic disc and deterioration of the field indicate inadequate control of the disease even if pressure is seemingly controlled. As is true of other field loss, glaucoma defects can be considered to be actively changing if the edges of the scotoma are not perfectly uniform and its boundaries are sloping when tested by quantitative perimetry. Arcuate defects that are well established and have steep edges are unlikely to progress rapidly. A sloping edge to a scotoma may mean a media change such as a cataract, preventing the patient from seeing a small object. It also characterizes the edge of a progressing scotoma. In general, the presence of a pink optic disc without any cupping is an excellent prognostic sign. The more extensively cupped the disc and the more advanced the field loss, the more grave becomes the prognosis. The use of topical corticosteroids has shown that field defects can be produced by increased pressure in sensitive individuals. These defects are completely reversible if the pressures are normalized promptly by antiglaucomatous therapy or by stopping the steroid medication. In a few cases of open-angle glaucoma, early field defects recorded with the Goldmann perimeter have disappeared with subsequent tension reduction by medical or surgical means (Fig. 11-6).

Dilation of the pupils of glaucomatous eyes with widely open angles every year is wise. This permits better evaluation of the discs and may reveal other ocular changes such as cataracts, macular degeneration, and retinal detachment, which might easily escape detection or lead to field changes that could be mistaken for progression of glaucomatous field loss. Posterior synechias often form after prolonged miosis and may be broken by 10% phenylephrine (Neo-Synephrine). Obviously, no unoperated narrow-angled eye should be dilated without full realization of the risk of angle closure.

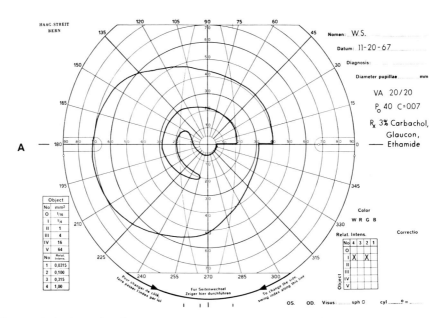

Fig. 11-6. A, Example of a young patient, W. S., with elevated pressure, progressive field loss, and disc cupping, who showed gradual recovery of field, **B** and **C,** over a period of sixteen months after filtering surgery.

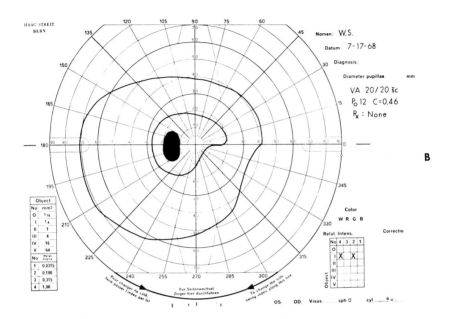

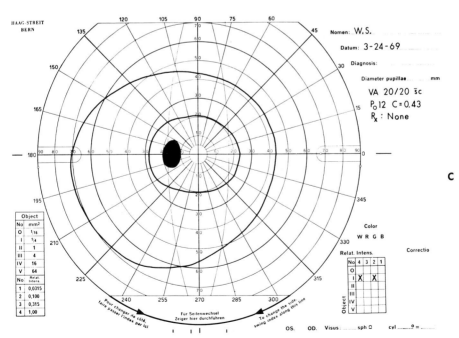

Fig. 11-6, cont'd. For legend see opposite page.

Field loss with good pressure control

In some cases of apparently well-controlled glaucoma, field defects continue to progress. Such cases require particularly careful evaluation. The following factors must be considered.

1. *Inadequate control of the intraocular pressure.* Severely damaged optic nerves may require pressure control at lower levels than usual, to prevent continuing damage. Tension below 16 mm Hg is desirable.

2. *Diurnal tension variations.* When the facility of outflow is low, diurnal pressure changes are exaggerated. Pressures found to be normal during office hours may become elevated into the pathologic range at other times. Highest levels of intraocular pressure occur usually in the early morning, but there are individual variations. The determination of 24-hour tension variations can be most helpful in planning therapy.

3. *Decreased ocular rigidity.* If the tension is being followed by Schiøtz tonometry, the physician must be sure that the ocular rigidity of the eye is normal. Particularly in myopic eyes, the Schiøtz reading may be normal because of low ocular rigidity, but the true intraocular pressure as measured by applanation will be elevated.

4. *Unsuspected use of corticosteroid medications.* The patient should be questioned to be sure that another physician has not prescribed corticosteroids either locally or systemically in an interval between visits to the ophthalmologist.

5. *Changes in the blood supply to the optic nerve.* Interference with the blood supply of the optic nerve may produce or aggravate glaucomatous defects. Blood studies should be made to rule out anemia. One should keep in mind that the profound drop in systemic blood pressure that may accompany antihypertensive therapy and the local ischemia that accompanies arteriosclerotic changes, carotid artery occlusions, severe injury, bleeding ulcers, and temporal arteritis can endanger the visual field. A bruit detected over the carotid area may reveal carotid stenosis as the etiology of a low-tension glaucoma.

6. *Epinephrine therapy.* In some eyes macular lesions may be related to the use of topical epinephrine. This should be remembered when there are progressive changes in a residual central island, especially in aphakic eyes.

7. *Retinal detachments.* These are clearly associated with the use of strong miotics. The accompanying pressure reductions with field loss are characteristic.

8. *Artifacts.* In a subjective test such as perimetry, one must always keep in mind the many artifactual errors that are possible (p. 163). In particular, alterations in pupil size and lens transparency must be considered.

THERAPEUTIC IMPORTANCE
Progression of field defects

As previously stated, evaluation of changes in visual fields depends on strictly comparable examinations. This means that the same examiner, if possible, should take the field, using identical technique, illumination, object size, and distance, and that the patient should be completely cooperative. Progression of field changes and disc cupping obligates the physician to increase therapy until tension is reduced to a level compatible with continuing integrity of the nerve. If full medical therapy has already been given, if increased therapy is not well tolerated by the patient, or if the patient is unreliable in the use of medications, a clear indication is present for prompt surgery.

The greater the degree of disc excavation and the more extensive the field defect, the more urgent is the need for control of the disease. Although perfect control is desirable at all times, less heroic treatment is justifiable when discs and fields are still normal. Once cupping has occurred, the nerve may not resist intraocular pressures that were long tolerated before.

Since progressing field defects and disc cupping are the major indications for surgery in open-angle glaucoma, the surgeon must be certain that an apparent progression is valid. The appearance of the optic disc should correlate with the field defect and provide additional objective evidence of progression. The surgeon should always keep in mind the various artifacts described.

Residual central island

A particularly difficult problem faces the surgeon when only a small central visual field remains or when a dense arcuate scotoma lies close to fixation. In general, every effort should be made to maintain medical control, but this must be judged mainly by the level of intraocular pressure because further progression of the field defect will obliterate macular vision. The macular fibers are relatively resistant to deterioration from pressure but will certainly not stand markedly elevated pressures for prolonged periods of time. If filtering surgery is performed, the central island will usually not be lost. Occasionally the resultant hypotony can cause macular edema or hemorrhage that can snuff out central vision, to the dismay of the surgeon and the patient alike. If the visual field defect splits fixation, the chances of visual acuity loss are much greater. Nevertheless, if tension is high, the risk should be taken rather than wait for inevitable blindness. Unfortunately, even with perfect control of pressure, a tiny central field may continue to deteriorate. As is so often the case, prevention of the problem by early diagnosis and energetic therapy is still the most desirable form of treatment. Every effort should be made to impress each patient with this point of view as soon as the diagnosis of glaucoma has been made.

PROBLEMS FOR CONSIDERATION

Although the anatomic and physiologic changes occurring in the anterior segment of the eye are responsible for the elevated intraocular pressure of glaucoma, the changes resulting in visual loss take place in the posterior segment. The exact mechanism of these changes and better ways of preventing them are among the least understood facets of glaucoma.

Detailed anatomic, physiologic, and metabolic studies of the ganglion cell layer of the retina and optic nerve should be undertaken. Additional detailed information is badly needed about the blood supply of the optic nerve head and particularly about the changes induced by glaucoma. Further clinical and experimental research is needed to determine the role of blood pressure and blood flow in the production of nerve damage and field loss. The availability of fluorescein angiography and ophthalmodynamography has not as yet provided these answers. More sophisticated techniques will be needed to determine accurately the effects on blood flow. The exciting studies on axoplasmic flow raise numerous investigative possibilities as to the role of this process in glaucomatous optic nerve damage. Whether permanent inhibition of axoplasmic transport leads to cellular destruction should be investigated, as well as the determination of neuronal conduction during periods of inhibition. Further data are required to determine whether elevated IOP blocks axonal transport at the disc as a primary mechanical effect, with neuronal dysfunction resulting from the blocked transport, or whether axonal transport is one of the physiologic functions affected secondary to ischemia produced by primary action of intraocular pressure on the vascular bed.

Ways of evaluating the pharmacologic effects of various substances on optic nerve function must be developed. The effects of vitamins, amino acids, drugs, and other agents on blood flow and visual function have to be determined. Phenytoin (diphenylhydantoin, Dilantin), long used as an anticonvulsant, has been evaluated in the treatment of early glaucomatous optic nerve damage. In vitro studies suggested that phenytoin might protect the optic nerve from the effects of hypoxia and perhaps reverse early field loss. Preliminary results indicate no significant effect of phenytoin when compared with a placebo. The concept that optic nerve function may be made more resistant to pressure or ischemic damage deserves further study.

Perhaps the most important area for intensive study is the susceptibility of the individual eye to pressure damage. Elevated intraocular pressure is a clue, but it does not define the disease. Ideally, the susceptible eye should be recognized and treated before irreversible damage occurs.

A major question is whether damage is pressure induced in all eyes or whether nutritional, vascular, and/or genetic factors are the major determinants of field loss. Careful studies of progressive glaucomatous field loss at lower-than-expected intraocular pressures should provide important clues. The tendency for elevated intraocular pressure appears to be genetically determined. It is probable that susceptibility to field loss is also genetically determined if we consider the fact that disc cupping can be genetically determined with steroid testing.

Better methods are necessary for evaluation of disc changes and early field changes. Although static perimetry is time-consuming, it provides a most accurate method of determining threshold sensitivity in selected meridians. It is necessary that this method be made available in more glaucoma centers and, more important, that the technique and instrumentation be made practical for the ophthalmologist treating the glaucoma patient.

References—Section IV

Anderson, D. R.: Ultrastructure of the optic nerve head, Arch. Ophthal. **83:**63, 1970.

Anderson, D. R., and Hendrickson, A.: Effect of intraocular pressure on rapid axoplasmic transport in monkey optic nerve, Invest. Ophthal. **13:**771, 1974.

Anderson, D. R., and Hoyt, W. F.: Ultrastructure of intraorbital portion of human and monkey optic nerve, Arch. Ophthal. **82:**506, 1969.

Armaly, M. F.: Genetic determination of cup/disc ratio of the optic nerve, Arch. Ophthal. **78:**35, 1967.

Armaly, M. F.: Ocular pressure and visual fields, Arch. Ophthal. **81:**25, 1969.

Armaly, M. F.: The genetic problem of chronic simple glaucoma, presented at the International Congress of Ophthalmology, March, 1970.

Armaly, M. F., and Sayegh, R. E.: The cup/disc ratio: the findings of tonometry and tonography in the normal eye, Arch. Ophthal. **82:**191, 1969.

Aulhorn, E., and Harms, H.: Early visual field defects in glaucoma. In Leydhecker, W., editor: Glaucoma; Tutzing Symposium, Basel, 1967, S. Karger.

Becker, B.: The cup/disk ratio and topical corticosteroid testing, Amer. J. Ophthal. **70:**681, 1970.

Brais, P., and Drance, S. M.: The temporal field in chronic simple glaucoma, Arch. Ophthal. **88:**518, 1972.

Dollery, C. T., Henkind, P., Kohner, E. M., and Paterson, J. W.: Effect of raised intraocular pressure on the retinal and choroidal circulation, Invest. Ophthal. **7:**191, 1968.

Drance, S. M., and others: Symposium on effect of glaucoma on visual functions, Invest. Ophthal. **8:**84, 1969.

Drance, S. M., and Reid, H.: The essentials of perimetry: static and kinetic, ed. 2, London, 1972, Oxford University Press.

Dubois-Poulsen, A.: Le champs visuel: topographie normale et pathologique de ses sensibilités, Paris, 1952, Masson & Cie.

Elliot, R. H.: The yielding of the optic nervehead in glaucoma, Brit. J. Ophthal. **5:**307, 1921.

Ernest, J. T., and Potts, A. M.: Pathophysiology of the distal portion of the optic nerve. I. Tissue pressure relationships, Amer. J. Ophthal. **66:**373, 1968.

Ernest, J. T., and Potts, A. M.: Pathophysiology of the distal portion of the optic nerve. II. Vascular relationships, Amer. J. Ophthal. **66:**380, 1968.

Gafner, F., and Goldmann, H.: Experimentelle Untersuchungen über den Zusammenhang von Augendrucksteigerund und Geischsfeldschadigung, Ophthalmologica **130:**357, 1955.

Goldmann, H.: Problems in present-day glaucoma research. In Streiff, E. B., and Babel, E., editors: Modern problems in ophthalmology, Basel, 1957, S. Karger.

Greve, E. L.: Single and multiple stimulus static perimetry in glaucoma: the two phases of perimetry, Docum. Ophthal. **36:**1, 1973.

Harrington, D.: The visual fields, ed. 3, St. Louis, 1971, The C. V. Mosby Co.

Hayreh, S. S.: Anatomy and physiology of the optic nerve head, Trans. Amer. Acad. Ophthal. Otolaryng. **78:**240, 1974.

Hayreh, S., and Walker, W. M.: Fluorescent fundus photography in glaucoma, Amer. J. Ophthal. **63:**982, 1967.

Henkind, P.: New observations on the radial peripapillary capillaries, Invest. Ophthal. **6:**103, 1967.

Henkind, P.: Radial peripapillary capillaries of

the retina. I. Anatomy, human and comparative, Brit. J. Ophthal. **51:**115, 1967.

Henkind, P., and Levitzky, M.: Angioarchitecture of the optic nerve. I. The papilla, Amer. J. Ophthal. **68:**979, 1969.

Hoyt, W. F., Frisen, L., and Newman, N. M.: Fundoscopy of nerve fiber layer defects in glaucoma, Invest. Ophthal. **12:**814, 1973.

Kalvin, N. H., Hamasaki, D. I., and Gass, J. D.: Experimental glaucoma in monkeys. II. Relationship between intraocular pressure and cupping of the optic disc and cavernous atrophy of the optic nerve, Arch. Ophthal. **76:**82, 1966.

Kornzweig, A., Eliasoph, I., and Feldstein, M.: Selective atrophy of the radial peripapillary capillaries in chronic glaucoma, Arch. Ophthal. **80:**696, 1968.

Levitzky, M., and Henkind, P.: Angioarchitecture of the optic nerve. II. Lamina cribrosa, Amer. J. Ophthal. **68:**986, 1969.

MacKenzie, W.: In Cant, J. S., editor: Centenary symposium on the ocular circulation in health and disease, London, 1969, Henry Kimpton.

Michaelson, I. D.: Retinal circulation in man and animals, Springfield, Ill., 1954, Charles C Thomas, Publisher.

O'Day, D., Crock, G., and Galbraith, J. E. K.: Fluorescein angiography of normal and atrophic optic discs, Lancet **2:**224, 1967.

Ourgaud, A. C., and Etienne, R.: L'exploration functionnelle de l'oeil glaucomateux, Paris, 1961, Masson & Cie.

Pickard, R.: A method of recording disc alterations and a study of the growth of normal and abnormal disc cups, Brit. J. Ophthal. **7:**81, 1923.

Richardson, K. T.: Optic cup symmetry in normal newborn infants, Invest. Ophthal. **7:**137, 1968.

Scott, G. I.: Traquair's clinical perimetry, ed. 7, St. Louis, 1957, The C. V. Mosby Co.

Shaffer, R. N., and Hetherington, J.: The glaucomatous disc in infants, Trans. Amer. Acad. Ophthal. Otolaryng. **73:**929, 1969.

Shaffer, R. N., and Richardson, K. T.: Optic nerve cupping in congenital glaucoma, Amer. J. Ophthal. **62:**507, 1966.

Shaffer, R. N., Ridgway, W. L., Brown, R., and Kramer, S. G.: The use of diagrams to record changes in glaucomatous discs, Amer. J. Ophthal. **80:**460, 1975.

Snydacker, D.: The normal optic disc; ophthalmoscopic and photographic studies, Amer. J. Ophthal. **58:**958, 1964.

Vrabec, F.: The temporal raphe of the human retina, Amer. J. Ophthal. **62:**926, 1966.

Weekers, R., and others: Symposium: The genesis of functional symptoms in an eye with raised tension, Acta XVIII Concilium Ophthalmologicum, Belgica **1:**873, 1958.

Zimmerman, L. E., de Venecia, G., and Hamasaki, D. I.: Pathology of the optic nerve in experimental acute glaucoma, Invest. Ophthal. **6:**109, 1967.

CHAPTER **12**

Angle-closure glaucoma with pupillary block

PRIMARY ANGLE CLOSURE

Patients with potential pupillary-block glaucoma have essentially normal eyes with the exception of a shallow chamber and a narrow entrance to the anterior chamber angle. The angle configuration is inherited from parents. Some population studies have shown that in whites, angle closure occurs three times more commonly in females than in males, whereas in blacks, the sex incidence is approximately equal. With increasing age the lens becomes bigger, the anterior chamber shallower, and the angle narrower.

The rarity of a truly shallow anterior chamber and narrow angle is not appreciated sufficiently. In over 2500 consecutive refractions of all ages, only approximately 5% of the patients had anterior chambers shallow enough to arouse the suspicion of narrow angles. In this series only 0.64% of the patients could be said to have critically narrowed angles. Therefore it is essential that the eye physician should recognize and carefully evaluate any patient with shallow chambers. This is best recognized by slit-lamp microscopy, but the convexity of the iris-lens diaphragm usually can be demonstrated by a flashlight directed horizontally toward the eye (Fig. 12-1). Since primary angle-closure glaucoma is a bilateral disease, a unilateral shallow chamber should lead to a search for secondary factors. The incidence of Grades 1 to 4 angles among 2500 unselected refraction patients is as follows: Grade 1, 0.64%; Grade 2, 1%; Grade 3, 60%; and Grade 4, 38.36%.

Törnquist has shown that shallow anterior chambers and narrow angles are genetically determined. Also, from the genetic point of view it is of interest that there is a significant decrease in the prevalence of nontasters of phenylthiocarbamide (PTC) in patients with proved angle-closure glaucoma compared with nonglaucomatous populations and in contrast to patients with primary open-angle glaucoma. The significance of this association is not known (Chapter 14).

183

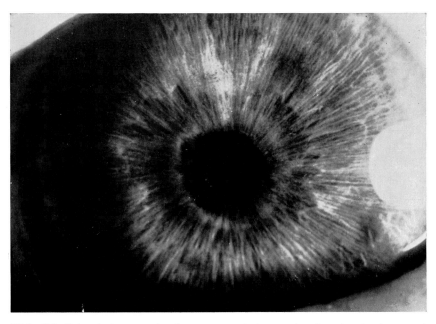

Fig. 12-1. Side-lighted photograph of narrow-angled eye, showing the shadow produced by the convexity of the iris-lens diaphragm.

The difference in chamber depth is the result in part of a somewhat smaller cornea than usual and in part of an anterior position of the lens. The forward position of the lens stretches the iris snugly across its surface. An increased pressure is needed to push aqueous through this iris-lens apposition, resulting in a relatively higher pressure behind the iris than in the anterior chamber. The peripheral iris is thus bowed slightly toward the trabecular wall. The extent of this forward movement depends on the laxity of the iris root. Since the angle between the iris and trabecular meshwork is less than 20° in these eyes, a rather small forward movement of peripheral iris will produce angle closure and an acute glaucoma.

Anatomic factors in narrow-angled eyes

Anatomic factors contributing to the shallowness of the anterior chamber and narrowness of its angle can be summarized as follows.

1. The eye, particularly its anterior segment, is often small with hyperopia, a small cornea, and well-developed ciliary body. The iris may insert on the anterior edge of the ciliary body.

2. The lens position is nearer the cornea than in myopic eyes and most emmetropic eyes.

3. Relative pupillary block is present because of these anatomic factors.

4. In the normal aging process, the lens thickens, the anterior chamber shallows, and the pupil becomes smaller. All these factors increase the relative pupillary block.

5. Pupillary dilation relaxes the peripheral iris, permitting it to be pushed against the meshwork more easily. The iris is also crowded into the angle.

6. A thicker iris, such as is found in brown eyes, may further compromise the angle.

Physiologic factors in relative pupillary block

How is an attack of acute angle-closure glaucoma triggered? Most of the factors enumerated previously are only slowly progressive, and any significant change such as an increase in lens thickness takes years to develop. The crucial variable factor is an alteration that can cause a sudden change, such as varying pupillary size. When the pupil is very small, there is a large arc of contact between iris and lens, and the two surfaces are held tightly together. This increases the pupillary block and the amount of aqueous humor trapped behind the iris. Thus, paradoxically, a miotic used for the treatment of glaucoma tends to aggravate the pupillary-block mechanism and can trigger an attack of angle-closure glaucoma. Actually, the miotic usually helps to prevent or to stop an angle-closure attack because the pull of the sphincter puts the iris on stretch and pulls the periphery away from the trabecular surface. At the same time the taut iris cannot be pushed as easily against the meshwork by the pressure in the posterior chamber.

When the pupil is completely dilated, there is little pupillary block because the iris-lens apposition is so much shorter. Pupillary dilation has been advocated by some as a method of breaking an attack of angle-closure glaucoma. This would seem risky, but it has proved successful in a number of cases. Two factors, however, favor angle closure: (1) loosening of the iris allows the aqueous humor to push the periphery forward more easily and (2) physical bunching of the dilated iris at its periphery may block the narrowed angle. Chandler believes the most dangerous position for the iris is in mid-dilation when the pupillary block is not yet broken but the iris is loosened (Fig. 12-2).

Diagnosis of primary angle-closure glaucoma
Narrow-angled eye before an attack of angle-closure glaucoma

The shallow-chambered, narrow-angled eye should be recognized by routine eye examination. The examiner can easily see the convex iris-lens diaphragm by sidelighting with a flashlight or by noting with the slit lamp that the iris periphery is very close to the cornea. Usually the whole chamber is shallow, but occasionally, particularly in younger patients before the lens has become so large, only the periphery is involved. Such eyes are particularly in danger because the physician is likely to use a mydriatic for refraction without realizing that he is dealing with a narrow-angled eye. It must be stressed that the finding of a normal pressure by tonometry before dilation is no protection against mydriatic glaucoma. The tension will be perfectly normal until mydriasis permits the iris to drop against the trabecular surface, which results in an abrupt rise of pressure. A careful examination, including gonioscopy in suspected cases, is the only way of anticipating such a complication.

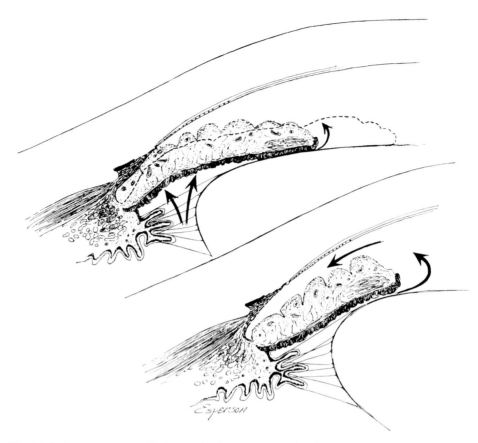

Fig. 12-2. In a narrow-angled eye, the lens is anteriorly placed in relation to the ciliary body and to the iris root. When the pupil is miotic (dotted line in top drawing), the iris is held against the lens and produces a maximum amount of pupillary block. In mid-dilation this pupillary block is not yet broken, but the relaxation of the sphincter may permit the lax peripheral iris to drop against the trabecular meshwork. With further dilation the pupillary block may be broken, aqueous humor escapes into the anterior chamber, and the iris drops away from the trabecular meshwork in some eyes.

Angle closure

Prodromal or intermittent angle-closure symptoms. Narrow-angled eyes capable of angle closure and angle reopening have symptoms caused by the rapid increases and decreases of intraocular pressure. A steaminess of the cornea is produced by the abrupt rise of pressure as a result of sudden angle occlusion. This is caused by epithelial edema and stretching of the corneal lamellas, which disrupt their optical continuity. The patient notices foggy or hazy vision with rainbow-colored halos around lights. Often the pressure level is not high enough to cause ocular congestion or severe pain, producing only mild discomfort and one-sided headache. All these symptoms subside in ½ to 2 hours if the pupillary block is relieved. This results from the miosis that occurs when the patient goes from a dimly lit to a brighter environment or is produced when the patient goes to sleep. The block can also be broken by pressure-induced dilation of the pupil, which may be sufficient to break the pupillary block. There may also be a decrease in aqueous production under the influence of a sudden rise of pressure.

Tonography sometimes shows a steep drop in spite of elevated pressure. Pressure of the tonometer on the central cornea forces aqueous between the iris and the trabecular surface. This results in a temporary increase in aqueous outflow and an apparently good facility of outflow. Gonioscopically, the angle is closed during attacks and open when the attack terminates. The longer the period of iris apposition to the meshwork and the more congestion present, the more likely it is that permanent peripheral anterior synechias will be formed.

As in the true acute attack, symptoms are often precipitated by any circumstance that will produce pupillary dilation, such as mydriatic drops, dim light, and sympathetic nervous system stimulation (emotional upsets, etc.) and very rarely by parasympathetic suppressants (e.g., atropine used for gastrointestinal symptoms or anesthesia). Miotics may also precipitate angle closure when used in treatment of concomitant open-angle glaucoma or in prophylactic management of narrow-angle glaucoma. Hyperemia and edema of the iris and uveal tract may occasionally be blamed. The very narrow angle is ready for closure in the same way that the loaded, cocked gun is ready to fire: many different circumstances can trigger the explosion. It is only a matter of time before one of these transient attacks becomes a permanent angle closure.

Attacks of angle closure can also occur in subjects placed in a prone or semi-prone position. Tasks that require a narrow-angled patient to lean forward (as in reading or sewing) are apt to cause symptoms of angle-closure glaucoma. An anterior displacement of the lens and iris diaphragm due to gravity or increased vascularity in the posterior segment appears to be responsible for shallowing of the anterior chamber and angle closure.

Acute angle-closure symptoms. When angle closure has become established, the symptoms of the intermittent attack become more severe and permanent. A sudden, high rise of pressure will induce more dramatic symptoms than a more gradual rise to the same pressure level. Any or all of the following signs and symptoms will be present.

1. *Angle closure* (Fig. 12-3 and Reel I-4). By definition, angle closure is always present. With the slit lamp, the iris is seen to be in apposition to the peripheral cornea, and this can be confirmed by gonioscopy. If the cornea is too hazy, it can be cleared by 2 or 3 drops of topical glycerin, by normalizing the tension, or by surgically removing the superficial epithelium if it is edematous.

2. *Blurred, foggy vision with colored halos around lights.* An abrupt rise of intraocular pressure stretches the corneal lamellas and disrupts their optical continuity, causing steaminess of the cornea. If the pressure remains elevated, actual edema of the corneal epithelium will appear, with vesicle formation. When the

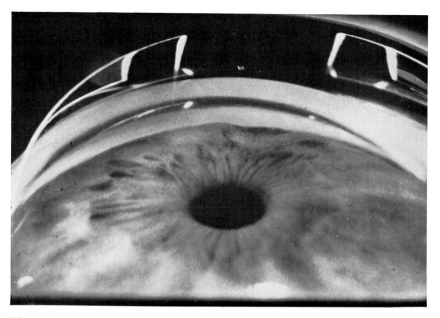

Fig. 12-3. Goniophotograph of closed angle. The iris root is against Schwalbe's line at the left of the photograph. The angle opens to a slit at the right of the photograph.

patient looks at a bright light, the hazy cornea acts like a diffraction grating, splitting the white light into its rainbow components and producing the typical colored halo (the blue-green component being nearest the light source). Any hazing of the ocular media, such as that caused by mucus on the cornea in front of the pupil, corneal scars, Krukenberg's spindles, or lens and vitreous opacities, can give a halolike glow around lights, but generally there is no color present.

3. *Mydriasis.* An increasing paralysis of the pupillary sphincter caused by the pressure elevation results in pupillary dilation, which is one of the differential points between glaucoma and iritis, the pupil being small in iritis. With high, long-continued pressures the pupil assumes a vertically oval, mid-dilated, fixed position. There is actual damage to the sphincter of the pupil, and subsequently it may not react even to direct stimulants.

4. *Venous congestion.* When the intraocular pressure exceeds that of the intraocular veins, increasing congestion occurs. The iris blood vessels become engorged, as do those of the conjunctiva. This occurs an hour or more after the onset of the acute attack.

5. *Aqueous flare.* With a vascular congestion some protein leaks out into the aqueous humor, causing an aqueous flare. This usually is not more than one plus. The excess protein and congestion can cause posterior synechias, but they tend to be fragile and less extensive than those in iritis. At first no cells are seen in the aqueous humor, but later pigment floaters appear. The iris surface will often be dusted with pigment after an acute attack.

6. *Pain.* Pain varies from a feeling of discomfort and fullness around the eye to one of the severest of pains. Usually the more congested the eye, the more severe the pain. The pain follows the trigeminal distribution and may be limited to the eye or may spread reflexly to the forehead, ear, sinuses, and teeth. In some unfortunate patients, teeth have been mistakenly extracted because of this severe referred pain.

7. *Autonomic stimulation.* Nausea and vomiting usually accompany the acute attack and may so overshadow the pain and dim vision that the patient may be treated for any of a number of abdominal disorders ranging from "stomach flu" to intestinal obstruction. In addition, the oculocardiac reflex produces bradycardia, and there is often profuse sweating.

8. *Disc and field changes.* With the generalized vascular congestion the optic nerve head becomes hyperemic and edematous. The disc can become swollen within 24 hours. The field is not diagnostic, merely showing generalized constriction. Actual total loss of vision can occur in a very few days if pressures are permitted to remain high. Normalization of pressure can sometimes result in surprising improvement of vision. Therefore energetic therapy is indicated even when only light perception is apparent at the initial examination. Cupping is seldom seen except in cases of chronic angle closure.

9. *Peripheral anterior synechias.* During the time of the acute attack, the iris is pressed solidly against the trabecular meshwork. In the first few hours of an attack, it is almost certain that permanent synechias have not formed, and an iridectomy will permit the angle to open completely. In a few more hours this opportunity may be lost forever, and even if the acute attack is broken, the eye will probably have permanent impairment of its outflow facility caused by permanent peripheral synechias. The iris is glued to the meshwork by exudate. The greater the congestion and the longer the iris is pressed against the angle wall, the more certain is the permanence of that union.

10. *Posterior synechias.* The same iris congestion that produces peripheral anterior synechias can also result in posterior synechias.

11. *Tonographic changes.* Before the angle closes, the otherwise normal narrow-angled eye will have a perfectly normal facility of aqueous outflow. During the period of occlusion the facility drops practically to zero. If the angle opens completely after the attack, the facility may again be normal. However, iris apposition to the meshwork seems to damage its permeability, and after repeated attacks or after prolonged iris–trabecular meshwork contact, the facility of outflow is decreased even when the angle opens completely. Peripheral anterior synechias decrease the facility in direct proportion to the area of the meshwork blocked by them.

12. *Sector atrophy of the iris.* At sufficiently high pressures there may be localized interruption of the arterial supply to the iris, resulting in ischemia and iris atrophy. This usually occurs in the upper half of the iris. Atrophy of this sector of the iris releases pigment from the pigmented epithelium, so that a fine

pigmentary dusting of anterior iris and posterior cornea is common. The sector-shaped iris atrophy is diagnostic of previous acute angle closure. Only herpes zoster ophthalmicus commonly causes a similar appearance.

13. *Lens changes* (Fig. 12-4). The high pressure can produce small anterior subcapsular lens changes that Vogt called *Glaukomflecken* or *cataracta disseminata subcapsularis glaukomatosa*. They are multiple, gray-white, oval to dotlike opacities at the ends of the lens fibers, which tend to follow the suture lines. These are diagnostic of a previous attack of angle closure. Senile cataracts frequently are precipitated by an attack of acute glaucoma.

Chronic angle-closure symptoms. In some narrow-angled eyes there may never be a sudden, total angle occlusion. Instead, there is a gradual increase in the area of contact between the iris and the meshwork, usually starting at the upper angle and spreading downward. When there is closure of nearly two thirds of the angle, a progressive rise in pressure begins and can slowly progress to heights of 40 to 60 mm Hg without the association of discomfort, pain, halos, or congestion. Therefore the angle-closure mechanism is capable of causing a loss of vision indistinguishable symptomatically from that of open-angle, chronic simple glaucoma.

More commonly, these eyes run an increased pressure with intermittent spikes. During the periodic elevations the eye may become slightly congested, and some

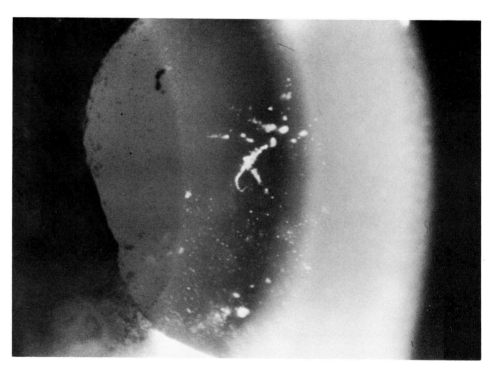

Fig. 12-4. Slit-lamp photograph of anterior lens with *Glaukomflecken*. (Courtesy Dr. K. Richardson and Dr. F. Cignetti, Pittsburgh.)

pain and halo formation may be noticed. Chandler calls this "subacute angle-closure glaucoma." The symptom complex is quite different from that of an unrelieved acute, congestive attack of angle-closure glaucoma. Usually the eye is clear, white, and comfortable without corneal edema, congestion, or mydriasis. Gonioscopically, the angle is usually occluded in most of its circumference, but a slitlike area of open angle remains, which is often found in the lower temporal region. Tonographically, the facility of outflow is decreased in direct relation to the area of angle occlusion. Over a period of many months or years, these eyes develop the cupped discs and field defects typical of the open-angle glaucomas.

Peripheral anterior synechias may not form until very late in this type of angle closure. In the absence of congestion, no fibrin leaks from the vessels to glue the iris to the trabecular meshwork. Some of these eyes can actually lose all vision from the prolonged increased intraocular pressure, and yet the iris will sometimes drop free of the trabecular meshwork if an iridectomy is performed. Unfortunately some eyes will form firm peripheral anterior synechias even though the clinical course has been identical to that of eyes that form no synechias. After an iridectomy it can be determined whether the iris is being held against the meshwork by the posterior aqueous pressure or whether the iris is glued to the meshwork with peripheral anterior synechias. This can be determined by gonioscopy with a Zeiss gonioprism (Chapter 2) and pressure on the cornea, or at the time of surgery (Chapter 23) with operating-room Koeppe lens gonioscopy.

Provocative tests. Any eye with a narrow angle deserves investigation of its actual capacity to occlude. Angle closure can be seen if gonioscopy is done in a dim light, avoiding pupillary constriction from the gonioscopic light source, or if the pupil is dilated by a mydriatic. If enough of the angle occludes, a pressure elevation will occur. However, it is well to remember that only 50% of eyes that have actually had an attack of angle closure in the past or whose companion eye has previously occluded will have as much as an 8 mm Hg rise of pressure after dilation. Some 85% of these same eyes will show a significant reduction (25% to 30%) in outflow facility under the same circumstances.

Dark room test. The time-honored method of provoking angle closure is by keeping the patient in a dark room for 60 to 90 minutes and then promptly measuring the tension. A rise of 8 mm Hg or more is considered positive. The patient must be kept awake because the miosis of sleep might prevent angle closure. Gonioscopy may reveal a closed angle under dim light, but often the pupil constricts, widening the angle. This test is more physiologic than other provocative tests, and the acute angle closure produced can be easily reversed with miotics.

Prone provocative test. This test is also performed under physiologic conditions. Patients are in the prone position for 30 to 45 minutes, and a pressure rise of 8 to 10 mm Hg with angle closure is considered positive. The test helps confirm angle closure and pressure rises, particularly in cases with a history of symptoms related to this position. Patients describing these symptoms should certainly be subjected to the test. The prone position permits a gravitational forward shift of the lens-iris diaphragm and closure of the narrow-angled eye. Gonioscopy performed immediately after the test may show angle closure. There are, however, occasional patients with widely open angles who will have a pressure elevation.

Combined dark room–prone test. To increase the effectiveness of physiologic provocative testing, it seemed logical to combine the dark room test, which is positive in a small percentage of narrow-angle glaucoma patients, with the prone provocative test. Combining these tests markedly increases the number of positive responders. The test is performed in a dark room with the patient lying face down or by sitting with the head forward, resting on the arms or hands placed on a table. A positive test is determined by a 10 mm Hg or greater pressure rise in 45 minutes. Gonioscopy performed immediately in dim light should reveal a closed angle.

Mydriasis test. The mydriasis test consists in instilling 2 drops of 5% eucatropine or 0.5% cyclopentolate (Cyclogyl) into the conjunctival sac. This will produce moderate pupillary dilation. An 8 mm Hg rise of pressure by the end of 1 hour is considered positive if gonioscopy shows that there has been an actual angle closure. It should be remembered that a few open-angle glaucomatous eyes will have tension elevations and decreases in facility of outflow either in the dark or after instillation of a mydriatic, but their angles will remain definitely open. In narrow-angled eyes the pupil of only one eye should be dilated at a time because of the danger of precipitating an acute episode of angle closure. At the conclusion of the test, 2% pilocarpine should be administered until the pupil is miotic. It should be remembered that the pupil may redilate after the pilocarpine effect begins to diminish. If the angle is at all narrow, the patient should continue pilocarpine drops every 4 hours for two or three doses to avoid angle closure.

Pupillary dilation plus tonography and gonioscopy. After the pupil of one eye is dilated with 5% eucatropine, tonography is done in dim light to avoid pupillary constriction. A decrease in outflow facility of 25% to 30%, if coupled with gonioscopic evidence of increased angle closure, is considered a positive test even in the absence of an actual rise in tension. This test will be positive in over 80% of proved angle-closure glaucomas.

Pilocarpine provocative test. This test is useful in narrow-angle glaucoma patients with closure and elevated pressures to rule out the possibility of an open-angle glaucoma component. Instillation of a weak miotic solution opens a closed angle and causes the pressure to fall markedly. If the angle is open gonioscopically and the pressures normalized, there is no significant open-angle glaucoma component. A peripheral iridectomy would then be the surgical procedure of choice rather than filtering surgery.

Other provocative tests. Kirsch has advocated the use of three procedures to provoke angle closure in susceptible individuals. The pupil is first dilated with mydriatics, then the patient is given a water-drinking test, and later miotics are used to induce pupillary block. Limited experience with this form of testing prevents advocating its general use. Some clinicians believe the test is unphysiologic and may produce acute glaucoma in angles unlikely to close under normal conditions.

Reliability of provocative tests. Unfortunately a negative provocative test does not rule out the possibility of angle closure in the future. Gonioscopic evidence of a narrow angle is the most important finding. The narrower the angle, the more imminent is angle closure and the more closely the patient should be followed.

Clinical evaluation of the tests. If the dark room or prone tests are positive or if there has been an attack of angle closure in the eye in question or its mate, an indication for iridectomy exists. Although a positive mydriatic provocative test indicates capacity for angle closure under the conditions of the test, there is no evidence that conclusively demonstrates that eyes with positive mydriatic provocative tests will develop spontaneous acute attacks of angle closure if not treated by iridectomy. Studies to provide such data are in progress. Occasionally a positive result may be obtained in an untreated eye; yet this same eye may have a 20° open angle (Grade 2) under miotic therapy. As long as miotics are used, such an eye is unlikely to develop occlusion, and therefore it may be justifiable to permit a reliable patient to continue on such a regimen, particularly if age and general health make surgery unwise.

If the patient has nuclear cataracts with Grade 2 angles and vision is greatly diminished by a miotic, it may be justifiable to avoid miotics. If visual deterioration or glaucoma potential necessitates surgery, cataract extraction is the procedure of choice, since both the opacity and the narrow angle are eliminated at the same time.

In general, the younger the patient and the narrower the angle, the more closely the patient must be watched and the more desirable peripheral iridectomy becomes to prevent an attack of acute glaucoma.

Therapy for primary angle-closure glaucoma
Medical therapy

The medical therapy for angle-closure glaucoma is useful only as a prelude to surgery. Glycerol, acetazolamide (Diamox), and pilocarpine may be used simultaneously to obtain prompt normalization of pressure. If the iris is not pulled away from the trabecular meshwork, peripheral anterior synechias may become permanent in a few hours.

When pressure has become normalized, the status of the outflow system can be evaluated by gonioscopy and tonography. It is of utmost importance that the eye should be operated on promptly. Too often the patient and the doctor are lulled into a false sense of security by the normalized pressure and lose the opportunity of effecting a safe cure by iridectomy.

Acute angle closure. The principal aim of medical therapy is to pull the iris from its contact with the meshwork, thus avoiding permanent peripheral anterior synechias. The more quickly this is accomplished the better, for synechias may form in a very few hours. All medical measures should be used simultaneously.

The necessary surgery can be performed much more safely if the pressure is normalized.

Hyperosmotic agents. Hyperosmotic agents are now available to accomplish prompt lowering of intraocular pressure.

1. *Oral glycerol.* A supply of glycerol should be available in every ophthalmologist's office. It is administered in a 50% solution, the dosage being between 0.7 to 1.5 ml/kg body weight or approximately 1 ml of the 50% glycerol solution per pound of body weight. If the patient is nauseated, one must resort to intravenous hyperosmotic agents.

2. *Oral isosorbide (Hydronol).* Emesis occurs less often with this medication than with glycerol. It is used in doses of 1 to 2 Gm/kg and can be used with greater safety in diabetics as a metabolically inactive agent.

3. *Urea (Urevert).* Urea is administered intravenously in a dose of 1 to 1.5 Gm/kg body weight.

4. *Mannitol, 20%.* This agent is administered intravenously in a dose of 1 to 2 Gm/kg body weight, usually when oral glycerol has failed or is contraindicated.

The latter two substances should be given at a maximum rate of 60 drops per minute. With all three of these medications the dose must be individualized for each patient to minimize vascular, central nervous system, and renal complications.

Oral glycerol should be given in the doctor's office as soon as the diagnosis of angle-closure glaucoma has been made. This is the quickest method of lowering pressure and will help the effectiveness of miotic therapy. Acetazolamide (Diamox) should be given if glycerol is not available. If the patient is nauseated, miotics and intravenous acetazolamide should be employed, and the patient should be sent to the hospital promptly for intravenous hyperosmotic therapy. Catheterization may be required, especially if general anesthesia is used, because of the diuresis that ensues after intravenous therapy.

The intraocular pressure usually falls in 20 to 90 minutes and remains down for 4 to 10 hours or longer. The angle may not open at all, but a safe period is provided during which miotics are more effective and surgery can be performed more safely. If the eye is congested, it may be best to hold tensions under control for 1 or 2 days by repeating the hyperosmotic medication so that surgery may be performed on a less irritated eye. (A discussion of the side effects of hyperosmotic drugs is given in Chapter 20.)

Miotics. Miotics are used to pull the iris away from the peripheral angle. Unfortunately, in an eye with a high pressure, the sphincter is often partially paralyzed and will not react to miotics effectively until pressure has been reduced by other measures. For this reason oral glycerol and topical miotics should be given as emergency office treatment. A miotic not only pulls the iris away from the trabecular meshwork but also adds to the relative pupillary block. This accounts for some of the paradoxical effects of miotics, the use of which may precipitate or worsen an acute attack. Nevertheless, miotics are still a most effective method of temporary control of acute glaucoma.

PILOCARPINE, 2% TO 4%, OR CARCHOLIN, 1.5%. One or 2 drops should be instilled in the affected eye five times, 1 minute apart. For the next 25 minutes the drops should be continued, with 1 or 2 drops given every 5 minutes, and then three or four times an hour until the angle opens or until surgery. The unaffected eye should be given 3 drops and continued on therapy four times a day to avoid a bilateral attack.

ESERINE, 0.5%, NEOSTIGMINE (PROSTIGMIN), 5%, OR METHACHOLINE (MECHO-LYL), 20%. One or 2 drops may be alternated with the pilocarpine if desired. These drops have the disadvantage of adding somewhat to the congestion of the eye and tend to increase nausea. Methacholine must be freshly prepared, for it is unstable in solution.

The stronger miotics such as demecarium bromide (Humorsol) and echo-thiophate iodide (Phospholine iodide) exaggerate both the pupillary block and the congestive components and therefore should not be used.

THYMOXAMINE. This adrenergic blocking agent, at present unavailable in the United States, has been used effectively to break attacks of acute angle closure. Applied topically every 15 minutes in a 0.5% solution, Thymoxamine inhibits contraction of the dilator muscle. Mechanically the vector forces created by Thymoxamine tend to open a closed angle more effectively than pilocarpine, which increases the pupillary block by constricting the sphincter muscle.

Carbonic anhydrase inhibitors. Acetazolamide is the carbonic anhydrase in-hibitor that is commonly used. If the patient is not nauseated, 500 mg of acetazola-mide may be given by mouth at once, and 250 mg repeated every 4 hours. If nausea is present, 500 mg of acetazolamide sodium in a sterile ampule can be dis-sovled in 10 ml of sterile water. Five milliliters should be given intravenously and 5 ml intramuscularly for a prolonged effect. Although effective for lowering pressure preoperatively, acetazolamide should never be used for continuing therapy lest the normalization of pressure and suppression of symptoms of angle closure en-courage both the doctor and the patient to continue medical therapy instead of proceeding with the definitive cure of pupillary block by iridectomy.

Retrobulbar anesthetic agents. Approximately 1.5 ml of 2% lidocaine (Xylo-caine) or 2% procaine may be given as a retrobulbar injection. This blocks the ciliary ganglion, reducing aqueous production, stopping pain, and decreasing con-gestion by eliminating the reflex arc. It is to be remembered, however, that the action of cholinesterase inhibitors like eserine and neostigmine is thereby blocked. Only pilocarpine, carbachol (Carcholin), and methacholine will remain effective as miotics. The use of lidocaine also risks retrobulbar hemorrhage, which might delay definitive therapy. Retrobulbar injection is seldom used since hyperosmotic agents have become available.

General measures. Morphine sulfate, 15 mg subcutaneously, is helpful in re-lieving pain and apprehension. Its central stimulation is of value in adding to pupillary constriction but is likely to make nausea worse. Meperidine (Demerol), 50 to 100 mg subcutaneously, is also useful for relieving pain and is less likely to produce nausea.

Chronic angle closure. Since the eye is not congested and the iris has been against the angle wall for many months, there is less urgency for therapy than in acute angle-closure glaucoma. Since there is no pain, morphine and retrobulbar injection are of little value. Miotics and acetazolamide are still most valuable in lowering tension. The addition of hyperosmotic agents preoperatively should be employed if normal levels of pressure have not been attained. The choice of iridectomy or a filtering procedure will depend on both tonography and gonioscopy. As a general rule, iridectomy is the procedure of choice.

Surgical therapy

Surgery is indicated in all cases of pupillary-block glaucoma. Exceptions to this statement can be found, but it is the best general rule to follow. Until an iridectomy provides a bypass for aqueous flow, the pupillary block remains as a continuing threat to the eye even if pressure has been normalized and the angle can temporarily be held open by miotics. Almost 50% of eyes whose fellow eyes had previously suffered an attack of angle closure themselves developed angle closure within a period of five years even though treated with miotics. When the patient was not faithful with the drops, the incidence of acute attack rose to 89%.

Intensive medical therapy will normalize the pressure and often will open the angle. If pressures cannot be normalized, a posterior sclerotomy and vitreous aspiration should be considered before iridectomy is performed. If tonography shows a normal facility of outflow and the angle is shown open by gonioscopy, one may be reasonably sure that control after iridectomy will be curative, with the exception of plateau iris. The principles of the surgery are discussed in Chapter 23.

Iridectomy (Reels I-4 and I-5) *and filtering operations.* When the decision of management by iridectomy versus filtering surgery is uncertain, the procedure of choice should be the less complicated iridectomy. If necessary, filtering surgery can be performed at a later date. Primary factors that help make this decision are the presence or absence of preexisting open-angle glaucoma, the duration of the attack (if any) of acute angle closure, and the extent of synechia formation in relation to the level of intraocular pressure. Tonography helps little in the choice of procedure.

Postoperative complications of peripheral iridectomy are uncommon but include flat anterior chamber, persistent fistula, hyphema, posterior synechia, cataract, malignant glaucoma, and infection. Surgical complications such as flat anterior chamber, hypotony, or lens injury are known to produce cataracts. Angle closure may predispose an eye to lens opacities. The question of a relationship between uncomplicated peripheral iridectomy and cataract is debatable. Because of inadequate controls and limited follow-up, reports conflict. An extensive, well-controlled study is being carried out by Kirsch, who has followed 100 iridectomized eyes an average of about 15 years and found no evidence of cataractogenesis when compared to spontaneous lens opacities in matched control eyes. In 18 cases of unilateral iridectomy the incidence of cataract formation did not differ significantly from the fellow eye. Other investigators, however, have found a slightly higher incidence of cataract formation after uncomplicated iridectomy, especially in eyes that have had an attack of angle closure.

Management of the fellow eye

While the acute glaucoma is being treated, the fellow eye should be treated with 1% pilocarpine solution every 6 hours to avoid angle closure. Gonioscopy needs to be performed after the pupil is small, to guard against those rare cases in which the angle is made narrower by miotics. A prophylactic iridectomy should be done after the first eye is out of danger. Only rarely is it justifiable to continue miotics in the second eye indefinitely. Unless there is marked asymmetry in the angle appearance and the second eye has a nonoccludable angle, it is safer to do a prophylactic iridectomy than to follow the patient on long-term miotics.

SECONDARY ANGLE CLOSURE

In all eyes with glaucoma due to pupillary block, free access of aqueous humor to the anterior chamber must be obtained promptly. This can occasionally be accomplished medically, but usually surgical intervention will be needed.

Miotic-induced

Miotic medications, particularly the strong miotics such as echothiophate iodide (Phospholine iodide), cause shallowing of the anterior chamber and narrowing of the angle. The mechanism of shallowing is due to relaxation of lens zonules, an increase in pupillary block, and congestion of iris and ciliary body. In this regard the actions of miotics will produce the opposite effect to that of atropine-like medications on the ciliary body. Strong miotics will progressively shallow the chamber during a period of several weeks or months. A review of gonioscopic findings prior to treatment is a clue to the etiology of iatrogenically induced narrow angles. If there is further question of this cause for narrowed angles, the miotic should be cautiously discontinued while the patient is under close observation.

Swollen lens

Except for the presence of a cataract, the glaucoma produced by a swollen lens is indistinguishable from that of angle-closure glaucoma with pupillary block. The lens can become intumescent, slowly with a senile cataract or rapidly when the cause is traumatic. There is the same shallow chamber with convexity of the iris and the same symptoms (except those visual symptoms that the lens opacity would obscure). Of course, it is usually unilateral (Fig. 12-5).

Medical treatment

Medical therapy is identical to that of angle-closure glaucoma described in this chapter. Its purpose is to reduce pressure to a safe level for surgery.

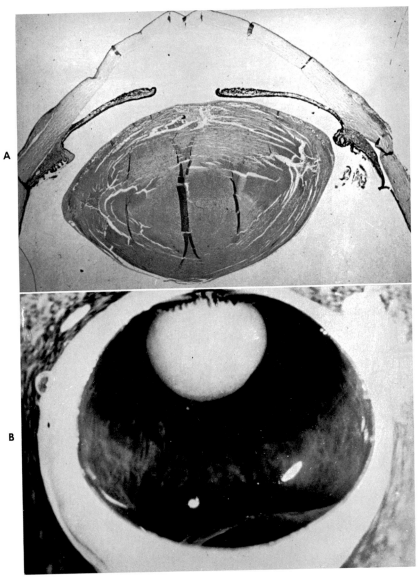

Fig. 12-5. A, Photomicrograph of swollen lens. **B,** Whole mount of a swollen lens. (Courtesy Dr. L. E. Zimmerman, Washington, D.C.; AFIP collection.)

Surgical treatment

Although an iridectomy would break the acute attack in most instances, the proper therapy is intracapsular lens removal. The resultant deepening of the chamber prevents future angle closure and should cure the glaucoma if damage to the trabecular meshwork has not occurred or peripheral anterior synechias have not formed. Thus one obtains both glaucoma control and visual improvement by the one procedure.

Posterior synechias to lens (iris bombé)

When iritis has caused complete adhesion of the iris to the lens, so that aqueous humor is unable to get through the pupil, the iris is ballooned forward in all areas where it is not attached to the lens. Usually the adhesion is greatest near the pupil. At the pupil the anterior chamber depth is normal, but elsewhere it is shallowed by the iris balloon. In some long-standing cases of iritis, the iris may be bound to the lens everywhere except at the extreme periphery. Only careful slit-lamp biomicroscopy or gonioscopy will demonstrate the peripheral balloon that reveals the true nature of the pupillary block.

Medical treatment

Since the posterior synechias are the key to the etiology, treatment is directed toward breaking them and minimizing the iritis that produced them.

Mydriatics. The combined use of cycloplegic and sympathomimetic agents aids in breaking posterior synechias.

ATROPINE, 2% TO 4%. One or 2 drops of 2% to 4% atropine should be given every minute for 5 minutes. The patient should be protected from the toxic effect of parasympathetic inhibition by holding the canaliculi closed for several minutes after the medication has been applied. For continuing therapy, 2% atropine should be used one to four times daily.

SCOPOLAMINE HYDROBROMIDE, 0.2%. This may be used in the same way as atropine.

PHENYLEPHRINE (NEO-SYNEPHRINE), 10%. To gain the added effect of sympathetic stimulation, 1 drop may be given every minute for 3 minutes, using the same precautions to occlude the tear duct. For continuing therapy, it may be used one to four times a day. It is a more effective dilator of the pupil than is epinephrine but affects secretion less.

EPINEPHRINE, 2%. This drug is often helpful. It not only aids pupillary dilation but also helps to lower intraocular pressure by suppressing aqueous production.

Corticosteroids. If iritis is at all active, one of the corticosteroids should be used topically in adequate dosage to suppress activity. In severe cases oral dosage may be advisable. An increase in intraocular pressure can occur after corticosteroid treatment. This may be due to a restoration of aqueous production before there has been corresponding improvement in facility of outflow, or the patient may happen to be one who responds to corticosteroids with a significant increase in intraocular pressure. Sub-Tenon's injection of steroids has been recommended in some severe, unresponsive, inflammatory problems. Extreme care should be exercised in administering sub-Tenon's or retrobulbar corticosteroids. Intraocular injection with severe damage and loss of the eye has been reported.

Hyperpyrexia. The use of typhoid vaccine intravenously has fallen into disuse since the advent of corticosteroid therapy. It is still a useful therapy in stubborn cases. Ten million organisms given intravenously will usually give a good febrile response. Depending on the response, treatment can be repeated every day or every other day for three to six times. It is usually necessary to double the dosage each time.

Salicylates. Aspirin and other salicylates add to the patient's comfort and decrease the inflammatory response.

Carbonic anhydrase inhibitors. A discussion of the use of carbonic anhydrase inhibitors in the treatment of glaucoma is given in Chapter 19.

Surgical treatment

Preoperatively, tensions should be reduced by the use of carbonic anhydrase inhibitors, osmotic agents, and retrobulbar anesthesia.

Iridectomy. An ab externo incision should be used to enter the anterior chamber. A spatula is sometimes needed to free the iris from the cornea. It is usually wise to do a sector iridectomy to create the generous opening necessary to prevent recurrence. The large opening may facilitate subsequent surgery such as lens extraction. As a rule, iridectomy is safer and surer than transfixion.

Transfixion. This is accomplished by passing a Graefe knife across the anterior chamber from limbus to limbus, transfixing the ballooned-up iris two to four times in its passage. Obviously, great care must be taken to keep the knife in the true plane of the iris to avoid damage to the lens. The procedure is useful in a congested eye when it is thought that an iridectomy would be too hazardous. The large iris vessels can usually be avoided, so that dangerous bleeding is prevented.

Lens subluxation

Anterior dislocation of the lens into the anterior chamber is a surgical emergency. The lens should be removed at once by an ab externo incision. It is wise to use miotics preoperatively to prevent the lens from dropping back into the vitreous humor (Fig. 12-6).

Posterior dislocation of the lens into the vitreous humor is often associated with glaucoma due to angle recession, but in some instances aqueous humor collects behind or in the vitreous humor, lifting it and the lens forward in a form of pupillary block. Although mydriatics may temporarily break this block, it is usually best to remove the lens, even though such surgery is hazardous. When posterior dislocation of the lens does not cause pupillary block, the lens should not be removed. The open-angle glaucoma should be treated in the same manner as primary open-angle glaucoma.

Panretinal photocoagulation

Panretinal photocoagulation, now frequently used for the treatment of diabetic retinopathy, transiently narrows the anterior chamber angle. Shallowing of the anterior chamber occurs within hours after treatment and is presumably caused by fluid increase in the subchoroidal space. The accumulation of subchoroidal fluid forces the ciliary body inward and forward on its attachment at the scleral spur, and also displaces the vitreous and the lens anteriorly. An element of pupil-

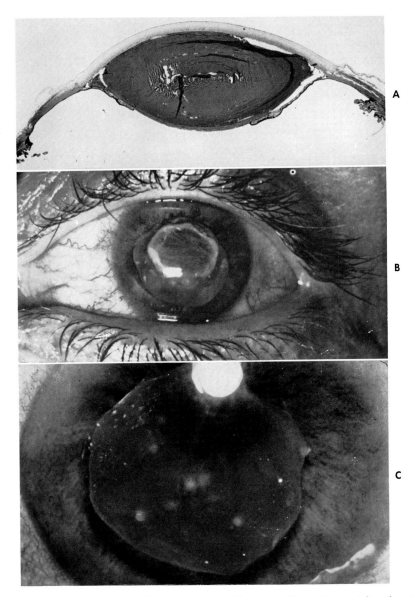

Fig. 12-6. A, Photomicrograph of anterior lens dislocation. Note the peripheral anterior synechias caused by aqueous humor pushing the iris forward against the posterior lens and cornea. **B,** Anterior dislocation of the lens with overlying corneal opacification. **C,** Anterior lens dislocation showing the nucleus of a morgagnian cataract prolapsed into the anterior chamber. (**A** courtesy Dr. L. E. Zimmerman, Washington, D.C.; AFIP collection.)

lary block is partly responsible for angle closure. The anterior chamber will, in 2 to 3 days, gradually redeepen, so that it is prudent to be as conservative as possible. Medical management by pilocarpine, acetazolamide (Diamox), and hyperosmotic agents will tide over most of these patients until the angle reopens. However, unresponsive patients with high pressures will require a posterior sclerotomy to drain the choroidal edema, or an iridectomy to break the pupillary block.

Scleral buckling

Buckling procedures for retinal detachments, particularly when the buckle is excessively tightened, will produce angle-closure glaucoma, sometimes necessitating iridectomy. The cause is reportedly a forward and inward rotation of the ciliary body, hinged at the scleral spur. This rotation moves the iris root, zonules, and lens forward and narrows the angle. Buckling the eye decreases the volume of the posterior globe, displacing the vitreous and secondarily the lens-iris diaphragm forward. Angle closure therefore is probably a mixture of pupillary- and nonpupillary-block mechanisms. The surgeon treating retinal detachment may elect to correct the problem by loosening the scleral buckle by draining the choroidal fluid or by iridectomy. Awareness of this entity helps prevent the problem during retinal surgery. A similar problem may occur if the scleral buckle slips posteriorly and compresses the vortex veins. Reoperation with reattachment of the buckle further forward is necessary.

Posterior synechias to vitreous humor in aphakia

One of the serious complications of lens extraction is the formation of posterior synechias to the vitreous humor or to the posterior capsule in extracapsular extractions. If there is a postoperative wound leak with a flat anterior chamber, posterior synechias as well as anterior synechias are sure to form in time, particularly if the eye is inflamed. A full iridectomy is less likely to be entirely sealed off but is by no means immune to this complication.

In the immediate period after a cataract has been extracted, it is important to tell whether a flat chamber is due to a wound leak or to pupillary block. Ordinarily, the differential diagnosis is easily made by taking the tension with a tonometer. If the eye is so soft that the intraocular pressure barely registers on the tonometer, a wound leak is present whether or not a fluorescein test is positive. If, however, the tension is nearly normal or above, a pupillary-block glaucoma or ciliovitreal-block (aphakic malignant) glaucoma is present and must be dealt with promptly.

Symptoms (Figs. 12-7 and 12-8)

The clinical appearance of aphakic pupillary block depends on the integrity of the anterior hyaloid membrane of the vitreous humor. If it is a solid membrane, the entire iris-vitreous diaphragm moves forward, which results in an irregularly shallow anterior chamber or in a flat chamber, whose nature is easily diagnosed. However, if the hyaloid membrane is weaker, a solid mushroom of vitreous humor

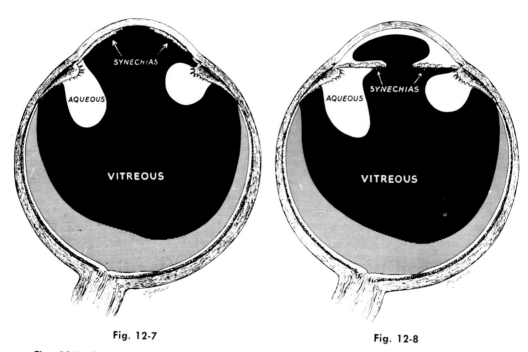

Fig. 12-7   **Fig. 12-8**

Fig. 12-7. Diagram of aphakic pupillary block, showing posterior synechias to anterior vitreous humor, closure of peripheral iridectomy, and aqueous humor trapped in the vitreous chamber. The anterior chamber is collapsed.

Fig. 12-8. Diagram of aphakic pupillary block, showing posterior synechias and closure of peripheral iridectomy with herniation of the anterior hyaloid membrane. The anterior chamber is partially full of vitreous humor. Aqueous humor is trapped in the vitreous chamber. This aqueous may be in pockets or may diffusely infiltrate the vitreous body. Often the anterior chamber is irregularly shallowed.

will be pushed into the anterior chamber. Miotics constrict the pupil around this herniation and increase the pupillary block. Peripheral iris is lifted forward, resulting in angle closure in spite of a centrally deep anterior chamber filled with vitreous humor. Where this hyaloid membrane is pressed against the posterior cornea, damage to the endothelium occurs, resulting in a corneovitreal adhesion and a corneal opacification.

If the entire vitreous face breaks, most of the anterior chamber will be filled with loose vitreous humor with no well-defined hyaloid surface. This type of vitreous humor in the anterior chamber does not cause corneal opacification but may produce an open-angle glaucoma.

The symptoms may be similar to those of acute or chronic angle-closure glaucoma, depending on the rapidity and height of the pressure rise and the ability of the eye to compensate for that rise without becoming congested. An incomplete pupillary block can be present for a considerable length of time without becoming clinically manifest, particularly if the rate of aqueous production is so low that it does not overbalance the poor outflow.

Medical treatment

The posterior synechias to the vitreous humor should be treated in the same way as posterior synechias to the lens. Every attempt should be made to dilate the pupil and break the synechias. This is hard to accomplish in the aphakic eye because the vitreous humor stretches and follows the dilating pupil without tearing loose from the iris. Often a subconjunctival injection at the limbus of 0.1 ml of a combination of 1% atropine, 4% cocaine, and 1:1000 epinephrine will dilate a pupil that does not dilate with topical mydriatics. The use of hyperosmotic agents may also help to break the pupillary block by reducing vitreous volume and causing the vitreous face to move posteriorly.

Surgical treatment

When the pupillary block is not broken by medical measures, iridectomy should be done promptly. By slit-lamp examination it is often possible to locate an optically clear area in the vitreous humor that corresponds to the area of aqueous collection. It is logical to perform the iridectomy in this area. Fortunately there is usually sufficient aqueous pressure that aqueous humor will break into the area of iridectomy wherever it is performed.

The iridectomy should be peripheral, an ab externo approach with a preplaced McLean suture and a conjunctival flap being the safest method. If extensive peripheral anterior synechias are also present, one can combine the iridectomy with either a synechialysis or a cyclodialysis done through the same or a separate scleral incision. A less formidable procedure is transfixion of the iris, which can be performed if sufficient anterior chamber is present. It is sometimes possible to combine such a transfixion with discission of the pupillary membrane, thus breaking the pupillary block and improving the visual status of the eye. *If iridectomy fails, the patient should be treated surgically for ciliary-block (malignant) glaucoma.*

Epithelial ingrowth

Usually glaucoma is produced by epithelial ingrowth covering the trabecular surface. Occasionally a pupillary block can be produced if the pupil is sealed to the vitreous humor by epithelium or by associated inflammatory posterior synechias.

Treatment is not very satisfactory when the process has extended to the pupil. A full iridectomy should be performed, including all areas of probable epithelial growth. An attempt to remove all islands of remaining epithelium should be made, using curettage and alcohol rub of the posterior cornea. Destruction of the epithelium by cryotherapy has been reported. Whatever the method, useful vision is seldom retained. Epithelial ingrowth is discussed further in Chapter 15.

Ciliary-block glaucoma (malignant glaucoma) (Fig. 12-9) (see also Chapter 23)
Characteristics

Ciliary-block glaucoma is a rare surgical complication in which the anterior chamber either fails to form or collapses, usually shortly after glaucoma surgery,

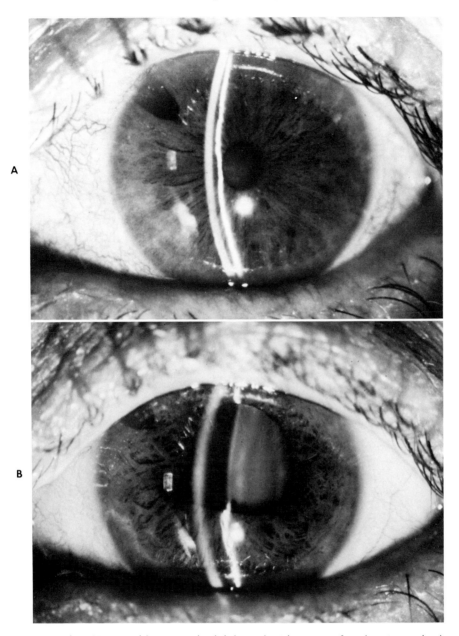

Fig. 12-9. This 60-year-old patient had bilateral iridectomies for chronic angle-closure glaucoma. Postoperatively the limbal incision leaked, and the patient developed ciliary block (malignant) glaucoma in the right eye. This was eventually controlled by lens extraction. During long-term follow-up, tensions in the left eye became more difficult to control on pilocarpine, epinephrine, and acetazolamide. In spite of iridectomy, the anterior chamber was shallow, **A,** and the angle measured grade 1 to closed. When pilocarpine was discontinued, the anterior chamber deepened slightly. Tropicamide (Mydriacyl) caused a marked increase in anterior chamber depth, **B,** and widening of the angle. When pilocarpine was again added, the pressure increased from 22 to 30 mm Hg, and the anterior chamber shallowed. This case clearly demonstrates the mechanical response of the predisposed ciliary-block glaucoma eye.

and tension elevation occurs. The lens or vitreous prolapses into the scleral ring, trapping aqueous humor behind it. A block then occurs that can defy the usual efforts at control; a high intraocular pressure and flat chamber are typical of the condition. The pressure may, however, register normal or slightly below normal. If ciliary-block glaucoma has followed filtering surgery in the first eye, it is almost sure to follow similar surgery in the second eye.

In almost all instances this complication occurs after external filtering operations on hyperopic, shallow-chambered, narrow-angled eyes. It is rare for the complication to occur if pressure can be normalized by miotics before surgery and is less likely to occur in any eye that is normotensive at the time of surgery. For this reason, it is now less common than in the days before hyperosmotic agents and acetazolamide became available. The eyes most in danger are those with chronic angle closure. Iridectomy or cyclodialysis can initiate the complication, but procedures that empty the anterior chamber, such as trephining, sclerostomy, and iridencleisis, are the most common offenders. Ciliary-block glaucoma has been known to occur several years after surgery. Pupillary-block glaucoma must be considered in the differential diagnosis particularly in the aphakic eye.

Medical treatment

It is now possible to break the malignant course by the use of the hyperosmotic agents. With the reduction of pressure, sometimes the anterior chamber will reform, but it is seldom retained without additional help. As advised by Chandler, Simmons, and Grant, instillation of 4% atropine and 10% phenylephrine (Neo-Synephrine) solutions 3 or 4 times a day results in posterior movement of the ciliary body away from the angle. The zonular ligaments tighten and pull the lens posteriorly away from the corneoscleral ring where it has been incarcerated. The filtering procedure that precipitated the malignant course will sometimes remain functional. For some patients, medical management may be necessary for the lifetime. If atropine is stopped, the lens may drop forward, with recurrence of the malignant course. In eyes with re-formed anterior chambers but insufficient filtration, acetazolamide (Diamox) should be used to decrease the intraocular pressure.

Surgical treatment

When medical therapy fails, the most effective surgical procedure in phakic ciliary-block glaucoma is prompt vitreous aspiration with restoration of the anterior chamber. The technique is described in Chapter 23. If this procedure is unsuccessful, a lens extraction may be necessary. Most cases will respond to this second procedure. It may, however, be impossible to re-form the anterior chamber after the lens has been removed, or the anterior chamber may collapse in the following days because of continuing ciliary block. Evidently, aqueous is capable of being trapped in the vitreous body itself or just behind it, lifting the hyaloid membrane or the whole vitreous body forward to produce aphakic malignant glaucoma, thus keeping the chamber collapsed and the pressure high. The anterior hyaloid membrane in these eyes has a fibrous appearance that is more dense than that of the usual hyaloid membrane.

With the lens removed, this continuing block is not unlike aphakic pupillary-block glaucoma except that iridectomy is unlikely to break the block. The eye with aphakic malignant glaucoma requires a broad discission of the hyaloid membrane in the pupillary area, after which the chamber usually deepens gratifyingly. If aqueous is collecting entirely behind the vitreous body, an actual Wheeler knife incision completely through the detached vitreous may be needed. Before incising the vitreous face, the surgeon should make an attempt to locate an optically clear space filled with aqueous.

Usually these eyes will have peripheral anterior synechias as the result of the original chronic angle closure, or they will have added synechias as the result of the collapsed chamber that accompanies the malignant course. These synechias can be removed by cyclodialysis after the pupillary block has been relieved if tension normalization is impossible by medical means.

When one eye has had malignant glaucoma following filtering surgery, vitreous aspiration in the second eye may prevent a malignant course. In a critically shallow-chambered eye, primary lens extraction may be the safest procedure. Even so, malignant glaucoma may in rare instances ensue.

CHAPTER **13**

Angle-closure glaucoma without pupillary block

PRIMARY ANGLE CLOSURE (PLATEAU IRIS)
Diagnosis of plateau iris (Fig. 13-1)

Plateau iris refers to an iris abnormality that may be associated with angle closure but in which a relative pupillary block plays little or no significant role. Because of an anterior insertion of the iris on the ciliary body, the iris is so close to the trabecular meshwork that dilation of the pupil bunches up the iris peripherally and presses it against the meshwork, triggering an attack of angle-closure acute glaucoma that is indistinguishable from that produced by pupillary block. The only help to the clinician is the observation that the central anterior chamber depth is greater than usual for an eye with acute glaucoma and that the iris has a less convex bulge than usual. Instead, the iris plane is quite flat, running directly toward Schwalbe's line. When the acute attack is broken by miotics, the peripheral iris can be seen to angle sharply backward to the ciliary body, leaving a very narrow angle entrance.

Treatment of plateau iris

In all primary angle-closure glaucoma there are two antagonistic factors operating: the pupillary-block mechanism, which is aggravated by miosis, and the compaction of the iris against the trabecular meshwork when the pupil is dilated. This latter factor predominates in plateau iris, but since there may still be some element of pupillary block, iridectomy is still the procedure of choice.

In spite of iridectomy, a patient may continue to have angle-closure symptoms. The usual postoperative cycloplegic medication is contraindicated. It is disconcerting to examine the iridectomized eye and find little or no opening of the angle. Usually there will have been sufficient increase in angle width to allow miotic therapy to prevent future acute attacks (Fig. 13-2).

208

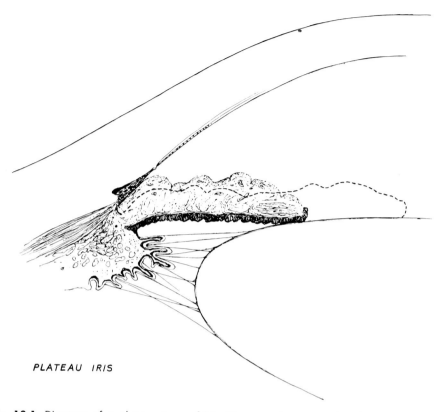

PLATEAU IRIS

Fig. 13-1. Diagram of a plateau type of iris. The central anterior chamber is deeper than in the usual narrow-angled eye. Pupillary block is minimal.

SECONDARY ANGLE CLOSURE

Peripheral anterior synechias decrease the facility of aqueous outflow in direct proportion to the area of trabecular meshwork blocked. A few small peripheral anterior synechias or those in the angle recess behind the scleral spur will interfere little with outflow. Thus the glaucoma potential of such an eye will depend on both the extent of angle closure and on the facility of outflow of the available meshwork. Since there is no pupillary block, the therapy of these eyes is essentially the same as that of open-angle glaucoma with emphasis on medical control, if possible, and surgery only if medical therapy fails.

There are only two ways by which the iris can become attached to the trabecular meshwork. Either it must be pushed against the meshwork as in pupillary block or anterior chamber collapse, or it must be pulled up onto the meshwork by contraction of inflammatory exudates or fibrous tissue as occurs in iritis.

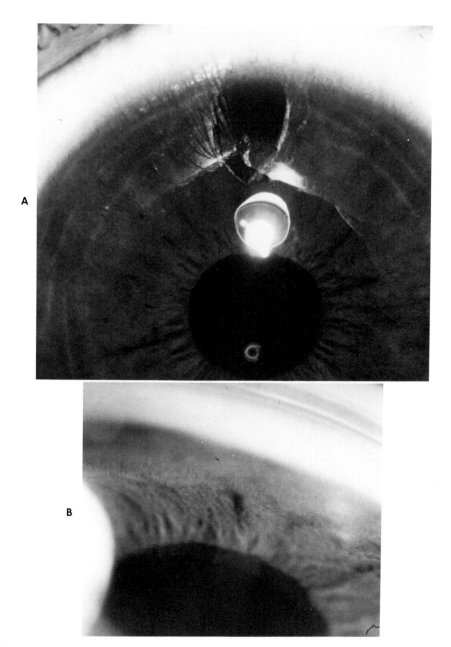

Fig. 13-2. S. C., a 32-year-old urologist, had frequent symptoms of hazy vision, halos, and discomfort in both eyes, at night and during surgery. **A,** After iridectomy preoperative symptoms continued, and dark room and prone provocative tests were highly positive. **B,** Plateau iris was diagnosed postoperatively by gonioscopy. Pilocarpine, 1% q.i.d., was prescribed for long-term use.

Peripheral anterior synechias from iris pushed against the meshwork

By previous pupillary block

An attack of primary angle-closure glaucoma or an iris bombé may have the pupillary block broken by iridectomy. However, during the period of iris apposition, permanent peripheral anterior synechias may have formed.

By anterior chamber collapse (Fig. 13-3, Plate 1, F, and Reel 1-3)

Most collapsed anterior chambers are caused by aqueous humor draining through fistulous tracts. This may be intentional as in glaucoma surgery, unintentional as after cataract surgery, or accidental as in lacerations of the cornea. There may be a gross leak of aqueous humor through a conjunctival incision, or it may flow out under the conjunctival flap with too little resistance to re-form the chamber. In the absence of an anterior chamber the Seidel fluorescein test is frequently negative. To identify the area of a wound leak, fluorescein-stained saline solution should be injected under pressure into the anterior chamber.

The longer the anterior chamber is collapsed, the more probable it is that there will be a decrease in facility of aqueous outflow due both to inflammatory damage to the trabecular meshwork and to permanent peripheral anterior synechias. In lacerations of the cornea, leakproof suturing should be done as soon

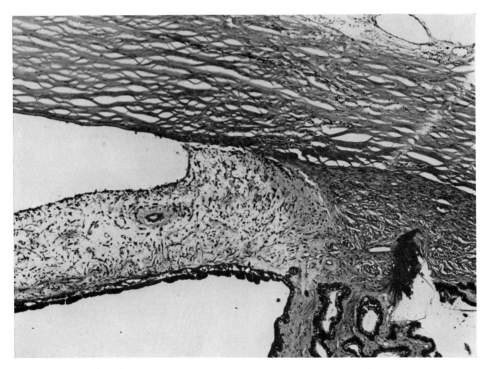

Fig. 13-3. Peripheral anterior synechias after a flat anterior chamber. (Courtesy Dr. S. Joe, Oakland, Calif.)

as possible. In cataract surgery, the prevention of a flat chamber by accurate and adequate suturing is better than any treatment. When delayed re-formation occurs, anterior chamber fluid injection should be combined with subchoroidal fluid drainage. In surgery for fistulizing glaucoma, many eyes have delayed re-formation due to the large limbal opening. A delay of 7 days may be tolerated before anterior

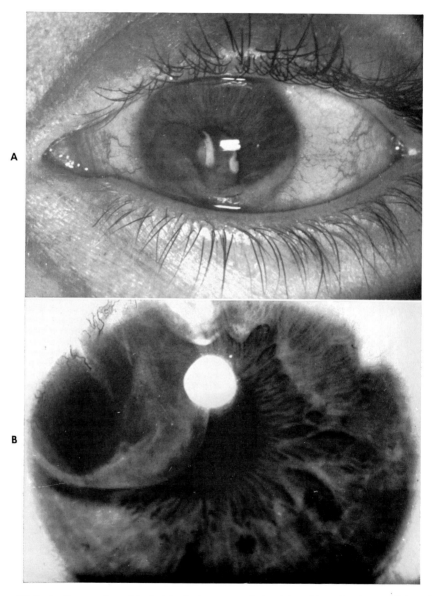

Fig. 13-4. A, Traumatic epithelial inclusion cyst of the iris with extensive peripheral anterior synechias and glaucoma. **B,** Postoperative epithelial inclusion cyst of the anterior chamber.

chamber re-formation and subchoroidal drainage must be performed. A congested eye will form peripheral anterior synechias quickly and should be operated on sooner than a quiet, white eye.

By tumors or cysts (Figs. 13-4 and 13-5 and Reels III-3 and III-4)

Cysts or tumors involving the ciliary body or the peripheral iris can push the iris up against the trabecular meshwork. Usually there is not sufficient involvement

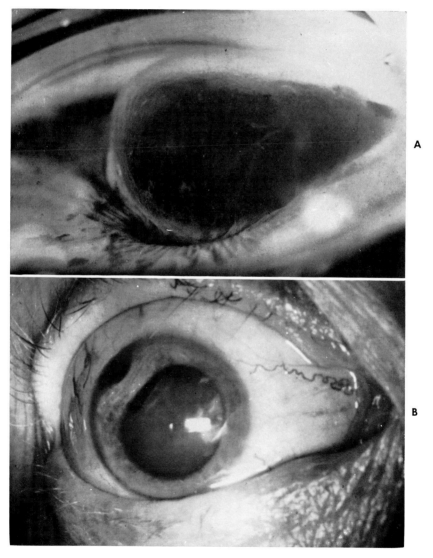

Fig. 13-5. A, Goniophotograph of anterior chamber cyst. **B,** Malignant melanoma of the ciliary body with invasion of the angle. The tumor not only displaced the lens but also pushed the iris against the trabecular meshwork for almost one half of the angle.

to produce glaucoma from the cyst or tumor alone, but associated peripheral anterior synechias further impair outflow.

Epithelial cysts are probably best handled by excision if they are small and by electrocoagulation if they are large. Light coagulation of iris tissues releases large amounts of debris into the anterior chamber. During the ensuing iritis, a devastating secondary glaucoma can occur. If angle closure is due to peripheral pigment cysts of the iris, rupture of the cysts by peripheral iridectomies is safer than light coagulation.

Peripheral anterior synechias from iris pulled up onto the meshwork

By iritis (Fig. 13-6 and Reel I-7)

In the majority of eyes with iritis no peripheral synechias are formed, and the decrease in facility of aqueous outflow is based on decreased permeability of the trabecular meshwork (Chapter 15). In some chronic iritis the inflammatory process causes transudation from the capillaries and the formation of exudates in the angle recess. As these exudates organize and shrink, the iris can be pulled up toward the cornea. Similarly, large pillarlike keratic precipitates can form a bridge between the peripheral iris and the cornea, which later shrinks, causing a localized peripheral synechia.

The synechias resulting from iritis are seldom as uniform in the height of their trabecular attachment as are the synechias of pupillary block, in which whole segments of the iris are usually attached in a straight line parallel to Schwalbe's line. Instead, there will be moundlike areas of synechias alternating with areas of

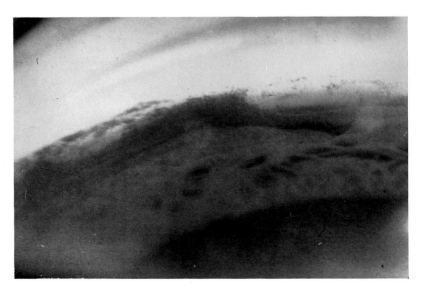

Fig. 13-6. Peripheral anterior synechias from iritis. The iris has been pulled up in irregular mounds as high as Schwalbe's line, which is covered by considerable pigment to the left of the large central synechia.

completely open angle. The decrease in facility of outflow will be dependent both on the block caused by the synechias and on the inflammatory damage to the trabecular meshwork (Chapter 15).

By neovascularization (rubeosis) (Figs. 13-7 to 13-10 and Reel II-2)

Early in the course of rubeosis, there is angle coverage by a fibrovascular membrane, which later shrinks, pulling peripheral iris up against the meshwork and

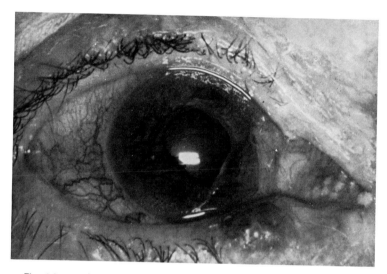

Fig. 13-7. Rubeosis iridis after occlusion of the central retinal vein.

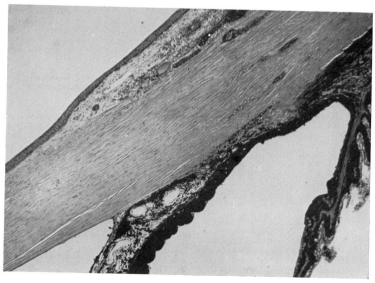

Fig. 13-8. Angle closure by rubeosis iridis after an occlusion of the central retinal vein.

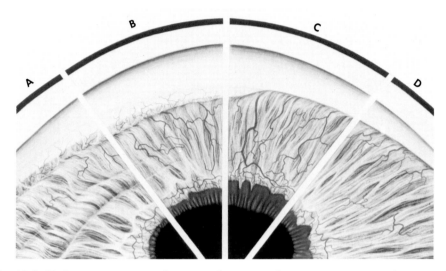

Fig. 13-9. Various appearances of neovascularization of anterior segment. Earliest vessels, A, usually arise at collarette of iris and are often accompanied by tiny twigs in chamber angle. Vessels may become more prominent and cover more of the iris, B. Contraction of fibrovascular membrane, C, exerts pigmented border of pupil and closes the angle. Often in later stages or following therapy, diminution in size and number of vessels may occur, D. (From Hoskins, H. D., Jr.: Trans. Amer. Acad. Ophthal. Otolaryng. **78:**330, 1974.)

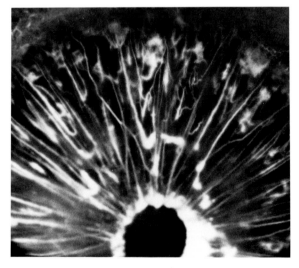

Fig. 13-10. Fluorescein angiogram of a patient with neovascular glaucoma secondary to central retinal vein occlusion. There is congestion of vessels, neovascularization, and fluorescein leakage. (Courtesy A. Vannas, Helsinki.)

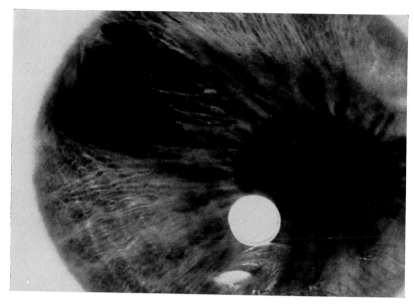

Fig. 13-11. Essential iris atrophy.

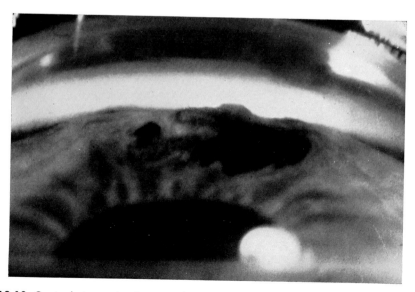

Fig. 13-12. Goniophotograph of essential iris atrophy. The angle is open on either side of the peripheral anterior synechia.

eventually resulting in total angle closure. The causes of neovascular glaucoma are discussed in Chapter 15.

By essential iris atrophy (Figs. 13-11 and 13-12 and Reel II-3)

Essential iris atrophy, a rare, usually unilateral disease, is an abiotrophy that involves the iris, the trabecular meshwork, and the corneal endothelium. Initially, the angle is wide open. Thinning and eventual hole formation begin in the mid-periphery of the iris. The pupil is displaced away from this area. Soon peripheral anterior synechias begin to form on both the side of the holes and the opposite side toward which the pupil is displaced. In the course of one to three years the synechias gradually extend in both directions, closing the angle in a zipperlike fashion. The base pressure of the eye begins to rise when the angle is half closed.

There is definite irregularity of the corneal endothelium seen by both bio-microscopy and gonioscopy. This is evidence of increased permeability of the endo-thelium, which leads to corneal edema at very low pressure levels. Often halos and hazing of vision will appear at tensions of 25 to 30 mm Hg.

Since the etiology is unknown, no definitive therapy is possible, nor does any palliative therapy seem to slow the progression. When glaucoma has developed, medical therapy is preferred as long as possible, and then cyclodialysis or a filtering operation is recommended. Too few cases have been treated surgically to allow evaluation as to which procedure is best. Prophylactic complete iridectomy has been suggested, but its efficacy remains unproved. One case reported by Hogan developed glaucoma four years after a radical iridectomy. At the base of the large iridectomy the peripheral anterior synechias were less dense than elsewhere, and successful cyclodialysis was performed in that area. Iridocycloretraction surgery recently described has not been successful.

CHAPTER 14

Primary open-angle glaucoma

Primary open-angle (simple) glaucoma is characterized by elevations of intra-ocular pressure sufficient to produce damage to the optic nerve. There must be gonioscopic evidence of the absence of angle closure at the time of pressure eleva-tion. The diagnosis of primary glaucoma can be made at the time of the initial examinations only when both eyes are affected and there is no evidence of antece-dent ocular disease (scars, synechias, surgery, inflammation, etc.). In its most common form, the outflow facility is reduced (Fig. 8-1).

PATHOLOGY AND DISORDERED PHYSIOLOGY

In over 99% of primary open-angle glaucoma the obstruction to outflow of aqueous humor is in the trabecular meshwork–Schlemm's canal system. Most evidence favors the trabecular meshwork bordering Schlemm's canal as the site of major resistance to outflow in both normal and glaucomatous eyes. This has been verified in several eyes of each category by microdissection. Material has become available from autopsy eyes and from trephine or sclerectomy biopsies of the filtration angle, demonstrating the early pathology of primary open-angle glaucoma. Correlation of the degree of impairment of outflow facility (perfusion or tonography) with the degenerative changes noted offers possibilities for a much better understanding of the type of pathologic alterations in the individual eye. The finding of gamma globulin and plasma cells more frequently in eyes with primary open-angle glaucoma raises questions of immunogenic mechanisms (Chap-ter 6). Obstructed outflow and normal or near normal secretion result in a rise of intraocular pressure. Cupping of the optic disc, optic atrophy, and field loss appear to be direct or indirect consequences of the elevated pressure.

CLINICAL PICTURE

Primary open-angle glaucoma is a chronic, slowly progressive, bilateral disease. It is insidious in onset and progresses imperceptibly without symptoms until late in the disease, when characteristic field loss occurs. Although it is usually described as progressing constantly, more careful evaluation reveals exacerbations and remissions of the outflow impairment and pressure elevation. These are seen more commonly in the earlier stages of the disease process. The disease may proceed to absolute glaucoma (blindness) without pain or other symptoms. There is, however, a relatively high incidence of vascular occlusion in glaucomatous eyes, which may be complicated by neovascularization of the iris and angle (rubeosis iridis) and a secondary, very painful, neovascular (hemorrhagic) glaucoma.

Age

Primary open-angle glaucoma occurs predominantly in people over 50 years of age but is found to have a significant incidence in the third and fourth decades of life and even in the teens, as revealed by newer diagnostic methods. The term *juvenile open-angle glaucoma* has been applied to patients under the age of 40 years. There appears to be little reason at present, however, for separating this group from other cases of primary open-angle glaucoma. No sex predominance has been noted in primary open-angle glaucoma.

Prevalence

The disease is the commonest of all the glaucomas, comprising 60% to 70% of adult glaucomas. The prevalence varies with the criteria used for making the definitive diagnosis, but most population surveys demonstrate a prevalence of approximately 2% of people over the age of 40 years. These statistics are based on intraocular pressure, usually indicating prevalence of ocular hypertension above an arbitrary pressure level. If one insists on the presence of visual field loss to make the diagnosis, the prevalence of glaucoma *with visual damage* is about 0.5%. Higher prevalence rates are reported in diabetics, high myopes, older age groups, and glaucoma families. Glaucoma accounts for 12% to 20% of blindness in the United States.

DIAGNOSIS

Presented with the classic findings of cupping and atrophy of the optic discs, characteristic field loss, elevated intraocular pressure, and open angles, the diagnosis is easy. However, since visual loss from glaucoma is usually nonrecoverable and effective treatment can avoid such loss, early diagnosis of primary open-angle glaucoma is imperative.

Elevated intraocular pressure

The measurement of intraocular pressure remains the most important means of glaucoma detection. Since elevated intraocular pressure precedes the loss of field by a number of years, routine tonometry on *all patients who are old enough to cooperate* is essential if one is to detect early glaucoma. The ophthalmologist has an ideal opportunity and an obligation to make such measurements on all patients seen for refractive problems.

Significance

Elevation of intraocular pressure is a relative term and can be considered abnormal only on a statistical basis. Nevertheless, the higher the intraocular pressure, the greater the likelihood of the patient having visual field loss. Ideally, one would like to know the particular intraocular pressure that will result in damage to the individual eye. Unfortunately this information is only available retrospectively at present. Also, in many glaucomatous eyes intraocular pressure is elevated only intermittently. Thus it is possible not to recognize glaucoma simply because the patient is seen at a time when his intraocular pressure is within normal limits.

If Schiøtz readings alone are used, an increased pressure may be masked by low ocular rigidity (Figs. 29-7 to 29-9). This is especially true in patients with myopia and thyrotropic exophthalmos and after ocular surgery. Applanation tonometry reveals the true pressure. In such eyes the tonographic tracings are flat, raising the suspicion of a diagnosis of glaucoma.

The significance of an elevated intraocular pressure in a patient with no other evidence of ocular abnormality is still uncertain. The fact that most patients with abnormal cupping and visual field loss have elevated intraocular pressure does not mean that most patients with elevated intraocular pressures will get visual damage if not treated. The prevalence of ocular hypertension is at least 10 to 15 times greater than the prevalence of glaucomatous visual field loss. Several studies (Table 14-1) indicate that patients with normal visual fields and intraocular pressures between 22 and 30 mm Hg have no greater than a 5% likelihood of developing field loss in periods up to ten years. The inability to accurately identify the eventual glaucoma patient before damage develops is one of the major gaps in our present understanding of the disease process.

Diurnal measurements

Patients with glaucoma demonstrate greater diurnal variations in intraocular pressure than do normal individuals, and this may prove helpful in making the diagnosis. But, of course, this presupposes that sufficient suspicion has been aroused in the first place to warrant round-the-clock pressure measurement. More

Table 14-1. Prospective studies of untreated ocular hypertension

Investigators	Intraocular pressure (mm Hg)	Years followed	Field loss	
Linner and Stromberg	22-26	5	3/152*	2%
Linner	22-26	10	3/95*	3.2%
Graham	≥ 21	4	1/232*	0.4%
Perkins	> 21	7	4/124*	3.2%
Norskov	20-25	5	0/72†	0%
Armaly	> 23	5	1/102†	1%
Wilensky and Podos	> 21	5-14	5/100†	5%

*Patients; †eyes.

helpful is the fact that in early glaucoma, tonography may reveal impaired outflow facility even when pressure elevations are only intermittent.

Cupping and field loss

Cupping of the optic disc and characteristic field loss in the presence of pressure elevations establish the diagnosis, but these are late consequences of the disease. The earliest changes in the optic nerve head may be very difficult to differentiate from physiologic cupping. Yet such changes may be accompanied by diagnostic field defects. The availability of improved techniques of visual field testing, as pointed out in Chapter 9, has reemphasized the importance of this procedure in glaucoma diagnosis. Early field changes, sufficiently characteristic to indicate the diagnosis yet minimal enough to be functionally inconsequential, can be routinely evaluated in glaucoma suspects. Although most ophthalmologists will treat extreme ocular hypertension, there has been an increasing tendency in recent years to follow moderate degrees of ocular hypertension without therapy, using careful perimetry as the diagnostic procedure.

Evidence suggests that progressive optic disc changes often precede the development of visual field loss. This is particularly true in young patients. The availability of fundus cameras in most medical centers makes yearly fundus photography of the optic discs a practical adjunct to careful perimetry in following glaucoma suspects. Progressive cupping of the discs may constitute the earliest evidence of impending damage.

Tonography

At the present time the best method available for early detection of the abnormalities associated with primary open angle glaucoma is the use of applanation tonometry and tonography. As indicated in Chapter 8, progressive decrease in outflow facility with time may precede the development of marked ocular hypertension and field loss. A P_0/C ratio over 100 after water drinking is found in over 90% of eyes with known open-angle glaucoma. Although most eyes with this abnormality will not develop field loss, the percentage is sufficiently high (about 10%) to warrant careful, continuous follow-up. Although tonography is not essential for the diagnosis or management of glaucoma, it does provide worthwhile information. The following findings should arouse suspicion:

1. Applanation reading, 21 mm Hg or higher
2. Schiøtz scale reading, 4.0/5.5 or 6.25/7.5 or less
3. Visual field changes
4. Prominent cupping of the optic disc
5. Family history of glaucoma
6. Intraocular pressure elevation after use of topical corticosteroids
7. High myopia
8. Thyrotropic exophthalmos
9. Central retinal vein occlusion
10. Retinal detachment

11. Krukenberg's spindle and/or dense trabecular pigment band
12. Endothelial dystrophy of the cornea
13. Exfoliation syndrome (pseudoexfoliation of the lens capsule)
14. Diabetes mellitus
15. Evidence of inflammation

GENETIC ASPECTS
Glaucoma inheritance

Primary open-angle glaucoma has been demonstrated repeatedly to be a familial and hereditary disorder. Most observers have considered it to be inherited in dominant fashion. Evidence supporting this mode of inheritance was also derived from newer methods of testing. Studies of the offspring of patients with proved open-angle glaucoma demonstrate a remarkably high prevalence of glaucoma (15% to 20% of those over 40 years of age). Even among younger offspring, a 40% to 50% prevalence of positive water-provocative tonograms ($P_0/C > 100$) was found. Some few of these offspring have been followed through the development of spontaneously elevated intraocular pressure and ultimately to cupping of the optic disc and field loss (Fig. 29-10). This agrees well with the 50% prevalence of the glaucoma gene among the offspring of glaucoma patients, predicted by dominant inheritance. However, a large number of patients with proved primary open-angle glaucoma failed to give a family history of glaucoma and had parents and siblings who were entirely normal to all testing. This was explained on the basis of lack of penetrance of the genetic trait or variations in the expressivity of the gene in the individual.

Corticosteroid response

Studies with topical corticosteroids have reopened the question of the inheritance pattern of primary open-angle glaucoma. It was found that essentially all patients with primary open-angle glaucoma (and even those with so-called normotensive glaucoma) responded to topical corticosteroids with dramatic elevations of intraocular pressure. In selected volunteer populations (negative family history and negative water tonograms) the pressure response to topical corticosteroids appeared to be biphasic or triphasic; that is the pressure values that prior to corticosteroid applications demonstrated a single Gaussian distribution, afterward fell into two or three separate and discrete distributions. It has been demonstrated that the type of response to topical corticosteroids was also genetically determined. Family and population studies suggested that after six weeks of topical betamethasone or dexamethasone, there were homozygous poor responders (nn) who failed to reach applanation pressures of 20 mm Hg, homozygous dramatic responders (gg) whose applanation pressure exceeded 31 mm Hg, and a heterozygous population (ng) of intermediary responders (20 to 31 mm Hg). Furthermore, when the steroid-responsive state of parents is known, the responses to steroids in their offspring fit the predictions of Mendelian inheritance (Table 14-2).

Although studies by Armaly support the genetic determination of steroid re-

Table 14-2. Distribution of pressures after steroids* for offspring of various phenotypes

Phenotypes of parents	Number of offspring	Pressure (mm Hg)		
		< 20	20-31	> 31
nn × nn	21	95%	5%	0%
nn × ng	42	48%	52%	0%
ng × ng	25	20%	56%	24%
gg × gg	12	0%	0%	100%

*Topical betamethasone (six weeks).

sponsiveness, studies by Schwartz and associates cast doubt on the hypothesis. They found that monozygotic twins, who should have identical steroid responses, had a concordance of only 65%. These findings may be the result of a relative insensitivity of topical testing in separating the nn and ng populations. Retesting a series of nn and ng responders gave a concordance of only about 62%, whereas gg responders had 82% identical retest responsiveness. A population of identical twins, largely made up of nn and ng responders, would therefore not be expected to give a concordance of over 65%. Further work is needed to verify these findings.

Recessive inheritance of primary open-angle glaucoma

Since almost all patients with primary open-angle glaucoma fall into the homozygous dramatically responsive group (gg), the hypothesis has been proposed that the genes determining corticosteroid responsiveness and primary open-angle glaucoma are closely related if not identical. The hypothesis suggests that this type of glaucoma is recessively inherited and that the glaucomatous individual is homozygous. All offspring of glaucomatous patients should then either have glaucoma or at least be carriers of the gene. When a large series of such offspring were tested with topical corticosteroids, using the criteria just described, it was found that almost all of them fell into either the homozygous (gg) (20% to 30%) or the heterozygous (ng) (65% to 70%) responsive states. Only a few (5% to 10%) may have belonged to the homozygous nonresponsive (nn) population. This and the relatively large number of individuals in "normal" populations that respond to topical corticosteroids suggest the responder gene to be very prevalent (0.2 to 0.3) in our population.

A gene prevalence of 0.2 would mean a division of the normal population into three groups: 4% homozygous marked responders (gg), 32% heterozygous responders (ng), and 64% homozygous poor or nonresponders (nn). Among the offspring of a parent who was a marked responder, 20% would be gg responders and 80% ng responders. The corresponding values for a gene prevalence of 0.3 would be 9% gg, 42% ng, and 49% nn—offspring 30% gg and 70% ng. The findings presented in Table 14-3 fit the 0.2 gene prevalence closely, but it should be noted that the volunteer population was selected in a manner to eliminate glaucoma, glaucoma suspects, and persons with a family history of glaucoma. The offspring population was also selected to eliminate those with initial applana-

Table 14-3. Applanation pressure after topical betamethasone (six weeks)*

		Percent with pressure elevation	
Category	Number	≥ 20 mm Hg	> 31 mm Hg
Primary open-angle glaucoma (with field loss)	50	100	92
Offspring	100	90	22
Volunteers	100	30	4

*Betamethasone was discontinued when applanation pressure exceeded 31 mm Hg.

tion pressure greater than 23 mm Hg or evidence of glaucoma. A study in which topical dexamethasone drops were administered four times daily for six weeks by hospital personnel to prison volunteers demonstrated a gene prevalence of 0.25. Almost identical responses were found in a series of hospitalized American Indians similarly tested. Pathologic genes with such high prevalences are entirely possible when the gene does not interfere with survival in the reproductive years.

Recessive inheritance of a prevalent gene can simulate dominant transmission (so-called pseudodominance) because of the reasonably common mating of homozygous glaucomatous individuals with nonglaucomatous heterozygous carriers. Recessive inheritance can also explain the occurrence of glaucoma in offspring of two apparently normal carriers. To date, the testing with corticosteroids of the parents of patients with proved primary open-angle glaucoma has demonstrated almost all such parents to have glaucoma or to respond as either the heterozygous (ng) or homozygous (gg) responders.

It is important to know that patients with clear-cut secondary glaucoma do not all respond with marked pressure elevation to topical steroids. Although the prevalence of high steroid responders in secondary glaucomas is greater than in the general population, it does not approach the frequency found in primary open-angle glaucoma. This may mean that the presence of the responder gene, even when heterozygous (ng), makes an eye more prone to the development of glaucoma when an additional ocular insult occurs (e.g., traumatic angle recession). Nevertheless, the absence of steroid-induced response in the normal eye of a patient with unilateral open-angle glaucoma strongly suggests a secondary glaucoma.

Clinical significance of genetic aspects of glaucoma and the corticosteroid response

The validation of the hypothesis of recessive inheritance of glaucoma and its relationship to corticosteroid responsiveness is of more than academic interest. It emphasizes the importance of asking directly for a family history of glaucoma in all routine eye (and medical) examinations. It is equally important to inform all patients with established glaucoma about the familial aspects of the disease so that their parents, siblings, and offspring may be examined and followed. In fact, this has proved to be one of the most effective and efficient means of glaucoma detection.

As indicated previously, corticosteroid responsiveness may help to differentiate some secondary glaucomas from the primary open-angle variety.

The recessive hypothesis and corticosteroid tracing of the gene through families help us to delineate those patients who have a great probability of developing glaucoma. For example, the offspring of two patients with proved primary open-angle glaucoma would fall into this preglaucomatous state. Careful studies and follow-up of such individuals should provide much valuable and needed information about the stages of development of the disease. In addition, age and sex correction factors could be derived.

Knowledge of the genetic constitution of the individual will help in glaucoma research. It will make possible the evaluation and improvement of such current methods of detection as tonography, water provocative testing, and perimetry. Most important will be the discovery of those factors that prevent, delay, or alter the appearance of development of the disease in individuals known to harbor the genes. The genetic preglaucomatous patient who never develops glaucoma but is correctly recognized constitutes one of the most exciting sources of newer information of clinical significance. Clues to environmental, endocrine, dietary, and other contributing factors will be forthcoming from studies of such people. One might even be fortunate enough to stumble on the enzymatic defect underlying the glaucomatous process.

Last, it is clear that topical corticosteroids should be used in very limited fashion in patients with primary open-angle glaucoma, in glaucoma suspects, and in their families. If steroids are required, careful follow-up must be made of their effects on intraocular pressure. Suitable modification of dose and frequency of steroids as well as antiglaucoma therapy should be instituted as indicated.

Other relationships of corticosteroid response and primary open-angle glaucoma

The ultimate validation of the hypothesis that the homozygous high responsive state (gg) identifies the genetic predisposition to primary open-angle glaucoma will require many years of careful study. Some supporting evidence, however, has come from the comparison of certain physiologic and biochemical relationships in glaucoma patients with individuals categorized according to their steroid response.

Water-drinking provocative test. As noted in Chapter 8, a P_0/C ratio greater than 100 after water drinking is found in 94% of eyes with proved open-angle glaucoma. Individuals classified as homozygous high responders (gg) have a similar high percentage of positive water-drinking tests. The ng and nn populations, however, have significantly lower prevalences of this abnormality (Table 14-4).

Phenylthiocarbamide (PTC) taste testing. The ability to taste phenylthiocarbamide in dilute solutions is bimodally distributed in most populations. White populations demonstrate some 30% nontasters and 70% tasters. PTC tasting is genetically determined, the nontasters representing the homozygous recessive state.

Table 14-4. Water-drinking provocative test

	Corticosteroid response			Open-angle glaucoma (field loss)
	nn	*ng*	*gg*	
Number of patients	200	250	80	300
$P_0/C > 100$ after water	6%	32%	92%	94%

Table 14-5. Phenylthiocarbamide taste test (whites)

	Corticosteroid response			Open-angle glaucoma (field loss)
	nn	*ng*	*gg*	
Number of patients	140	200	72	250
Nontasters	25%	35%	50%	51%

A comparison of this genetically determined ability with the presence or absence of glaucoma demonstrates interesting correlations (Table 14-5). There is a much greater prevalence of nontasters (51%) among patients with primary open-angle glaucoma with field loss than is found in the normal population. The differences are highly significant. Furthermore, individuals who respond to topical corticosteroids as homozygous responders (gg) resemble the primary open-angle glaucoma population in their distribution when PTC taste-tested (50% nontasters). On the other hand, those individuals who respond poorly or not at all to topical corticosteroids (nn) have a low prevalence (25%) of nontasters for PTC. Blacks have a lower prevalence of nontasters than do whites but demonstrate similar associations between glaucoma and PTC tasting.

Interestingly, the prevalence of nontasters in patients with angle-closure glaucoma is lower than that found in the general population or in patients with primary open-angle glaucoma.

Thyroid function. Patients with low thyroid function as measured by serum protein-bound iodine (PBI) tend to be nontasters of phenylthiocarbamide. Patients with primary open-angle glaucoma, who have a high prevalence of PTC nontasters, also have a high prevalence of low PBI's. Furthermore, low PBI's occur with almost identical frequency in homozygous high responders to topical corticosteroids (gg) and patients with proved open-angle glaucoma and field loss. Both populations differ significantly from the nn and ng groups (Table 14-6).

Diabetes mellitus. Diabetes mellitus occurs more frequently in patients with primary open-angle glaucoma than in the general population. Even when known diabetics are excluded, glucose tolerance tests in patients with primary open-angle glaucoma reveal a high prevalence of diabetes (18%) (Table 14-7). Testing in individuals classified according to their steroid responsiveness demonstrates a similar prevalence of diabetes mellitus (16%) in homozygous high responders (gg) but much lower prevalences in poor (nn) and intermediate (ng) responders. The high steroid responders appear identical to the glaucomas by this testing,

Table 14-6. Thyroid function (PBI)

	Corticosteroid response			Open-angle glaucoma (field loss)
	nn	*ng*	*gg*	
Number of patients	40	41	38	44
PBI < 5.5 μg/100 ml	8%	12%	34%	34%

Table 14-7. Diabetes mellitus

	Corticosteroid response			Open-angle glaucoma (field loss)
	nn	*ng*	*gg*	
Number of patients	41	53	50	68
Positive glucose tolerance test*	2%	4%	16%	18%

*Sum of plasma glucose at 0, 1, 2, and 3 hours, ≥ 600 mg/100 ml.

and both groups are different in their frequency of diabetes from the remainder of the population.

Although diabetes mellitus is more common in patients with primary open-angle glaucoma, the presence of glaucoma in a diabetic seems to offer some protection from the development of proliferative diabetic retinopathy. Thus, whereas hemorrhages and microaneurysms may occur, disabling proliferative diabetic retinopathy is almost never seen in a diabetic with primary open-angle glaucoma. It is not known whether this protection is related to the mechanical effects of the elevated intraocular pressure on the retinal blood vessels or whether a genetic interrelationship accounts for the observation.

Cup/disc diameter ratio. The cup/disc diameter ratio is a genetically determined characteristic, with ratios greater than 0.3 found in about 17% of the general population. About 80% of eyes with glaucomatous damage have ratios above 0.3. In the opposite eyes of glaucomatous patients with unilateral field loss, a cup/disc ratio over 0.3 is found in about 54%. Ratios greater than 0.3 are found in 45% of high responders, but in only 13% of eyes classified nn and 20% of eyes classified ng by topical corticosteroid testing (Table 14-8).

Although the preceding relationships between corticosteroid response and primary open-angle glaucoma do not prove the hypothesis presented, they offer supporting evidence to its validity.

Even if the corticosteroid response is not genetically determined, the resemblance of high steroid responders to patients with primary open-angle glaucoma is striking and suggest that this marker may indicate those eyes with a greater risk of developing glaucoma.

Plasma cortisol suppression. Patients with primary open-angle glaucoma demonstrate hypersensitivity in intraocular pressure response to topically applied corticosteroids. These patients also demonstrate corticosteroid hypersensitivity in plasma cortisol suppression. When treated with a 1 mg oral dose of dexamethasone,

Table 14-8. Cup/disc diameter ratio

	Corticosteroid response			Open-angle glaucoma (opposite eyes without field loss)
	nn	ng	gg	
Number of patients	160	170	208	52
Cup/disc ratio > 0.3	13%	20%	45%	54%

Table 14-9. Plasma cortisol suppression*

	Corticosteroid response (nn + ng)	Open-angle glaucoma (field loss)
Number of patients	37	35
> 25% suppression		
1.0 mg dose	100%	100%
0.5 mg dose	62%	100%
0.25 mg dose	27%	83%

*Nine hours after oral dexamethasone.

Table 14-10. Inhibition of lymphocyte transformation by prednisolone

	Corticosteroid response			Open-angle glaucoma (field loss)
	nn	ng	gg	
Number of patients	22	15	27	36
Mean 50% inhibitory dose (ng/ml)	78.4%	59.0%	39.4%	37.2%

both glaucoma patients and the nn and ng corticosteroid responders show suppression of their plasma cortisol levels, as measured 9 hours later. With lower doses of dexamethasone most glaucoma patients continue to demonstrate suppression, but nn and ng patients do not (Table 14-9). Thus glaucoma patients appear to have both systemic as well as topical hypersensitivity to corticosteroids.

Lymphocyte transformation. Normal lymphocytes separated from a blood specimen can be stimulated to transform into a metabolically active state by exposure to phytohemagglutinin. The degree of transformation can be quantitatively assayed by measuring the uptake of tritiated thymidine into DNA. Corticosteroids inhibit this transformation. A 50% inhibition of lymphocyte transformation is produced by about half as much prednisolone in preparations from glaucoma patients as from nn individuals. High steroid responders (gg) resemble the glaucoma population (Table 14-10). These findings demonstrate an increased corticosteroid sensitivity in glaucoma patients at a cellular level completely separate from the eye.

HLA antigens. Numerous reports throughout the medical literature demonstrate a correlation between the presence of specific histocompatibility antigens and certain diseases, especially those believed to have an immunogenic basis. A correlation exists between two of these antigens, HLA-B12 and HLA-B7, and primary open-angle glaucoma. In one study, 88% of patients with glaucoma were found to have either HLA-B12 or HLA-B7 antigens. These antigens were found in only 30% of the nonglaucomatous population. Furthermore, of 30 ocular hypertensive, high steroid responders (gg) with either of the antigens, 43% developed visual field loss. Among 30 similar ocular hypertensive high responders without either antigen, field loss occurred in only 7%. These results are preliminary, but suggest that ocular hypertensive individuals with the specific HLA antigens are much more susceptible to the development of visual field loss.

Multifactorial vs. autosomal recessive inheritance of primary open-angle glaucoma

Armaly has proposed that primary open-angle glaucoma is determined by a multifactorial inheritance of several interacting genes, rather than by a single recessive gene as identified by the homozygous corticosteroid response (gg). At first glance, these hypotheses appear totally different. However, if one considers that many factors, some genetic and some environmental, may modify a genetic predisposition to a disease, some of these differences can be resolved. The fact that almost all patients (actually about 90%) with primary open-angle glaucoma are homozygous high responders (gg), and almost no poor (nn) and intermediate (ng) steroid responders have field loss, suggests that eventual cases of primary open-angle glaucoma are likely to be found in the gg population. It is entirely possible that other factors such as diabetes, cup/disc ratio, and systemic blood pressure may determine which individuals in the gg population ultimately develop damage. Further studies with lymphocyte transformation techniques and the cyclic AMP system, for example, may identify a yet unknown metabolic status that protects a genetically glaucomatous individual from developing field loss. The eventual hope is that such a modifying factor can be discovered and made clinically applicable, so that all patients with genetic glaucoma can be spared from ever having the disease. At the present time the concept of a single autosomal recessive gene, modified by other genetic and nongenetic factors, seems to be a reasonable and simple hypothesis.

THERAPY

The goal in the treatment of primary open-angle glaucoma is to avoid visual loss during the lifetime of the individual by lowering intraocular pressure. In contrast to the situation in angle-closure glaucoma, there is no method at present for curing open-angle glaucoma. Intraocular pressure may be lowered by increasing outflow facility or by depressing the rate of aqueous secretion.

When to start

It is difficult to state dogmatically when treatment of open-angle glaucoma should be started. It has been common practice to start therapy as soon as a clear-cut diagnosis is made. With more sensitive methods for earlier detection, such antecedents of glaucoma as decreased outflow facility are often discovered before elevation of intraocular pressure or loss of field. The disease may remain in this status for years (e.g., in families with a history of glaucoma) and may never progress. Since side effects of miotics are significant and are most prominent in young people, it is often elected to delay therapy until there is persistent elevation of intraocular pressure (e.g., to over 30 mm Hg) or until in the best judgment of the ophthalmologist the pressure is high enough to produce damage to the optic nerve. Delaying therapy also avoids the development of resistance or sensitization to various types of antiglaucoma medication. It is sometimes claimed that earlier treatment is more effective and can be maintained longer. However, it must be remembered that a better prognosis is to be anticipated in early stages of the disease and in persons who never develop the disease, whether or not medical or surgical treatment is instituted. Moreover, controlled studies in which only one eye was treated with miotics have offered no support for the hypothesis that such therapy alters the progression of the outflow defect or alters the ultimate status of the eye.

The time for starting therapy in the absence of field loss is an individual matter to be decided for a particular patient. It will depend on ease and reliability of follow-up, experience of the clinician, age of the patient, family history, rapport and understanding with the patient, side effects of the therapy, as well as the presence of other ocular diseases (e.g., cataracts, retinal detachment, etc.), height of the intraocular pressure, and degree of impairment of outflow channels. As noted previously, approximately 5% of untreated patients with intraocular pressures of 22 to 30 mm Hg will develop visual field loss within 10 years. It is fair to state that ocular hypertensives would be safer with their intraocular pressure lowered if this could be accomplished effectively and without side effects. A therapeutic trial with topical pilocarpine or epinephrine is sometimes undertaken. If medication causes no side effects and significantly lowers pressure, it may be continued. Even these medications, however, may occasionally produce severe side effects, which must be weighed against the potential therapeutic gain. Prolonged use of cholinesterase inhibitors and carbonic anhydrase inhibitors in ocular hypertension is rarely justified. Of course, all eyes that demonstrate pressure damage to the optic nerve must be treated.

In a recent and still preliminary study patients with marked ocular hypertension without field loss were placed on topical epinephrine in one eye. Eyes that responded with a significant fall in intraocular pressure were maintained on therapy for several years; when there was minimal effect on pressure, the medication was stopped within a month or two. Of 19 treated patients, 6 (32%) lost visual field in the untreated eyes and none developed field loss in the eye treated with epinephrine. This confirms the beneficial effect of lowering intraocular pressure in preventing field loss. Equally interesting were the findings in the patients in whom medication was discontinued because of lack of effect. Of 14 such patients, untreated in either eye, *none* developed field loss. This suggests that ocular hypertensives destined to develop field loss are responsive to topical epinephrine but those whose pressures do not respond are also resistant to optic nerve damage. These findings have subsequently been applied to a larger group of 80 ocular hypertensives, 20 (25%) of whom developed glaucomatous field loss when followed for five to ten years. Of 34 epinephrine responders, 17 (50%) developed visual field loss as compared to 3 of 46 (6.5%) nonresponders. Hypotensive response was defined as a pressure reduction of greater than 5 mm Hg in the treated eye. Epinephrine responsiveness in ocular hypertensives may provide a simple and valuable predictive test for development of visual field loss.

Follow-up of nontreated patients

If the decision is made not to treat the patient for a time, one may explain this to the patient as the beginnings of glaucoma or better still as "borderline pressure values that require watching but no therapy at present." Follow-up every three to six months should include careful checking of visual fields, fundus examination, and applanation tonometry. Yearly tonography, if available, may also be worthwhile. When possible, fundus photographs of the optic discs should be taken at yearly intervals. If reasonable follow-up proves impossible, then it is much safer to treat the patient. Remarkably, many of these borderline or early glaucomas are found to go through episodes of complete remission and then demonstrate recurrence of abnormal findings. When subjected to genetic evaluation, a number of patients with borderline pressure and facility values appear to be carriers of the trait rather than true instances of glaucoma.

Care should also be taken to remain cognizant of medical problems that the patient may develop. Myocardial infarction, cerebrovascular disease, medical therapy for systemic hypertension, or some other "hemodynamic crisis" may push the ophthalmologist to begin therapy or follow the patient more closely.

Medical treatment

Medical therapy is usually started with 1% to 2% pilocarpine hydrochloride or nitrate every 6 to 8 hours. If this is not tolerated, 0.5% concentration may be tried. If 2% proves inadequate, it may be increased in frequency or in concentration. Concentrations above 4% rarely afford greater benefit. If the patient cannot tolerate miotics (e.g., young persons or patients with cataracts), 1% to 2% topical epinephrine once or twice daily often proves most effective.

Diurnal pressures

Diurnal curves of intraocular pressure permit evaluation of the best time to administer therapy. *If intraocular pressure can be maintained below 20 mm Hg at all times of the day, it is very rare for additional field to be lost.* Although complete diurnal pressure curves are not needed in all, or even most, patients with glaucoma, measurement of intraocular pressure can be made at different times of the day.

Tonography

Although pressure may appear to be controlled at the time of the office visit in spite of reduced outflow facility, one of the best safeguards against loss of visual field is the maintenance of a normalized outflow facility. Thus, as summarized in Chapter 8, if the outflow facility can be increased to more than 0.18, over 80% of eyes will continue to be controlled for periods of over three years. If P_0/C can be maintained at 100 or less, continued control is found in over 90% of eyes.

Choice of therapy

If pilocarpine or epinephrine therapy proves inadequate, other miotics are used (carbachol [Carcholin], neostigmine [Prostigmin], eserine, demecarium bromide [Humorsol], echothiophate [Phospholine], etc.) (Chapter 18) as well as the addition of topical epinephrine and/or carbonic anhydrase inhibitors (Chapter 19). The choice of medication depends on the height of the intraocular pressure, the outflow facility, age of the patient, state of the lens, allergic reactions, and side effects. In some patients, conventional therapy becomes more acceptable or pressure is further reduced by the use of sedatives or tranquilizers.

Combinations of miotics

It is important to emphasize that, if miotics are used singly, it is often possible to return to the so-called "weaker" miotic with successful control after failure of a "stronger" miotic. Thus it is common to see patients who became resistant to pilocarpine and were controlled for periods of time on demecarium bromide or echothiophate. Because of subsequent failure of these stronger anticholinesterase agents, the patients are referred for surgery. In many instances, stopping the present medication and reinstituting pilocarpine therapy demonstrates the recovery of responsiveness to the drug and satisfactory pressure control (Fig. 29-17). Only occasionally is medical control better maintained with combinations of miotics. It is best to recheck visual fields very soon after changing miotics in order to get a new base line at the new pupil size. If this is not done, the field change due to the pupillary effects of the new miotic may be misinterpreted as failure of control with progression of field defect. Similar reevaluation of fields is essential after changes in refraction, cataract extraction, or glaucoma surgery.

Surgical treatment

Surgery is indicated only if there is proved progression of visual field loss on all variations of maximum tolerated medical therapy. The threat of surgery often alters the patient's tolerance to drugs. It must be established that the loss of visual field is not due to decreased size of the pupil, progression of lens changes, or vascular accidents.

Frequency of follow-up

Follow-up at first is usually more frequent (e.g., weekly or monthly) and at various times of the day. This is also true when control is not optimal. With ideal control, three to six months may be permitted to intervene between visits. Evaluation should then include symptoms and side effects of medication, visual acuity and central fields, applanation tonometry, ophthalmoscopy, and measurement of blood pressure. At least once a year the pupils should be dilated to evaluate the lens and the fundus periphery. Yearly tonography, when available, provides further information regarding the glaucoma control.

Ocular rigidity

It is important to emphasize that medical therapy, particularly with stronger miotics, may decrease ocular rigidity and lead to false assurances as to status of control when Schiøtz readings with one weight only are used (Fig. 29-16). At present this is best avoided by using applanation tonometry.

Instructions to patient

In the treatment of glaucoma it is important to instruct the patient as to the time and method of administration of drops, including pressure over the inner canthi to avoid systemic absorption. The physician should plan the time of medication with the patient and should specify that the name of the medication and its hours of administration appear on the label. In addition, the patient should be informed in simple terms of the mechanisms of glaucoma, the reasons for and goals of treatment, and, to the best of our understanding, how various treatments work and what their local side effects are. In this fashion the all-important confidence of the patient in the physician can be established. The use of booklets, sketches of the eye, and cartoons often prove helpful. The patient must be convinced of the necessity of lifelong follow-up of pressure and visual fields at regular intervals and the religious use of his drops as prescribed. There is little or no evidence that limitation of activities, diet, tobacco, alcohol, coffee, fluids, sleep, movies, television, reading, driving, etc. alter the course or control of glaucoma patients. There is also no evidence that nitrate or nitrite vasodilator drugs as used for angina pectoris are contraindicated for patients with glaucoma. It is wise for the patient to know the name and concentration of the miotic he is using. A glaucoma card carried by the patient may prove helpful. It is also important that the patient and his other physicians appreciate the systemic side effects and possible toxicity of the antiglaucoma agents he is using. Both should be warned against the hazards of unnecessary use of topical corticosteroids. Experience emphasizes that this is particularly important for physicians, nurses, and pharmacists who have more ready access to these agents and are likely candidates for self-medication.

Drug warnings

Numerous drugs commonly used systemically in general medicine carry a warning against their use in patients with glaucoma. Most of these medications are parasympatholytic agents (e.g., antispasmodics) or other agents that might produce pupillary dilation. Unless they are used in near-toxic doses, there is little evidence that these drugs will adversely affect intraocular pressure in patients on therapy for primary open-angle glaucoma. Parenteral atropine given preoperatively may partially reverse the effect of a miotic, but elevated intraocular pressure for the few hours that the drug is active will not alter the visual status of the patient. Such drugs can be potentially dangerous in the patient with anatomically narrow angles and may precipitate an attack of angle-closure glaucoma. Patients with known angle-closure glaucoma should have had bilateral iridectomies that would prevent acute closure from mydriasis. Since open-angle glaucoma is not adversely affected and angle-closure glaucoma after iridectomy is not affected, the only patient in potential danger is one who has undiagnosed angle-closure glaucoma. When questioned before administration of a drug, he, of course, would not know that he has glaucoma! For the most part, therefore, drug warnings concerning glaucoma are of little value except for medicolegal protection of the manufacturer.

PROBLEMS FOR CONSIDERATION

There is general agreement that primary open-angle glaucoma is associated with increased intraocular pressure and that reduction of pressure can retard or prevent visual damage. The progression of events, however, leading to field loss and optic nerve damage are not well defined. Present methods of detection and diagnosis are unsatisfactory, since many eyes with statistically elevated intraocular pressures may never develop field loss and other eyes with glaucomatous damage may have normal intraocular pressures due to spontaneous diurnal fluctuations. Until the life history of the disease can be accurately determined, it is impossible to establish diagnostic criteria short of visual damage. Using this as the criterion for diagnosis, however, defeats the purpose of early detection so that effective therapy can prevent the development of such damage. The ability to predict accurately the development of glaucoma in the individual patient before field loss has occurred is perhaps the major problem in glaucoma detection at the present time.

Some clues to the above-mentioned problem are available and are utilized now. Glaucoma relatives have a comparatively high probability of developing the disease. The degree of pressure response to topical corticosteroids appears to be genetically determined and closely associated with primary open-angle glaucoma. If this hypothesis is correct, it may be possible to identify the genetic glaucoma patient long before the actual disease develops. Long-term studies of these groups of patients are in progress in an effort to develop and evaluate better techniques of glaucoma diagnosis. The exciting studies demonstrating systemic hypersensitivity to corticosteroids in glaucoma patients, as well as cellular hypersensitivity of their lymphocytes, suggest a metabolic, enzymatic abnormality. The identification of this abnormality may make possible accurate and early detection of glaucoma.

The mechanism of steroid inhibition of lymphocyte transformation by phytohemagglutinin is unknown. However, the availability of an in vitro test of corticosteroid sensitivity outside of the eye that correlates with topical steroid testing provides exciting speculation for study of glaucoma patients. For example, cyclic AMP appears to provide the means of mediating many cell functions. It is generated from ATP by the enzyme adenylcyclase and is inactivated by phosphodiesterase. The concentration of cyclic AMP can be increased by compounds that stimulate adenylcyclase or inhibit phosphodiesterase. Cyclic AMP inhibits hemagglutinin-induced lymphocyte transformation. Theophylline, an inhibitor of phosphodiesterase, also inhibits lymphocyte transformation. Furthermore, the concentration of theophylline required for 50% inhibition of transformation correlates closely with that of prednisolone, and lymphocytes from glaucoma patients are more sensitive than those from nonglaucoma controls. This suggests that the cyclic AMP system may mediate the glucocorticoid effect in human lymphocytes. A genetic abnormality in this enzyme system could be responsible for the differential ocular response to glucocorticoids and perhaps for open-angle glaucoma. Further refinement of this system may permit separation of glaucoma patients from the normal population by the effect of cyclic AMP on lymphocytes—a test totally separated from the eye.

Whereas the capacity to respond to topical corticosteroids is genetically determined, the mechanism of this response is unknown. Various mechanisms have been proposed, such as effects of steroids on connective tissue, mucopolysaccharides, immunogenic mechanisms, and fibrinolytic activity. All these require thorough study. Unfortunately the material from responsive human eyes is not readily available for such experiments. These studies could be aided considerably by the availability of steroid-responsive laboratory animals. Efforts to find such animals have thus far been unsuccessful.

The anatomic changes in the eye induced by topical corticosteroid administration are virtually unknown. Thinning of the endothelial cells lining Schlemm's canal has been reported, as has thickening of the juxtacanalicular tissue with deposition of plaques and an unidentified material. Practically nothing is known about the biochemical abnormalities in the trabecular meshwork of glaucomatous eyes. The possibility of correlating biochemical changes with the degree of steroid responsiveness should be investigated. Ways of blocking these changes in steroid-responsive eyes may hold the ultimate key to the prevention of glaucoma. Again, the need for a responsive laboratory animal is obvious.

The need for new therapeutic approaches to glaucoma is equally as great as the need for better diagnostic techniques. At present all therapy in open-angle glaucoma is aimed at the reduction of intraocular pressure. It is perfectly possible that improving the nutrition and increasing the resistance of the optic nerve to pressure damage would be more effective than lowering intraocular pressure. There is relatively little known about the biochemistry and physiology of the optic nerve, and the potential rewards from research in this area are great.

CHAPTER **15**

Special considerations of open-angle glaucoma

OPEN-ANGLE GLAUCOMA WITH LOW TENSION

The finding of normal intraocular pressure in the presence of glaucomatous cupping and field loss has resulted in the term *low-tension glaucoma*. There is no question that such cases do occur and may represent examples of "weak" optic nerves that atrophy at normal intraocular pressures. If one assumes that the optic atrophy of glaucoma results from an ischemic process, it is not surprising that such a process could occur from poor vascular supply to the optic nerve unrelated to increased intraocular pressure. At least some of the "weak" discs may result from reduced blood pressure and blood flow impairing the nutrition of the nerve. Some of these patients give a history of an episode of severe blood loss, frequently from gastrointestinal bleeding, or an acute episode of systemic hypotension, such as may occur after a myocardial infarction. In other cases there may be evidence of carotid insufficiency with an audible bruit or low pressures by ophthalmodynamometry. Many of these patients have diabetes mellitus. Small hemorrhages at the disc margin may also be seen, representing another manifestation of the ischemic process.

Although the above-mentioned patients represent instances of low-tension glaucoma, most cases will fall instead into one of the following categories.

1. Low ocular rigidity, so that the Schiøtz reading is false. The truly elevated intraocular pressure is revealed by applanation readings (Figs. 29-7 to 29-9).

2. Large diurnal fluctuations in intraocular pressure, so that pressure elevations occur at times other than usual office hours. Such cases are not truly low-tension glaucoma, yet they make up the largest number of cases so classified. Diurnal pressure studies are mandatory whenever progressive field loss or cupping occurs in glaucomatous eyes seemingly well controlled.

3. Impaired outflow facility, but hyposecretion lowering intraocular pressure in spite of the obstructed drainage channels. The recognition of these eyes is an

237

important application of tonography (Fig. 29-3). Such eyes often develop intermittently elevated pressures with alterations in aqueous secretion.

4. Other causes of damage to retina and optic nerve (vascular, congenital, inflammatory, degenerative, traumatic, unknown).

5. Intracranial neoplasm, usually in the anterior chiasmal area, producing field defects and optic atrophy that may be confused with glaucomatous damage.

It should be emphasized that the first two categories account for well over 90% of cases classified as low-tension glaucoma. Patients with true low-tension glaucoma deserve a thorough and meticulous ocular, medical, and neurologic investigation for possible treatable conditions. When the field loss can be traced to some single acute episode, the prognosis for retention of the remaining field is good. In deteriorating cases, efforts must be made to keep the intraocular pressure as low as possible.

SECONDARY OPEN-ANGLE GLAUCOMA

Although it is conventional to confine the diagnosis of secondary glaucoma to eyes with peripheral anterior synechias, to postoperative or posttraumatic damage, or to obvious ocular inflammatory disease, more and more instances of secondary open-angle glaucoma without peripheral anterior synechias are recognized. These may be seen as consequences of inflammation, trauma, foreign body, hemorrhage, and other causes. Presumably the obstruction to outflow in these eyes is in the trabecular meshwork–Schlemm's canal–episcleral vein system. The block may be particulate (inflammation, hemorrhage, pigment, etc.) or may more closely simulate primary open-angle glaucoma (e.g., siderosis). At any rate, the entity of secondary open-angle glaucoma is probably more common than is usually considered and is often misdiagnosed as primary open-angle glaucoma. Certainly any patient with unilateral open-angle glaucoma should be strongly suspected of having glaucoma on a secondary basis.

Inflammation of the anterior segment of the eye and trauma account for the largest percentage of open-angle secondary glaucomas.

Corticosteroid-induced glaucoma

The astute observations of François, Goldmann, and others documented what was considered to be a very rare form of open-angle glaucoma that followed the topical use of corticosteroids. The availability of very potent topical corticosteroid preparations and their indiscriminate use have resulted in an "epidemic" of corticosteroid glaucoma. As discussed in Chapter 14, the open-angle glaucoma induced by steroids resembles closely primary open-angle glaucoma in mechanism (reduced outflow facility), damage to the optic nerve, and response to therapy. Furthermore, the steroid pressure elevation occurs more often in primary open-angle glaucoma patients and their families and appears to be genetically determined. The magnitude of the pressure elevation depends on the steroid used, its concentration, frequency of application, and length of time of administration. Systemic steroids only rarely induce pressure elevations, but instances of remarkably high pressures in very responsive individuals have been seen.

The diagnosis of corticosteroid glaucoma is much the same as of the primary variety, but it requires a careful history with direct questioning as to the use of corticosteroids. Consultants seeing referred glaucoma patients often find that they are using topical corticosteroids. In one office 26 patients with uncontrolled glaucoma due to corticosteroids were referred during one six-month interval. Most of these patients were using steroids for trivial reasons (contact lenses, conjunctival or lid irritation, vague discomfort, etc.). Often corticosteroids were being applied to alleviate irritation or injection produced by miotic or epinephrine therapy! Physicians, nurses, dentists, and pharmacists must be questioned with particular care, for many have used topical corticosteroids for years without their ophthalmologists being aware of it. In some of these individuals the glaucoma has been uncontrollable and has even required filtering operation. Some have lost extensive parts of the visual fields, with high pressures, no pain or symptoms, and entirely white eyes. In most instances discontinuing corticosteroids resulted in marked improvement of the glaucoma status. Seldom did this occur promptly (3 to 7 days); usually improvement took place very slowly over a period of weeks or months. Antiglaucoma therapy was commonly required during this period. In some instances complete normality of pressure and outflow facility (and even of water provocative testing) was achieved without need for any therapy. Unfortunately, extensive field loss usually persisted. In rare instances, corticosteroid-induced glaucoma has persisted for many months after cessation of use of steroids. Progressive field loss in several young patients in this category has led to surgical intervention.

It must be remembered that corticosteroids are of enormous value in suppressing ocular inflammatory reactions to various injurious agents. Knowledge of various undesirable side effects of such potent agents permits the clinician to recognize their early occurrence in an individual patient and to alter his therapy accordingly. Such information should not lead the competent physician to abandon the use of sight-preserving corticosteroids when they are indicated. On the contrary, an understanding of side effects permits careful evaluation of relative merits and potential risks of corticosteroid therapy. Obviously, corticosteroids should be used only when indicated, for the minimum time necessary, and with careful follow-up of intraocular pressure. Particular care must be taken in glaucoma patients and their families. Suitable antiglaucoma medication can be used, as well as the proper corticosteroid, concentration, and frequency of administration.

Availability of anti-inflammatory corticosteroids that do not elevate intraocular pressure, even in susceptible individuals, helps resolve the dilemma so frequently presented to the clinician today.

Prediction of steroid response

When topical corticosteroids are required to treat an ocular inflammation, it may be of considerable importance to be able to predict the likelihood of steroid-induced pressure elevation. In patients with normal intraocular pressure and no family history of glaucoma, approximately 4% to 6% can be expected to develop intraocular pressures over 30 mm Hg if treated with 0.1% dexamethasome four times daily for four to six weeks. The percentage of high responders will be greater if steroids are continued longer than six weeks. The percentage will also be much greater when the patient has a relative with open-angle glaucoma or when he has diabetes, high myopia, a Krukenberg's spindle, or borderline intraocular pressure before steroids. Such information is readily obtainable and may be of extreme importance, especially when one considers that the high steroid responder may represent "genetic glaucoma." As an example, the sibling or offspring of a glaucoma patient has a 20% to 30% likelihood of developing markedly elevated pressures (> 31 mm Hg). If such a patient also has diabetes, the percentage increases to almost 40%; when his pressure before steroids is > 22 mm Hg, the percentage is over 90%!

Inflammation
Anterior uveitis (Fig. 15-1 and Reel II-1)

During the course of anterior uveitis, the trabecular meshwork may become partially or completely obstructed by inflammatory debris, mutton-fat keratic precipitates, and particulate matter, and outflow facility may be further impaired by the increased viscosity of the aqueous humor. Blood is often seen in Schlemm's canal in inflammatory processes. The meshwork may be overgrown by fibrous tissue or endothelium and Descemet's membrane. In addition, the inflammatory disease may involve the trabecular meshwork itself and further impair its metab-

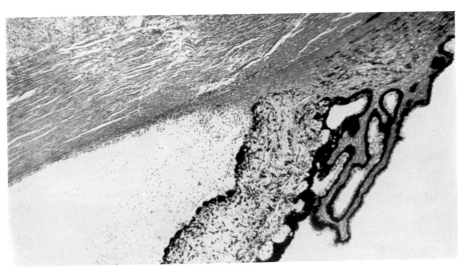

Fig. 15-1. Inflammatory cells, fibrin, and peripheral anterior synechias obstructing the trabecular meshwork after irradiation of an eye.

olism and function. The result is increased resistance to outflow of aqueous humor. However, inflammatory involvement of the ciliary body and iris often alters the secretory pump and blood-aqueous barrier in such fashion as to result in profound hyposecretion. Therefore eyes with anterior uveitis are often in hypotony, and the impaired outflow facility is not appreciated. The administration of steroids or the spontaneous subsidence of the inflammatory process may restore secretion when outflow facility is still impaired. This results in pressure elevation. In chronic anterior uveitis the damage to the trabecular meshwork may be more permanent but still not visible gonioscopically. In herpes zoster, for example, as many as 25% of affected eyes are found to have elevations of intraocular pressure, often unrecognized.

The treatment of secondary glaucoma due to active anterior uveitis is directed at the inflammatory process. Efforts must be made to dilate the pupil with mydriatics and cycloplegics and to decrease the inflammatory reaction so that damage, scarring, and visual loss are minimized. Corticosteroids are particularly useful for this purpose. Their prolonged use may prove necessary, and one must then try to differentiate possible elevations of intraocular pressure caused by the steroids rather than by the original disease process. In unilateral conditions, a corticosteroid provocative test *in the normal eye* may permit such differentiation. In some most difficult situations the intraocular pressure alternates between disease-caused and steroid-induced elevations. In all inflammatory processes, one hopes that the outflow mechanism will restore itself to normal. As long as the outflow facility is impaired, pressure should be maintained within normal limits by the addition of topical epinephrine, systemic carbonic anhydrase inhibitors, and osmotic agents. When the inflammatory process is no longer active, miotics may prove helpful.

Heterochromic iridocyclitis. Heterochromic iridocyclitis is one type of mild uveitis that often retains an open angle but demonstrates keratic precipitates. Insidious pressure rises are found in some 20% of the hypochromic eyes. Twiglike neovascularization of the iris periphery and trabecular meshwork in often seen in this condition. Hyphema is a frequent complication of minor trauma. Cataracts occur in about 85% of eyes with heterochromic iridocyclitis, and lens extraction is not always well tolerated. Therapy of the iridocyclitis is relatively ineffective. Most important in differential diagnosis are those instances of heterochromia with pressure elevation on the more pigmented side. This occurs in diffuse iris melanomas and in hemosiderosis or siderosis bulbi.

Glaucomatocyclitic crisis. The glaucomatocyclitic crisis is a reasonably discrete entity falling into this category of secondary open-angle glaucoma. It is characterized by minimal inflammatory signs and symptoms, and synechias are extremely rare. The inflammatory disease may be confined entirely to the trabecular meshwork. The process is usually unilateral with recurrent involvement of the same eye. Occasional bilateral cases are seen with both eyes involved at the same time or on different occasions. Bilaterality or more impressive inflammatory signs should suggest careful reexamination of the fundus, particularly the far periphery, for chorioretinitis, since inflammatory lesions can closely resemble the glaucomatocyclitic crisis picture in the anterior chamber. In contrast to the small pupil of anterior uveitis, eyes with glaucomatocyclitic crisis have a dilated pupil. The patients have remarkably few symptoms relative to the height of the intraocular pressure. Their first complaint may be blurring of vision on the basis of corneal edema. During the attack of pressure elevation the angles are open. The attack rarely lasts more than two weeks, and changes in visual field are unusual. During the attack, and often only after the pressure is normalized, one sees occasional cells and flare in the anterior chamber and few small discrete keratic precipitates. During the attack, the outflow facility is markedly depressed but usually returns to normal values between attacks. Rarely is there permanent alteration in outflow facility. Recent studies indicate elevated aqueous levels of prostaglandins during the acute crisis (p. 258). Because of the self-limited nature of the condition, surgery is usually contraindicated in glaucomatocyclitic crisis. It is best treated with mild mydriatics, topical steroids, topical epinephrine, and systemic carbonic anhydrase inhibitors.

The frequent association between glaucomatocyclitic crisis and primary open-angle glaucoma is generally not appreciated. In one study of 11 patients with glaucomatocyclitic crises, 8 had elevated pressures, and 5 had glaucomatous visual field loss in the *opposite* eye.

Lens-induced glaucomas

The lens plays an important role in many of the secondary glaucomas.

Subluxation (Fig. 15-2). Traumatic or spontaneous subluxation of the lens can result in glaucoma with angle closure due to pupillary block by vitreous or lens. In many instances of lens subluxation the outflow facility is decreased in both eyes without angle closure. Some of these are explained as congenital anomalies of the angle (e.g., in Marfan's syndrome) and are not necessarily a consequence of the lens dislocation. Other lens dislocations may be associated with inflammatory disease (e.g., syphilis) and secondary glaucoma. In some lens dislocations (e.g., homocystinuria), open-angle glaucoma has not been described, but anterior dislocation with acute pressure elevations has been seen (Chapters 13 and 17). Many eyes, particularly those with traumatic posterior subluxation of the lens, have impaired outflow facility, abnormally deep anterior chambers, and recessed angles (Fig. 15-5). The mechanism by which outflow facility is impaired in these instances is not clear. It appears to be related to the trauma rather than to the dislocated lens itself. Removal of the lens is indicated only if vision is impaired by the lens or a phacolytic inflammation ensues. Cryostatic methods often prove useful in removing such dislocated lenses. Peripheral iridectomy may prevent the development of pupillary block and is usually preferable to lens extraction. Removal of the lens usually does not reverse the glaucomatous process, and further medical or surgical therapy is necessary.

Phacolytic glaucoma (Fig. 15-3). In phacolytic glaucoma the trabecular mesh-

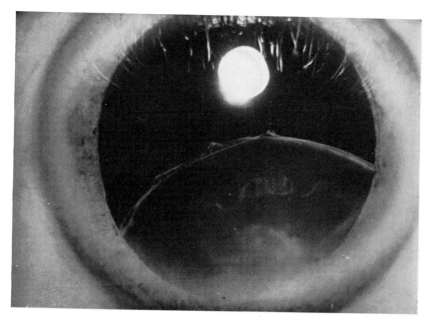

Fig. 15-2. Dislocated lens.

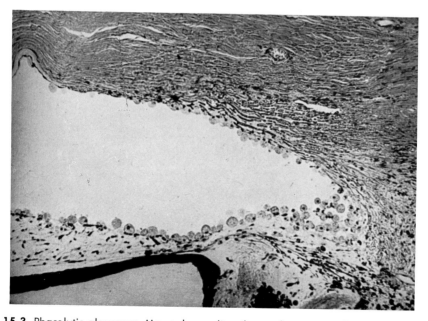

Fig. 15-3. Phacolytic glaucoma. Macrophages line the angle recess and trabecular spaces.

work is blocked by macrophages containing lens material. In these eyes the anterior chambers are deep, the angles are open, the cataract is often hypermature, and there may even be faulty light projection. Early in the disease process the inflammatory reaction is minimal, with a few clumps of macrophages on the back of the cornea and impaired outflow facility. As the disease progresses, there is marked elevation of intraocular pressure with corneal edema, congestion, and pain. In many instances phacolytic glaucoma is believed to result from leakage of lens material through the lens capsule into the anterior chamber. In some instances there may be rupture of the capsule. Macrophages filled with lens material are found not only in the trabecular area but also on the surface of the iris and the back of the cornea. It has been found that 25% or more of eyes with phacolytic glaucoma coming to pathologic examination have recessed angles. In the differential diagnosis of phacolytic glaucoma one must consider (1) a swollen cataractous lens that has induced angle closure, which is easily recognized by gonioscopy, and (2) lens-induced uveitis with glaucoma, in which the glaucoma is related to the inflammatory reaction or its sequelae.

The therapy of phacolytic glaucoma should consist of prompt measures to lower intraocular pressure (epinephrine, carbonic anhydrase inhibitors, and osmotic agents) and to decrease the inflammatory disease (steroids) and of prompt extraction of the lens after intraocular pressure is reduced. The removal of the lens often results in normalization of outflow facility and intraocular pressure, and no further therapy is required. Even with questionable light perception and projection preoperatively, surprisingly good vision may be obtained.

Lens-induced uveitis. Lens-induced uveitis results from reactions to lens material either through the intact capsule or after spontaneous rupture or extracapsular extraction of a mature cataract. The process is characterized by marked exudation of lymphocytes and plasma cells, invasion of the lens by leukocytes, much reaction in the anterior chamber, and conglomerate or lardaceous precipitates on the back of the cornea. The eyes are often soft at the time of the acute reaction, but after the development of synechias, membranes, and scarring, glaucoma may be a consequence. Cataract extraction or removal of cortical material is curative in these cases of uveitis and results in the avoidance or alleviation of the glaucomatous process.

Traumatic glaucoma
Penetrating injuries

Eyes are unhappily prone to suffer penetrating injuries from a variety of sharp objects such as toys, glass, wire, scissors, and knives. The glaucoma resulting from such an injury is dependent on the position and the extent of the injury, the skill of the surgeon in repairing the damage, and the posttraumatic reaction of the eye.

The initial repair of the injury is of greater importance in maintaining a useful eye than any subsequent operations to counteract secondary glaucoma.

Contusions (Figs. 15-4 and 15-5)

A blow of a blunt object to the eye results in a sudden increase in intraocular pressure and a variety of injuries to the intraocular contents. In the anterior segment, the iris is suddenly forced against the lens by the pressure of the aqueous humor and by the stretching of the posterior sclera. The valvelike action of the iris prevents aqueous humor from running back through the pupil, and the pressure may cause a blowout of the peripheral iris, called an iridodialysis. This causes flattening of the pupil on the side of the tear and displacement of the pupil away from that area. This is an important sign, in case diathermy is needed at a later date to stop recurrent bleeding. There may be a tear of the pupillary sphincter.

A more frequent, and potentially more serious, lesion is produced if the tear occurs back into the ciliary body. This is the usual source of the severe recurrent hemorrhages into the anterior chamber and vitreous humor that so often lead to loss of the eye. More often, tears into the ciliary body (Fig. 15-5) result in the gonioscopic picture of a recessed angle. Within 1 or 2 hours after severe blunt trauma, the intraocular pressure may increase markedly. This may result from red cells obstructing the trabecular meshwork or perhaps from acute edema of the outflow channels themselves. The glaucoma usually subsides in 24 to 72 hours and is followed by a period of marked hypotony, but the patient may require frequent doses of hyperosmotic agents to lower the pressure during the acute phase. In a few eyes with angle recession there is a secondary rise in intraocular pressure approximately one to two months after injury, which if controlled medically, may spontaneously subside within a year and disappear completely, requiring no further medication. In some instances, particularly when the recession is extensive, there is late (ten or more years) development of an open-angle glaucoma. It is usually readily differentiated from primary glaucoma by the appearance of the angle and its unilaterality. Gonioscopically, the most important characteristic sign is widening of the distance from the sceral spur to the iris root, resulting in a broadened ciliary band in the area of the recession. A localized deepening of the anterior chamber is frequent, and remnants of torn iris tissue and scattered pigment may be seen along the margins of the tear. Segmental disruption of iris processes is a helpful sign when present. Occasionally the signs are quite subtle, and only back-and-forth comparison between the two eyes reveals the abnormality.

Although angle recession is very common after traumatic hyphema, the vast majority of eyes with recessed angles fail to develop glaucoma or any evidence of outflow impairment. It is therefore apparent that a recessed angle is a symbol of trauma to the eye and a rough measure of the severity of the injury. It is not synonymous with glaucoma, nor is the recession necessarily causative in the development of the pressure elevation. Rather, the recessed angle, the glaucoma, and the lens dislocation, when present, are merely all consequences of the trauma. It is important to look specifically for recessed angles in all unilateral glaucoma and particularly in those with a history of blunt injury about the eye. Rarely, a blowout

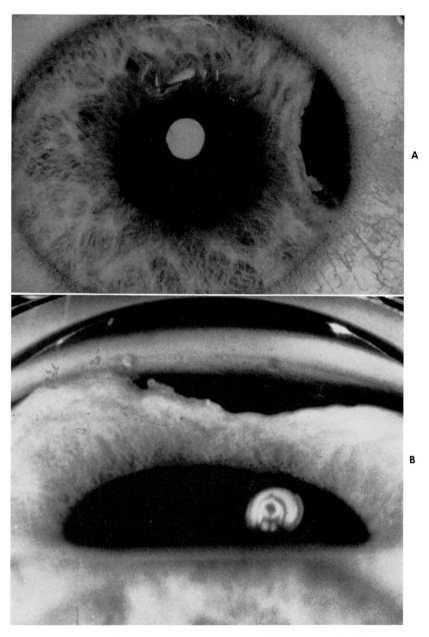

Fig. 15-4. A, Traumatic iridodialysis. **B,** Gonioscopic view of traumatic iridodialysis. Vitreous humor comes forward into the anterior chamber and occupies the area of the iridodialysis.

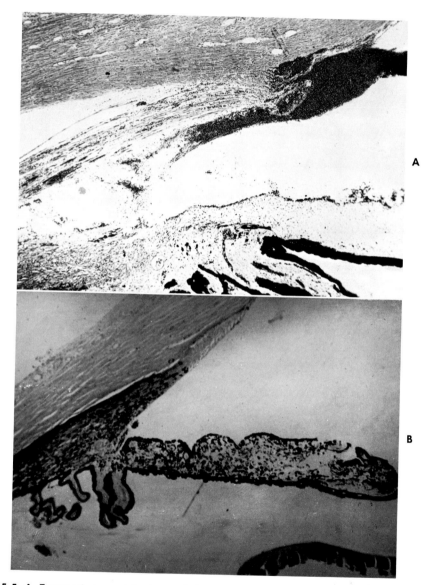

Fig. 15-5. A, Traumatic tear at the base of the iris, extending back into the ciliary body. **B,** Late results of a traumatic tear into the ciliary body. The iris now inserts halfway down the ciliary body, which results in an extremely deep angle recess.

into the suprachoroidal space can occur, producing a cyclodialysis. This may lead to severe hypotony and late cataract formation.

Hemorrhage (Figs. 15-5, A, and 15-6)

Spontaneous or traumatic hemorrhages into the anterior chamber, particularly if recurrent, are an important cause of secondary glaucoma. After many types of trauma there is often a rise in intraocular pressure for a short period. This is usually followed by more prolonged hypotony. If the trauma has resulted in sufficient hemorrhage into the anterior chamber to block the outflow channels, a marked rise in intraocular pressure may ensue when secretion recovers. If this is allowed to persist, blood staining of the cornea as well as severe damage to the optic nerve may occur. Even in the instances in which hemorrhage into the anterior chamber is less massive, breakdown products of the blood itself (perhaps iron) may result in permanent damage to the outflow channels (hemosiderosis). The impaired outflow facility may present a picture of unilateral chronic open-angle glaucoma that is most difficult to distinguish clinically or histologically from primary glaucoma. Finding of traumatic recession of the angle is an important differential point.

Early treatment. The usually recommended treatment of anterior chamber hemorrhage consists of bilateral patches and absolute bed rest with sufficient sedation to make the regimen tolerable to both the child and the parent. Recent studies indicate no difference in visual prognosis or recurrent hemorrhage between cases treated with bilateral patching and those permitted limited activity with only unilateral protection of the injured eye. With rare exception, the patient should be

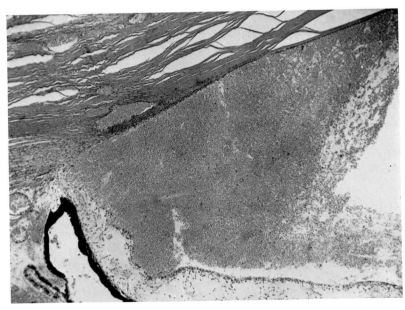

Fig. 15-6. Anterior chamber hemorrhage with red cells obstructing the trabecular meshwork.

hospitalized for close observation. Usually no drops are used unless signs of severe iritis are present, in which case mild mydriatics are indicated. The routine can be modified if there has been no hemorrhage after 5 days. A recent study suggests that the antifibrinolytic agent aminocaproic acid, given orally for 5 days after traumatic hyphema, significantly reduces secondary hemorrhage.

Recurrence of the hemorrhage is most common on the second to fourth day and is often accompanied by increased intraocular pressure. This is best treated by systemic acetazolamide (Diamox) and topical epinephrine. Acute elevations may require oral glycerol or even intravenous urea or mannitol. If possible, miotics are avoided for fear of pulling on the traumatized peripheral iris. A change in the color of the blood in the anterior chamber from bright red to black (the so-called eight-ball hemorrhage) is an ominous finding and indicates breakdown of the hemoglobin molecule. It is often a forerunner of blood staining of the cornea. If the intraocular pressure cannot be controlled by medical means or if the anterior chamber remains completely filled with blood, the blood should be washed out. Preoperative hyperosmotic therapy often simplifies the operation and makes it safer. Occasionally such lowering of intraocular pressure hastens blood resorption and avoids surgery. Needless procrastination results in more trabecular damage and anterior synechias with a chronic glaucoma that is most difficult to manage.

With the use of a 22-gauge needle on a syringe containing one of the highly purified fibrinolysins or kinases (e.g., urokinase) of human origin, most clots can be lysed and washed out. This may be accomplished by gentle irrigation back and forth into the syringe. After the anterior chamber is cleared of blood, an air bubble is introduced. If this fails to remove the blood, it is safest to turn down a conjunctival flap, place a McLean suture, and enter the anterior chamber by an ab externo incision. The blood should be washed out through a small incision if possible. Often the blood can only be removed by extending the incision and pulling out the clot with the forceps. In some eyes a small circle of diathermy coagulation points 3 mm. back of the limbus at the suspected site of the bleeding may be helpful in preventing recurrent hemorrhage.

Late treatment. In those eyes that have suffered sufficient trabecular damage or have formed sufficient anterior synechias, chronic glaucoma develops. These eyes should be treated like other chronic secondary glaucomas. Preference should be given to medical therapy, using even strong miotics and carbonic anhydrase inhibitors. Any persistence or recurrence of iritis should be treated by mydriatics and corticosteroids. The patient or his parents should be warned of the danger of chronic glaucoma occurring months or years after the initial injury. It is therefore important to have periodic examinations for many years.

Hemolytic glaucoma

Intraocular hemorrhage, particularly into the vitreous, may occasionally lead to acute pressure elevation that is presumably due to trabecular obstruction by breakdown products of red cells and macrophages containing blood pigment.

There is usually a moderate inflammatory reaction associated with the glaucoma. Topical corticosteroids and mydriatics, plus carbonic anhydrase inhibitors, may relieve the inflammation and normalize the pressure. Anterior chamber irrigation is occasionally necessary. In rare instances cyclocryotherapy may be used as a means of lowering intraocular pressure until the material is cleared from the angle and trabecular function restored.

Intraocular foreign bodies (Fig. 15-7 and Reel III-5)

Intraocular foreign bodies, particularly those that contain iron, produce considerable damage to the eye (siderosis). The damage is not confined to the lens, pars plana, and retina but also involves the trabecular meshwork (Fig. 15-8). The siderosis not only decreases outflow facility but also produces alterations in the structure of the trabecular meshwork that closely resemble those of primary open-angle glaucoma (Fig. 15-9). The resulting open-angle glaucoma is difficult to control. Therapy in these cases should consist of the prompt removal of the foreign body before there is damage to the outflow channels. When glaucoma exists, the treatment should be that of any other type of open-angle glaucoma.

Postoperative

After such surgical procedures as cataract extraction there may be impaired outflow facility without evidence of peripheral anterior synechias. Such cases may represent preexisting open-angle glaucoma or the consequences of the trauma and inflammatory reaction after surgery and their effect on the trabecular meshwork.

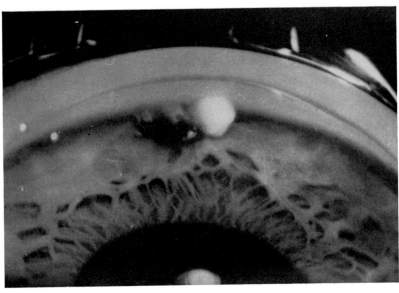

Fig. 15-7. Intraocular foreign body in chamber angle with exudate.

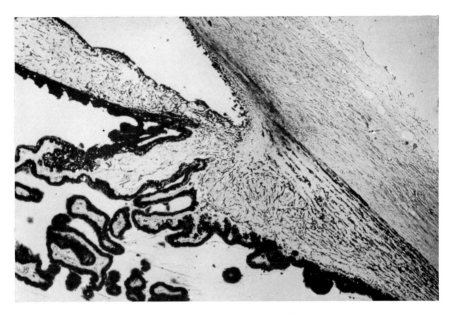

Fig. 15-8. Siderosis of the trabecular meshwork caused by an intraocular foreign body.

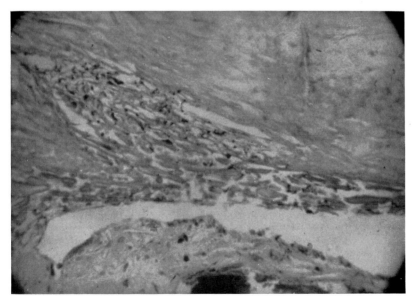

Fig. 15-9. Siderosis of the trabecular meshwork and unilateral open-angle glaucoma caused by an intraocular iron foreign body in the vitreous humor. Note the resemblance to primary open-angle glaucoma.

All patients with aphakic eyes should be followed carefully and studied for evidences of glaucoma.

Angle-closure glaucoma

As indicated in Chapter 12, many eyes suffer trabecular damage following acute or recurrent attacks of angle closure. Even after successful peripheral iridectomy these eyes demonstrate impaired outflow facility without sufficient anterior synechias to account for the defect. After iridectomy they require medical management, much as other chronic secondary open-angle glaucomas. Filtering surgery is reserved for those uncontrolled on intensive medical regimens.

Alpha-chymotrypsin–induced glaucoma

The use of alpha-chymotrypsin to facilitate cataract extraction results in easier extraction and permits intracapsular removal even in younger adults. Corneal edema and difficulties with wound rupture were noted soon after the introduction of this enzyme. Kirsch first recognized the sharp elevation of intraocular pressure that occurs in many eyes subjected to alpha-chymotrypsin. Scanning electron micrographs suggest that the pressure elevation results from acute mechanical obstruction of the trabecular outflow channels by particles of zonular material. The effect does not relate to preexisting glaucoma and can be demonstrated in

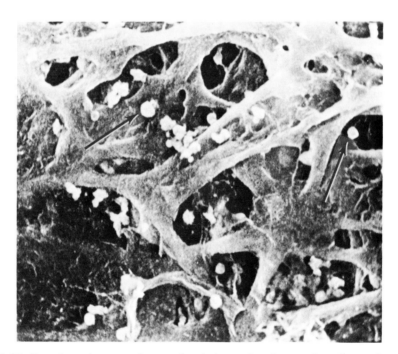

Fig. 15-10. Scanning electron micrograph of the trabecular meshwork (monkey) after alpha-chymotrypsin. The arrows point to zonular fragments embedded in the meshwork. (Courtesy Dr. D. Anderson, Miami.)

the animal eye (Fig. 15-10). Carbonic anhydrase inhibitors are usually not effective in avoiding the pressure elevation, but hyperosmotic agents such as oral glycerol help to blunt the pressure rise. Fortunately the effect appears to be self-limited and completely reversible. No permanent glaucoma has been reported as a consequence of alpha-chymotrypsin, but severe ocular damage may result from the effects of the elevated intraocular pressure in the early postoperative period.

Tumors (Fig. 15-11 and Reel III-3)

Neoplasms of the iris or ciliary body may directly invade the angle, or tumor cells may break loose and metastasize to the angle. When sufficient trabecular func-

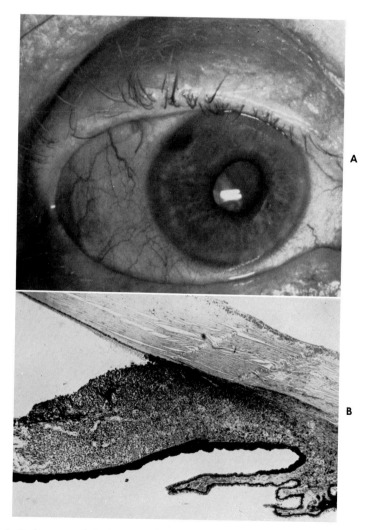

Fig. 15-11. A, Melanoma of the iris invading the angle. **B,** Histologic picture of malignant melanoma of the iris invading the trabecular meshwork.

tion is compromised, pressure will rise. Diagnosis is obvious on slit-lamp and gonioscopic examinations.

In eyes with glaucoma and retinal detachment a tumor should be suspected. Decreased outflow facility is found in some eyes with melanomas even when these lesions are in the posterior parts of the eye and there is no evidence of invasion of the trabecular meshwork. The mechanism for impaired outflow facility in such eyes remains unknown.

Epithelial ingrowth (Fig. 15-12)

Epithelization of the anterior chamber can follow perforating injuries or surgery. The epithelium spreads over the back of the cornea and the anterior surface of the iris. Glaucoma results when sufficient angle is covered to obstruct outflow. Epithelization is extremely difficult to treat. Occasionally epithelium can be removed with an alcohol sponge before the angle is compromised markedly, but not without considerable damage to the cornea. Proof of diagnosis by biopsy of the back of the cornea or of the iris must be available before such drastic therapy is attempted. When glaucoma has developed, the prognosis is very poor. Maximum medical therapy is often inadequate, and most of these eyes are lost.

If the condition is discovered before the entire angle is compromised, some eyes with epithelial ingrowth can be salvaged. The most effective technique consists of excision of all iris tissue covered with the epithelial membrane, excision of the fistula through which the epithelium entered the chamber, and treatment of the involved corneal endothelium with a cryoprobe. In one series of 40 eyes with epithelial ingrowth treated in this fashion, a permanent cure with vision of 20/50 or better was achieved in 11 (27.5%).

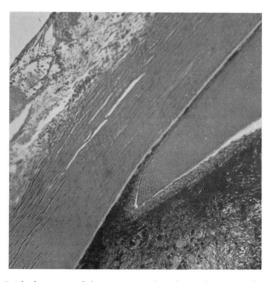

Fig. 15-12. Epithelization of the anterior chamber after a perforating injury.

Epithelium introduced into the anterior chamber may form cysts (Figs. 13-4 and 13-5). Large cysts may impair outflow and result in glaucoma. The cysts are amenable to surgical excision or to obliteration by chemicals, diathermy, or photocoagulation.

Neovascular glaucoma (rubeosis iridis) (Figs. 13-7 to 13-10 and Reel II-2)

Neovascular glaucoma results from a growth of fibrovascular tissue over the surface of the iris and trabecular meshwork. This produces marked impairment to outflow facility and dramatic elevations of intraocular pressure, often with recurrent hemorrhages into the anterior chamber (hemorrhagic glaucoma). Although the neovascular tissue usually leads to peripheral anterior synechias and a zipper-like pull of the iris to the cornea, one often sees stages of rubeosis iridis with impaired outflow facility and newly formed blood vessels arborescing over the wide open angle.

Rubeosis iridis is found in some eyes after central retinal vein occlusion, central retinal artery occlusion, diabetic retinopathy, malignant melanoma, and retinal detachment. Particularly in the groups that follow central vein occlusion or diabetic retinopathy, it is possible to recognize the newly formed vessels on the iris and angle structures at stages before there is measurable impairment of outflow facility or elevation of intraocular pressure. Tonography and gonioscopy can be correlated as the outflow facility becomes progressively impaired.

In the case of the rubeosis after central retinal artery or vein occlusion, there is often preexisting open-angle glaucoma. As indicated in Chapter 14, this association is most important to recognize, particularly for the sake of the contralateral "normal" eye. It is estimated that rubeosis iridis and hemorrhages occur in 10% to 30% of all central vein occlusions but almost never follow branch vein occlusions.

The rubeosis of diabetic retinopathy is almost always associated with retinitis proliferans and recurrent hemorrhages and often with renal damage. Occasionally it is seen in eyes with remarkably good vision.

The neovascular glaucomas respond poorly to miotics, secretory inhibitors, and surgery. The acute ocular congestion and severe pain are made worse by miotics but may be dramatically relieved in some instances by intensive topical corticosteroids and atropine. A trial of this therapy frequently makes the patient more comfortable but may not alter the intraocular pressure. Most of these eyes have little vision because of the underlying retinal vascular disease. When some useful vision is present, intensive cyclocryotherapy (eight to twelve applications at −80° C for 1 minute each) just behind the limbus appears to be the most effective treatment currently available. Disappearance of the rubeosis is impressive but often only temporary. Transient hyphema is frequent. In one series, 40% of patients who had vision of finger-counting or better retained this degree of vision one year after cyclocryotherapy.

Another mode of therapy, panretinal photocoagulation is much too recent to fully evaluate. Treatment with 1000 to 1500 argon laser applications to the retina has in some cases effectively controlled intraocular pressure and markedly reduced neovascularity in the anterior segment. It may be necessary to use oral glycerol to decrease pressure and clear the cornea in order to photocoagulate. An interval of two to three weeks is needed before the results of therapy are seen. The approach can be considered in eyes with some useful or potentially useful vision. Controlled studies are needed to determine the general success rate of this new treatment.

Retrobulbar pressure

Pressure on the globe as a consequence of infection, tumor, or hemorrhage in the orbit may result in impaired outflow facility and elevated intraocular pressure. This may be seen in the presence or absence of elevated episcleral venous pressure. The pressure elevation in these eyes is usually to the high twenties and low thirties. They respond to miotics and secretory inhibitors but not as impressively as eyes suffering from primary open-angle glaucoma. The impaired outflow facility may persist even after the orbital disease process has subsided.

Thyrotropic exophthalmos

Similar findings are also found in thyrotropic exophthalmos. Such proptosed eyes should be suspected of having low rigidity and should be measured with two Schiøtz weights or by applanation tonometry. With limitation of motility, marked variations in intraocular pressure may be recorded in the same eye as efforts are made to fixate in different positions. Thus a patient with thyrotropic exophthalmos and limitation of upward gaze may be recorded as having an intraocular pressure of 22 mm Hg in primary position, 17 mm Hg on looking down, and 50 mm Hg on attempted upward gaze. Positioning of the head for applanation tonometry will also induce marked pressure changes in these eyes.

Thus the secondary open-angle glaucoma of thyrotropic exophthalmos may be most complicated. Pressure elevations may result from increased episcleral venous pressure, impaired outflow facility, and contraction of extraocular muscles against inflammatory adhesions in the orbit. In addition, the exophthalmos may result in corneal damage from exposure and superimposed infection. Associated with the corneal inflammation, anterior chamber and iris reaction with synechias may develop and further impede the outflow of aqueous humor. The elevated intraocular pressure may be masked to Schiøtz measurement by reduced ocular rigidity or abnormalities of posterior indentation of the globe. Damage to the optic nerve in thyrotropic disease may be a consequence of the increased intraocular pressure or of direct or indirect damage to the nerve itself by the infiltrative process in the orbit.

Epidemic dropsy

Associated with so-called epidemic dropsy is an acute bilateral glaucoma with open angles. There is evidence that this is a consequence of the consumption of argemone oil (containing sanguinarine) as a contaminant of sesame oil or other cooking oils. *Argemone mexicana* is an herb of the poppy family indigenous to the West Indies and was known as "chicalotl" to the Aztecs. It was introduced into India, Africa, Australia, Philippines, and Southeast Asia where it grew well. The condition is associated with little pain or inflammation of the eyes, even though the pressures may be over 60 or 70 mm Hg. The patients note colored halos and blurred vision and may go on to extensive field loss or even blindness before they seek medical advice. Besides the elevated pressure, corneal edema in the presence of open angles helps in making the diagnosis. The mechanism of the pressure elevation has not been established but is believed to be a consequence of damage to outflow channels. Miotics are said to be of little help in treating this disease, and surgery is recommended. The response of this disease to secretory inhibitors is not known.

Prostaglandins

The prostaglandins are a family of metabolically active, lipid-soluble, 20-carbon unsaturated fatty acids that derive their names from the fact that they were originally extracted from vesicular glands. They exist in small amounts in virtually all mammalian tissues, and their actions are diverse. For example, they are involved in inflammation, pain, fever, smooth muscle contraction, gastric secretion, lipid and carbohydrate metabolism, cardiovascular responses, renal physiology, and blood coagulation. Ocular effects of certain topical or intracameral prostaglandins consist of elevation of intraocular pressure, hyperemia of the conjunctiva, miosis, and increased protein content of the aqueous humor. The precise site of prostaglandin synthesis is not known, nor is the exact mechanism of action. Increased production of cyclic adenosine-3′,5′-monophosphate (cyclic AMP) is apparently involved. Some prostaglandins are known to be present in iris where they are synthesized from fatty acid precursors.

The acute rise in intraocular pressure produced by prostaglandins or their precursors is associated with an increase in total outflow facility, an apparent increased aqueous production, a disruption of the blood-aqueous barrier, and a marked increase in protein in the aqueous humor. Recent studies suggest that the site of disruption of the permeability barrier is at the tight junctions of the nonpigmented epithelium of the ciliary body. Prostaglandins PGE_1 and PGE_2 have the greatest effect on intraocular pressure, with pressure changes from other prostaglandins less pronounced. There appears to be a transport mechanism in the ciliary body that removes prostaglandins from the eye. This may represent a natural protective mechanism.

The synthesis and release of prostaglandins in the eye can be inhibited and their effects prevented by aspirin and indomethacin. Topical corticosteroids, on the other hand, do not inhibit the intraocular pressure response. The anti-inflammatory, analgesic, and antipyretic effects of aspirin-like drugs appear to take place via inhibition of prostaglandin synthesis. Other agents such as polyphloretin phosphate directly block the actions of prostaglandins and so inhibit their effects.

Adenyl cyclase, the enzyme that generates cyclic AMP, and cyclic AMP phosphodiesterase, which converts cyclic AMP to inactive adenosine 5′-monophosphate, are present in ciliary processes and iris tissue. If the elevation of intraocular pressure induced by prostaglandins is due to the generation of increased levels of cyclic AMP, agents that increase phosphodiesterase activity should block prostaglandin effects. Imidazole increases phosphodiesterase activity and demonstrates this action.

Prostaglandins may have numerous etiologic and therapeutic implications in glaucoma, particularly in the management of some of the secondary glaucomas.

1. *Acute trauma.* Ocular compression, blunt trauma, paracentesis, mechanical and laser irritation of the iris, and alkali burns may produce increased intraocular pressure, elevated aqueous protein, and hyperemia. In experimental models, aqueous prostaglandin levels are elevated by these stimuli. These effects are blocked by prostaglandin-synthesis inhibitors such as aspirin and indomethacin. Use of these agents in acute traumatic glaucoma or glaucoma subsequent to ocular surgery may prove of considerable benefit.

2. *Acute uveitis.* Eyes with acute uveitis frequently demonstrate congestion, miosis, disruption of the blood-aqueous barrier and, on occasion, elevated intraocular pressure. Aqueous humor from such eyes contains increased levels of prostaglandins. The use of prostaglandin inhibitors in such cases appears warranted.

3. *Glaucomatocyclitic crisis.* Markedly increased aqueous levels of prostaglandins are also found in eyes with glaucomatocyclitic crises. The decreased outflow facility during the acute crisis suggests that prostaglandins per se do not account for the entire picture. One may postulate, however, increased trabecular resistance from the plasmoid aqueous related to breakdown of the blood-aqueous barrier. In any case, a trial of aspirin and/or indomethacin appears to be indicated in the management of acute glaucomatocyclitic crisis.

4. *Alpha-chymotrypsin glaucoma.* A transient elevation of intraocular pressure lasting several days may be seen after use of alpha-chymotrypsin for cataract surgery. This rise in pressure is thought to be due to trabecular obstruction by zonular fragments. A recent study in rabbits demonstrated that a second sustained rise in intraocular pressure may be maintained for more than a year after injection of alpha-chymotrypsin into the posterior chamber. Anterior-chamber injection of the enzyme had no effect. Pretreatment of the animals with indomethacin has no effect on the transient pressure rise but prevents the sustained increase of intraocular pressure. The sustained pressure elevation is postulated to be caused by an inflammatory reaction in the trabecular area consequent to disruption of the blood-aqueous barrier. This disruption is thought to be prostaglandin dependent and so blocked by indomethacin. These findings suggest that permanent trabecular damage and secondary glaucoma may result from repeated or prolonged defects in the blood-aqueous barrier.

5. *Primary open-angle glaucoma.* Since prostaglandins are physiologic constituents of uveal tissue that are capable of elevating intraocular pressure, a rela-

tionship to open-angle glaucoma can be envisioned. In one study, 6 of 8 eyes of patients with primary open-angle glaucoma had elevated PGE_1-like activity compared to nonglaucomatous eyes. These results have been denied in other studies.

6. *Epinephrine toxicity.* Prostaglandins have yet another action of possible importance related to therapy for glaucoma. Release of norepinephrine after sympathetic nerve stimulation causes synthesis of prostaglandins, which, in turn, antagonize the norepinephrine response. Prostaglandins thus play a negative feedback role as part of the mechanism that modulates transmission in the sympathetic nervous system. Superior cervical ganglionectomy causes release of norepinephrine from degenerating sympathetic nerves in the eye. This leads to prostaglandin synthesis, producing, among other things, hyperemia of the conjunctiva and iris. Inhibition of prostaglandin synthesis by indomethacin prevents this hyperemic response. The possibility exists that epinephrine-related hyperemia seen in glaucoma patients may be related to catecholamine-stimulated prostaglandin synthesis and release. Use of prostaglandin inhibitors such as aspirin may reduce the severity of this response.

OPEN-ANGLE GLAUCOMA ASSOCIATED WITH OCULAR
ABNORMALITIES OR DISEASES

Not all open-angle gluacoma associated with eye disease should be classified as secondary. It only serves to confuse classifications if such conditions as macular degeneration, xanthelasma, amblyopia, drusen of the optic nerve, retrobulbar neuritis, and cataracts are considered reasons to classify glaucoma as secondary. There remain a number of eye diseases that are actually associated or occur frequently with open-angle glaucoma. They are usually not causative of the glaucoma but instead either are a consequence of it or share with it a common or related pathogenic factor. Because they require special consideration and until further data are available, these open-angle glaucomas are considered under this admittedly noncommittal heading.

High myopia and glaucoma (Figs. 29-7 to 29-9)

The problem of making a diagnosis of glaucoma in a patient with myopia presents unusual difficulties. The low ocular rigidity in many of these eyes results in Schiøtz readings within normal limits. Their true status is revealed by applanation tonometry and flat tonograms. Furthermore, in patients with myopia it is difficult to interpret the appearance of the discs. Many of these discs look atrophic, and the myopic conus may add to the confusion. An enlarged blind spot and various irregular field losses may occur on the basis of myopic atrophy and lead to incorrect diagnoses. It is interesting to speculate on the role of intraocular pressure in the development and progression of posterior staphylomas and myopia. At any rate, in spite of the difficulties in diagnosing glaucoma in the high myope, the fact remains that glaucoma occurs more frequently in such individuals, and the presence of myopia (especially over 5.00 D) in adults should raise a suspicion of

Table 15-1. Glaucoma-associated conditions

Diagnosis	Number	Corticosteroid response		
		nn	*ng*	*gg*
Myopia > 5.00 D	30	14%	50%	36%
Krukenberg's spindles	15	27%	60%	13%
Diabetes mellitus				
Juvenile	86	38%	48%	14%
Adult				
No proliferative retinopathy	200	31%	49%	20%
Proliferative retinopathy	60	50%	42%	8%
Volunteers	300	58%	36%	6%

glaucoma. Topical corticosteroid testing in high myopes without glaucoma (Table 15-1) demonstrates a 36% incidence of high responders (gg), some six times the rate found in the general population. The open-angle glaucoma of high myopia is essentially identical with primary open-angle glaucoma as to both mechanism and genetic background (including response to topical corticosteroids). Therapy is identical with that for open-angle glaucoma in other eyes, but extra caution must be exerted in the use of stronger miotics because of the predilection of the highly myopic eye to detachment.

Vein occlusion

The detection of central retinal vein occlusion should suggest the presence of preexisting primary open-angle glaucoma. Most important is the often neglected consideration of the opposite eye. This may be the only seeing eye in individuals with painful hemorrhagic glaucoma. In a series of 40 consecutive patients with unilateral hemorrhagic glaucoma referred to one tonography laboratory, 26 (65%) had evidence of impaired outflow facility in the contralateral, "normal" eye. The presence of vein occlusion should lead to exhaustive studies for evidence of primary open-angle glaucoma in both the involved and contralateral eyes. Therapy does not differ from that for other open-angle glaucomas.

Pigmentary glaucoma (Fig. 15-13 and Reels II-5 and II-6)

Pigmentary glaucoma is a term used to describe a group of open-angle glaucomas associated with depigmentation of the iris, a Krukenberg's spindle, and marked pigmentation of the trabecular meshwork. In addition, there is often iridodonesis by gonioscopy and pigment deposition on the lens, zonules, and periphery of the retina. Iris processes seem to be more abundant in these eyes and frequently insert anterior to the scleral spur. This condition tends to occur in younger people and has a predilection for male myopes. Pressure elevations may be of sufficient magnitude to produce corneal edema and halo vision. Because of the dramatic slit-limp and gonioscopic findings, pigmentary glaucoma has frequently been considered a secondary glaucoma. Whether this should be classified apart

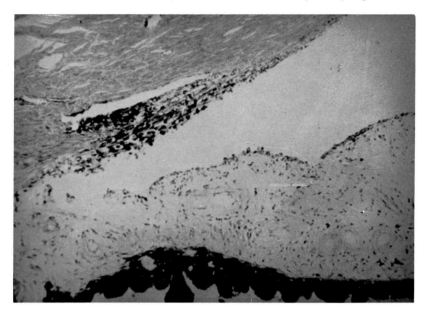

Fig. 15-13. Histologic picture of open-angle glaucoma with intense pigmentation of the trabecular meshwork.

from primary open-angle glaucoma is unclear. One finds so-called pigmentary glaucoma in the families of patients with primary open-angle glaucoma. In addition, topical corticosteroid testing demonstrates an increased prevalence of high responders in individuals with pigment spindles specifically selected to eliminate glaucomatous patients or those with a family history of glaucoma (Table 15-1). These findings suggest a possible genetic relationship between the pigment disturbance of pigmentary glaucoma and primary open-angle glaucoma. On the other hand, patients with pigmentary glaucoma (and visual field loss) do not demonstrate markedly increased cellular sensitivity to corticosteroids as determined by inhibition of lymphocyte transformation. This suggests that pigmentary glaucoma may differ in its etiology from primary open-angle glaucoma.

Whatever the relationship to open-angle glaucoma, all patients with Krukenberg's spindles should be considered glaucoma suspects. The diagnosis is established in much the same way as for open-angle glaucoma. Floating pigment and a flare in the anterior chamber may simulate uveitis. The treatment is the same as that for primary open-angle glaucoma, although many ophthalmologists believe that pigmentary glaucoma is more difficult to control, particularly in women.

Glaucoma and diabetic retinopathy

As noted in Chapter 14, diabetes mellitus occurs more frequently in patients with open-angle glaucoma. The reverse is also true—primary open-angle glaucoma is seen more often in diabetics than in nondiabetics. When tested with topical corticosteroids, both juvenile and adult diabetics demonstrate an increased prevalence of high responders (gg) as compared with the general population (Table 15-1). Patients with proliferative diabetic retinopathy, however, do not share this greater likelihood of high steroid response but more closely resemble the general population. Thus the presence of diabetes mellitus increases the likelihood of primary open-angle glaucoma by about three times. When glaucoma is present, however, there is less likelihood of the patient developing proliferative diabetic retinopathy.

Exfoliation syndrome (pseudoexfoliation, glaucoma capsulare)
(Figs. 15-14, 15-15, and Reel II-4)

In glaucoma capsulare, a variety of open-angle glaucoma, blue-white or grayish flecks are seen at the pupil margin. Conglomerates of the same material appear on the anterior surface of the lens, and flakes are found on both surfaces of the iris, on the trabecular meshwork, on the zonules, on the ciliary body, and on the hyaloid membrane. Some observers (Vogt) have interpreted this material as originating from the lens capsule and called the condition "senile exfoliation of the lens capsule." Others (Malling; Busacca) considered it to be a deposition of material on the lens capsule (pseudoexfoliation), for the lens capsule itself was found to be of normal thickness. This latter view was generally accepted until electron microscopic studies demonstrated similar deposits within and beneath the lens capsule. It was assumed the deposits were fibrillar secretions of the lens epithelium. Recent electron microscopic findings, however, demonstrate similar fibrillar material intimately associated with the basement membranes of the epithelium of iris and conjunctival vessels, and trabeculum. Because of this, the exfoliative syndrome has been described as a more generalized ocular basement membrane disease. Continued formation of exfoliative material after lens extraction fails to support the concept of the lens as the sole source of these deposits. In addition, these deposits were found in the conjunctival vessels of the opposite, clinically uninvolved eye.

The diagnosis of exfoliation syndrome is usually made by the finding of typical deposits under the pupillary border. The pathologic depositions on the anterior lens capsule produce three discrete areas: a translucent central disc, a peripheral band, and a clear intermediate zone separating the two affected areas. It is often necessary to dilate the pupil to make the major sites of deposition on the anterior lens capsule more obvious, by demonstrating the edge of the central disc and the intermediate zone.

The dandrufflike deposits on the trabecular meshwork are often associated with increased trabecular pigment, even extending anterior to Schwalbe's line, and have been suggested as a causative mechanism for the impaired outflow and elevated intraocular pressure. The incidence of narrow angles in this group of patients (about 20%) is considerably higher than the general population. It has been reported that some 30% to 80% of eyes with exfoliation have glaucoma. Furthermore, these deposits are found in about 50% of cases of open-angle glaucoma in Scandinavian countries, with some estimates ranging as high as 80% to 90%. In

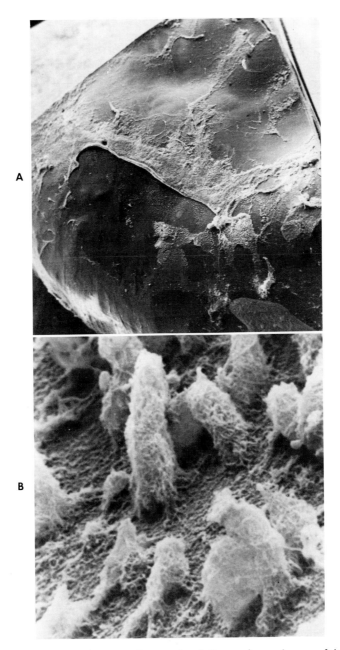

Fig. 15-14. A, Scanning electron micrograph of the surface of an exfoliative lens. **B,** Capsule is covered by a network of fine fibrillar material, together with random bushlike excrescences of coarser fibrils. (**B** x7900, from same lens as **A.**) (Courtesy D. H. Dickson, Halifax, Nova Scotia.)

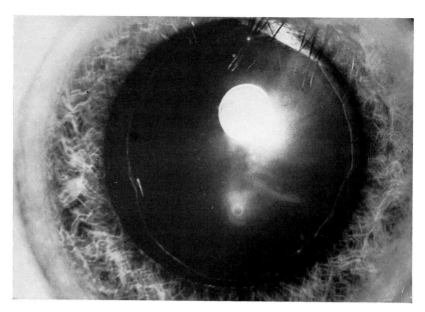

Fig. 15-15. Exfoliation of the lens capsule.

the United States, England, and Germany exfoliation is seen in under 5% of the glaucoma population and is also found in a very small percentage of eyes in non-glaucoma populations over the age of 50 years. The frequency of exfoliation in the elderly nonglaucoma population in Scandinavian countries is 5% to 8%.

In opposite eyes of patients with unilateral exfoliation and glaucoma, the incidence of glaucoma is about 15%, considerably less than would be predicted for primary open-angle glaucoma. The frequency of high pressure response to topical corticosteroids in these cases is also less than predicted for primary glaucoma. Furthermore, topical corticosteroid testing in patients with exfoliation but without glaucoma fails to demonstrate an increased prevalence of high responders as found in eyes with high myopia or Krukenberg's spindles. These findings suggest that glaucoma capsulare might truly be a secondary glaucoma and not genetically related to primary open-angle glaucoma. Exfoliation is thought to be hereditary, but other factors such as climate, occupation, and diet might also be related. It is important to differentiate exfoliation from true splitting of the lens capsule such as seen in glassblowers' cataract, which is usually not associated with glaucoma.

The diagnostic tests and treatment of glaucoma capsulare are much the same as that for primary open-angle glaucoma, although most authors emphasize a poorer prognosis for the former. The condition is not alleviated by lens extraction.

Glaucoma and retinal detachment

Most eyes with retinal detachments have a decreased intraocular pressure. This is a consequence of the hyposecretion of aqueous humor. Hyposecretion may be causative in producing the detachment but is more probably a consequence of the detachment. An unusually large number of patients with retinal detachments have decreased outflow facility. This may be explained by a common cause of both the detachment and the impaired outflow, such as trauma, uveitis, cataract extraction, or degenerative processes. In some eyes glaucoma may be a consequence of the retinal detachment, the inflammatory process it may set up, the surgery used in its treatment, or even vascular occlusion and rubeosis iridis. An interesting unusual variety of open-angle glaucoma is that seen in small peripheral retinal tears with little or no detachment. The glaucoma is cured by sealing the break.

On the other hand, one may have preexisting primary open-angle glaucoma. This situation appears to be more common than was previously recognized. The evidence for this is based on testing of the contralateral eye with tonography and water drinking. Here, one often finds evidence of early primary open-angle glaucoma, suggesting that the glaucoma and retinal detachments in these patients are two associated defects. An interesting sidelight of this correlation is the occurrence of retinal detachment after the use of miotic therapy. Again, this may be a consequence of the contraction of the ciliary muscles by the miotic, an effect of the pressure lowering, or merely the pulling free of an already weakened retina.

In one clinic 530 consecutive patients with retinal detachment were subjected to repeated tonometry, tonography, gonioscopy, and visual field examinations. Glaucoma as defined by two out of three of the criteria selected (repeated pressures over 23 mm Hg, outflow facility less than 0.13, or cupping and glaucomatous field loss) was found in 65 patients. In 26 patients, the glaucoma was believed to be secondary to trauma (10), to uveitis (2), to cataract extraction (8), or to the retinal detachment and its therapy (6). The remaining 39 patients were found to have bilateral primary open-angle glaucoma. In 19 of these, the glaucoma had been unrecognized and involved the opposite eye as well as the hyposecreting eye with the detachment. Six of the 19 had cupping and field loss.

In the management of patients with retinal detachments, particularly after reattachment, intraocular pressure may remain low in spite of markedly impaired outflow facility for some period of time. However, secretion is usually reestablished, and eyes with impaired outflow facility should be watched closely for subsequent pressure rises. The management of open-angle glaucoma in patients with a history of detachment presents additional problems; in particular, there are the hazards of causing recurrence or of hastening the development of a detachment in the eye by the use of strong miotics.

Fuchs' dystrophy

There is a high incidence of open-angle glaucoma in patients with Fuchs' dystrophy, estimated at 10% to 15% of such eyes. In a study of 16 patients with this condition, Waltman found that 2 (12%) had lymphocyte hyperresponsiveness to corticosteroids as determined by inhibition of lymphocyte transformation. It is interesting to speculate as to whether the endothelial dystrophy involves the endothelium of the trabecular meshwork and results in obstruction to outflow. In one study, 82% of the patients with dystrophy had outflow facilities below 0.18, and 35% were less than 0.11. The disease process does not appear to differ from that of primary open-angle glaucoma. Glaucoma should be suspected in all patients who have endothelial dystrophy. When corneal edema and bullous keratopathy appear, some dehydration of the cornea can be obtained by the use of hypertonic ointments such as saline or EKG sol. It is particularly important in these patients to keep intraocular pressure down. The edema of the cornea is related to the height of the intraocular pressure as well as to the inability of the endothelium to deturgesce the cornea.

Glaucoma with retinitis pigmentosa

It is estimated that about 3% of patients with retinitis pigmentosa have glaucoma. There is no evidence that such glaucoma differs from other open-angle primary glaucoma. These patients present problems in follow-up because it is difficult to evaluate progression of glaucomatous changes in the presence of ring scotomas or loss of peripheral field. Furthermore, they often have posterior subcapsular lens changes, so that the use of miotics reduces vision markedly.

GLAUCOMA WITH NORMAL OUTFLOW FACILITY
Hypersecretion glaucoma (Figs. 29-4 and 29-19)

Hypersecretion glaucoma is a rare type of open-angle glaucoma characterized by a normal outflow facility in the face of an elevated intraocular pressure. It is of historical interest in the evolution of tonography, but its identification has rather limited clinical importance. The mechanism of pressure elevation appears to be increased production of aqueous humor. The pressure tends to be elevated intermittently to values in the high twenties to midthirties. The disease occurs particularly in women 40 to 60 years of age with neurogenic systemic hypertension. With sufficient elevation of intraocular pressure, field loss may result without the development of impaired outflow facility (as verified by tonography, perfusion, and histologic examination).

The diagnosis of hypersecretion glaucoma cannot be made by tonometry alone but requires tonographic demonstration of a normal outflow facility at the time the pressure is elevated. At other times these patients have perfectly normal tonograms. It is necessary to rule out artifactual tracings, use of inadequate weight for tonography, elevated episcleral venous pressure, elevated ocular rigidity (by applanation tonometry), and angle closure (by gonioscopy) with opening of the angle when the tonometer is applied (Figs. 29-5 and 29-6). At present it is more difficult to rule out the possibility of primary open-angle glaucoma with impaired outflow facility but with a marked decrease in aqueous secretion when the tonometer is applied. This constitutes a form of pseudofacility. In fact, Goldmann's review of many of the original patients with "hypersecretion" glaucoma revealed that they were instances of high pseudofacility. When the tonographic facility was corrected for pseudofacility, these glaucomas also demonstrated reduced "true" facility. Nevertheless, their high pseudofacility appears to protect them from excessive intraocular pressure elevation and from optic nerve damage. True hypersecretion glaucoma thus becomes exceedingly rare, but the name remains useful as a tono-graphic classification and for its prognostic significance. When therapy is required in these patients, it has proved most efficacious empirically to begin with topical epinephrine. The true hypersecretor tends to respond poorly to miotics but dramatically to topical epinephrine or carbonic anhydrase inhibitors (Figs. 29-4 and 29-19). Because of the intermittency of the hypersecretion, eyes with this variety of glaucoma tend to sustain optic nerve damage and lose field much more slowly and to a much lesser degree than those with open-angle glaucoma and impaired outflow facility. Hypersecretion is a relative term, and so any definition of hypersecretion must be arbitrary. The resultant intraocular pressure is still dependent on the outflow capacity of the individual eye. Thus, at secretory levels of 4 to 5 μl/min, many eyes will have pressures in the abnormal range. However, some patients have this degree of hypersecretion but with normal intraocular pressures. On the other hand, elderly people with outflow facilities in the low ranges of normal can develop pressures in the thirties at only moderately elevated secretory levels.

Elevated episcleral venous pressure (Figs. 15-16 and 15-17)

The episcleral venous pressure may be elevated in such conditions as superior vena caval obstruction, mediastinal tumor, and arteriovenous (carotid-cavernous) fistula. As is evident from Equation 1 of Chapter 5, under these circumstances intraocular pressure is elevated millimeter for millimeter with the rise in episcleral venous pressure. This may occur without abnormality of the gonioscopic appearance of the angle (except for the common occurrence of blood in Schlemm's canal) and with normal tonographic measurements of outflow facility. The condition is identified by recognizing the disease process itself that has caused the elevated venous pressure in the head. In addition, there are usually chemosis and prominent dilated tortuous vessels of the bulbar conjunctiva. There may also be exophthalmos and papilledema. In many instances there will be a marked increase in intraocular pressure when the patient lies down. Occasionally in arteriovenous fistula neovascularization of the iris and chamber angle leads to neovascular (hemorrhagic) glaucoma.

Therapy for glaucoma with elevated episcleral venous pressure is that for the primary condition. It has been demonstrated that ligation of the carotid artery in carotid-cavernous fistula will result in normalization of episcleral venous pressure and of intraocular pressure. In some eyes prolonged elevation of episcleral venous pressure results in reductions of outflow facility without gonioscopically visible changes in the angle. Unfortunately the decreased outflow facility may persist after episcleral venous pressure values are normalized.

A familial form of open-angle glaucoma associated with elevated episcleral venous pressure may also occur. In this condition, which may be unilateral or bilateral, there is no history of trauma, and efforts to discover the etiology of the elevated venous pressure have been unsuccessful. These patients have congested

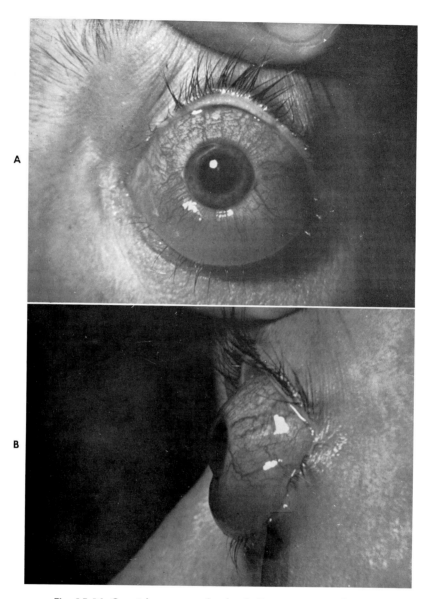

Fig. 15-16. Carotid-cavernous fistula. **A**, Front view. **B**, Side view.

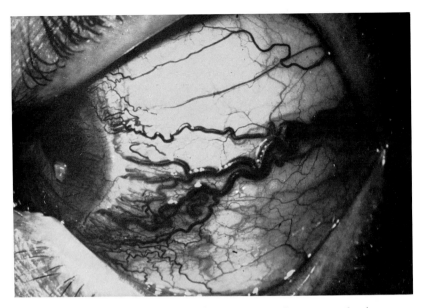

Fig. 15-17. Distended episcleral veins in carotid-cavernous fistula.

episcleral veins and elevated intraocular pressures, often with normal outflow facilities, and may develop field loss and cupping. Medical therapy cannot lower intraocular pressure below that of the episcleral veins, and filtering surgery becomes necessary if damage develops.

PROBLEMS FOR CONSIDERATION

The secondary glaucomas occur in conjunction with some recognizable ocular disease believed to be associated with, or causative of, the glaucoma. In some secondary glaucomas the cause is obvious. In most cases, however, our knowledge of the mechanisms responsible for the glaucoma is extremely limited.

The necessity of studying the mechanism of steroid-induced glaucoma and its implications in the etiology of primary open-angle glaucoma have been discussed. The anti-inflammatory properties of corticosteroids and their value in ophthalmology is unquestioned. The fact that such agents can produce glaucoma in susceptible eyes makes it necessary to find agents that will maintain the anti-inflammatory properties without the pressure-raising properties. Medrysone and tetrahydrotriamcinolone represent the initial efforts toward this goal. They should be valuable agents for external ocular inflammation. Unfortunately neither is sufficiently potent to suppress most intraocular inflammation. FML is more potent but can raise pressure in glaucomatous eyes after prolonged use.

Information is needed on the mechanisms of repair of the trabecular meshwork after traumatic or inflammatory damage. The tools for such study are available, including experimental animals (e.g., monkeys) whose eyes are similar to the human eye. The knowledge of such mechanisms and ways to provide optimum conditions for recovery are of considerable clinical importance. Clues obtained in such experiments could also be applied to the study of primary open-angle glaucoma, and biochemical or enzymatic abnormalities or deficiencies searched for.

Similar investigations should be carried out in monkeys on the factors involved in siderogenic glaucoma (hemosiderosis). We know that anatomic changes in the trabecular meshwork occur in this condition, and it seems likely that the iron molecule in some way interferes with the metabolic pathways of the cells of the meshwork.

Glaucomatocyclitic crisis is a rare type of glaucoma associated with mild inflammation and occurs in repeated, self-limited bouts. Histologic and histochemical descriptions of the trabecular meshwork in such eyes have never been made. The fact that such marked outflow impairment can completely regress in a matter of one to two weeks suggests that the cells of the trabecular meshwork possess considerable reparative properties.

Neovascular glaucoma presents many problems involving both etiology and therapy. Why retinal hypoxia or anoxia should stimulate neovascularization over the iris surface is not known. The elaboration of some vessel-stimulating "x" substance from hypoxic tissue has been postulated, but the nature of this substance is obscure. Efforts should be made to induce rubeosis in experimental animals, and biochemical studies should be made to find vessel-stimulating substances in hypoxic ocular tissues, especially retinal tissue. The rare occurrence of rubeosis iridis in eyes with choroidal malignant melanomas suggests that a product elaborated by the tumor is also able to stimulate neovascularization. Studies of such tumors might lead to the discovery of the substance. Therapy of neovascular glaucoma has been almost universally unsuccessful. More careful and thorough examination of patients susceptible to the development of rubeosis (those suffering from diabetes, central vein occlusion, etc.) has led to the discovery of neovascularization in the chamber angle of eyes before any pressure elevation or congestion develops. This neovascularization at times appears to arise from Schlemm's canal. In spite of early identification, no way to reverse the process is known. Such methods are badly needed, as are ways of treating the full-blown picture when it develops.

Glaucoma in association with recession of the chamber angle in eyes that have suffered blunt trauma has been well documented as a clinical entity. The mechanisms responsible for the anatomic changes in the trabecular meshwork are not known. Obviously the damage is related to the trauma, but why complete functional repair occurs in some cases and not in others is not understood. Even more baffling is why the glaucoma in some of these eyes does not develop for ten years or more after the trauma. Angle recession can be produced in experimental animals, and histologic and biochemical studies performed at varying time intervals. Such studies might answer many of the present questions about this condition. Studies have shown that the opposite eyes of patients with traumatic recessions in one eye have a remarkably high percentage of steroid responsiveness. Why steroid-responsive eyes should be more prone to develop angle recession with trauma is entirely unclear. Nevertheless, it appears that trauma is more likely to lead to glaucoma in eyes that respond to steroids with increased intraocular pressure.

Ideas about the relationship of lens dislocation to glaucoma have undergone considerable change in recent years. This has largely been due to the discovery of angle recessions in many of the eyes with glaucoma and dislocated lenses. This suggests that the subluxated lens per se is not the causative factor. Experimental studies are needed to demonstrate whether eyes with enzyme-induced lens dislocation are prone to develop glaucoma and whether surgical removal of the lens alters the course.

"Enzymatic" glaucoma is another entity that requires much further research. The frequent occurrence of elevated intraocular pressure in the early postoperative period in eyes in which alpha-chymotrypsin was used for zonulolysis has been well documented. The exciting scanning electron microscopic studies showing obstruction of the trabeculum by zonular fragments provide the answer to the etiology of this transient glaucoma. Long-term studies of the patients developing this condition are needed to determine whether any permanent trabecular damage results. The application of this investigative tool to other types of glaucoma (e.g., glaucomatocyclitic crisis, rubeosis) may provide equally valuable information.

Epithelial ingrowth, although much more rare than neovascular glaucoma, is equally as difficult to manage and very frequently results in loss of the eye. Numerous attempts to induce this condition in laboratory animals have been unsuccessful. The lack of an experimental model has greatly hampered therapeutic efforts, and new attempts must be made to reproduce the condition in animal eyes. Only then will it be possible to evaluate reliably therapeutic measures such as x-ray and corneal cryotherapy and develop better methods of prevention and cure.

The relationship between glaucoma and high myopia is not understood and needs to be investigated. The fact that buphthalmos develops in infant eyes when intraocular pressure is elevated suggests that slight elevations of intraocular pressure might be important in the progressive enlargement of eyes with myopia. The possibility of preventing progressive myopia by lowering intraocular pressure in young myopes is intriguing. If steroid-responsive laboratory animals can be found, the possibility of producing ocular enlargement by moderate degrees of pressure elevation can be studied. Electron microscopic, histochemical, and biochemical studies of the trabecular meshwork in myopic eyes are needed.

The relationships between glaucoma and retinal detachment require further study. The mechanism whereby eyes on miotics tend to develop retinal tears needs investigation. Laboratory animals can be used to determine how and where ciliary body contraction causes tension or strain on the choroid and retina. Common metabolic deficiencies or abnormalities in the choroid, retina, vitreous, and trabecular meshwork of eyes with glaucoma and eyes with retinal detachment should be searched for.

Metabolic studies of corneas of patients with endothelial dystrophy might provide clues to a possible metabolic abnormality of the endothelial cell related to a basic defect in primary open-angle glaucoma. Since corneal transplants are often performed on these patients, fresh human material for laboratory study is available.

The relationship between the pigment abnormality of Krukenberg's spindle and the development of glaucoma is not known. The commonly held belief that mechanical, pigmentary obstruction of the trabecular meshwork is the cause of the glaucoma in these patients has not been proved. The frequent occurrence of primary open-angle glaucoma in relatives of patients with pigmentary glaucoma should be further emphasized.

The glaucoma associated with the exfoliation syndrome has many unanswered questions. Evidence is accumulating that it may truly be a secondary glaucoma, but this is certainly not proved. Studies of the metabolic defect responsible for the abnormality in this condition are necessary. Better studies, both clinical and histologic, are needed of the prevalence of exfoliation in the United States and other countries where the reported incidence of glaucoma capsulare is low.

16

Combined-mechanism glaucoma

The classification of glaucomas into angle-closure and open-angle glaucomas is of enormous importance not only in the understanding of the mechanism but also in the approach to diagnosis and management of the individual patient with glaucoma. Unfortunately the glaucoma in some patients does not fit discretely into either category and appears to be a combination of both forms of primary glaucoma or of one or more forms of primary and secondary glaucoma. There are a large number of combinations possible. Only a few of the more common will be listed and briefly discussed.

COMMON TYPES OF COMBINED GLAUCOMAS
Open-angle glaucoma complicated by angle closure

The occasional eye with chronic simple glaucoma and an anatomically narrow angle is a common cause for confusion as to classification and therapy. With increasing age and an enlarging lens some eyes in this category develop progressive narrowing of the angle and may develop an acute episode of angle-closure glaucoma. Such an acute attack may occur in spite of reasonable control of the impaired trabecular function. In these eyes it is difficult to establish a diagnosis of impending acute angle closure unless significant pressure rises and occlusion can be demonstrated spontaneously or after a provocative test. Since miotic therapy is needed to maintain trabecular function, one cannot use the usual mydriatic provocative tests. Mydriatics, by reversing the effects of miotics, may lower outflow facility even without occluding the angle. In these patients therefore one must rely even more heavily on the gonioscopic appearance of the angle.

Rather than an acute attack, most eyes with this type of combined-mechanism glaucoma develop progressively greater difficulty in pressure control as partial angle closure is superimposed on the trabecular damage. The use of stronger miotics or epinephrine may induce further angle closure and may even precipitate an acute attack in such eyes. In patients seen for the first time with extremely narrow angles, glaucoma uncontrolled medically, and evidence of long-standing damage to the optic nerve, the differential diagnosis between chronic angle-closure glaucoma and this combined form of glaucoma may be most difficult. If gonio-scopic evidence of angle closure is confirmed, the treatment of choice is peripheral iridectomy. This eliminates the angle-closure element and often permits reestab-lishment of medical control of the open-angle glaucoma. Strong miotics and epi-nephrine can be safely used in such eyes after iridectomy. The use of strong miotics such as echothiophate iodide (Phospholine iodide) can slowly shallow the anterior chamber and narrow the angle. Gonioscopy prior to therapy should reveal true angle width.

Angle-closure glaucoma with trabecular damage

In patients with pure angle-closure glaucoma the trabecular meshwork may be damaged after repeated attacks with or without peripheral anterior synechias. This results in impaired outflow facility out of proportion to the gonioscopic evidence of angle closure. The management here is that of the angle closure, with prefer-ence given to peripheral iridectomy. After this procedure is done, the patient can be reevaluated, and attempts can be made to control outflow facility and pressure with miotics and secretory inhibitors much as in other secondary open-angle glau-comas.

Secondary glaucoma after a surgical procedure in primary glaucoma

After such surgical procedures as cataract extraction or a filtering procedure in primary glaucoma, either angle closure or open angle in type, the development of a flat anterior chamber may result in either peripheral anterior synechias or trabecular damage. One is then faced with a primary glaucoma complicated by postoperative secondary angle-closure or open-angle glaucoma. Such cases can be difficult to unravel, particularly if one does not have all the information required about the patient before the operation was done. Patients with this combination of disease processes are treated as secondary glaucomas, preferably with appro-priate medical therapy, unless pupillary block demands surgery. Filtering surgical procedures are reserved for those eyes that fail to be controlled on maximum medi-cal therapy.

Secondary glaucoma after an inflammatory process in primary glaucoma

In the category of primary glaucoma complicated by an inflammatory process must be included those patients who develop iritis after a surgical procedure or even the administration of miotics. The iritis may lead to peripheral anterior synechias or to trabecular damage without gonioscopic change, resulting in a com-bined form of glaucoma. The therapy here is directed toward improving trabecular function. If posterior synechias with iris bombé and angle closure are evident, it may be necessary to do a peripheral iridectomy.

Neovascular glaucoma after vein occlusion in open-angle glaucoma

The sequence of events in chronic open-angle glaucoma followed by vein oc-clusion, rubeosis, and hemorrhagic glaucoma is seen fairly often in ophthalmologists' offices. Immediate therapy is necessarily directed toward the difficult management of the hemorrhagic glaucoma. Particular attention, however, should also be given to the diagnosis and treatment of possible open-angle glaucoma in the contralateral eye. Central retinal vein occlusion occurs with increased frequency in glaucomatous eyes. This is especially true when a vein occlusion has occurred in the opposite eye.

Secondary open-angle glaucoma with superimposed secondary angle closure

In eyes that have been subjected to inflammation or trauma and have developed secondary open-angle glaucoma, recurrence of the inflammatory disease process or its progression, as well as iris bombé, may result in peripheral anterior synechias and angle closure. Therapy is directed at the inflammatory process. Secretory suppressants are used for control of intraocular pressure. When pressure is lowered, peripheral iridectomy may be needed to relieve the angle-closure aspects of the problem. After subsidence of the inflammatory process, trabecular function is reevaluated and the need for therapy is determined.

Glaucoma after elevated episcleral venous pressure with subsequent impaired outflow facility

In thyrotropic exophthalmos or retrobulbar tumors, episcleral venous pressure may be elevated and result in increased intraocular pressure in spite of normal values for outflow facility. Many of these eyes later develop decreased outflow facility with open angles, and this often persists even after the exophthalmos subsides or is corrected surgically. The resultant open-angle glaucoma is treated much as other such secondary glaucomas, with preference to medical therapy.

Absolute glaucoma

Absolute glaucoma is usually defined as any type of glaucoma that proceeds to no light perception. It may merely represent the terminal stages of open-angle glaucoma, or it may have various complicating factors (e.g., rubeosis iridis) or an admixture of various types of glaucoma. The management of these eyes is largely concerned with control of pain and the absolute necessity of ruling out intraocular neoplasm. Enucleation is the surest and best means of resolving both problems. When a tumor can be excluded with certainty, cyclocryotherapy, retrobulbar injection of alcohol, and other such procedures may be justified. Filtering surgery should not be considered because of the possibility of sympathetic ophthalmia. Sympathetic ophthalmia has also been seen after cyclodiathermy.

CHAPTER **17**

Congenital glaucoma

The term *congenital glaucoma* should be reserved for those cases of glaucoma in which developmental anomalies are manifest at birth. The most frequent is primary congenital, or infantile, glaucoma. Less frequent are those cases associated with other congenital anomalies such as aniridia and the Sturge-Weber syndrome. In patients with infantile glaucoma intraocular pressure is usually elevated at, or shortly after, birth, but in the others it may not become elevated for several decades.

PRIMARY CONGENITAL, OR INFANTILE, GLAUCOMA (Fig. 17-1)
Prevalence and genetic pattern

Over 60% of the cases of primary congenital, or infantile, glaucoma are diagnosed in the first six months of infancy, and more than 80% have their onset before the end of the first year. The condition is sufficiently rare that the average ophthalmologist is unlikely to see more than one new infantile glaucoma in five years of practice. The average pediatrician is even less likely to see a case. This adds greatly to the risk of a missed diagnosis in the early stages of the disease. Since successful management depends on early recognition, it is most important that both ophthalmologists and pediatricians be instructed in the early signs and urged to seek specialized care promptly.

The anomaly that results in congenital glaucoma is genetically determined and exhibits a recessive inheritance pattern in most cases. This means that both the parents are heterozygous (Ncg) and have a single defective gene (cg). Twenty-five percent of their offspring would be expected to have the two defective genes and thus exhibit infantile glaucoma. Fifty percent would have a single gene, and 25% would be completely normal (Ncg × Ncg = cgcg + Ncg + Ncg + NN). The pool of these defective genes in the general population is very small; thus a carrier is unlikely to mate with another carrier. This accounts for the rarity of the condition. Although sex linkage is not common in the inheritance pattern, over 65% of the patients are boys. The disease is bilateral in 75% of the patients. In the unilateral cases, there will sometimes be the full-blown gonioscopic appearance in the affected

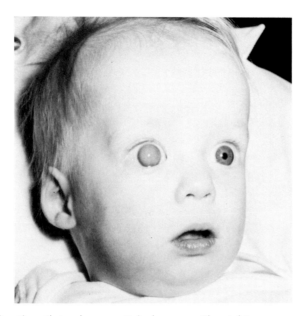

Fig. 17-1. Child with unilateral congenital glaucoma. The right cornea was enlarged and cloudy with an elevated intraocular pressure.

eye and an incomplete pattern in the seemingly normal eye, with areas of angle-recess formation alternating with a flat insertion of iris into the trabecular mesh-work. Sporadic cases of congenital glaucoma can be caused by interference with fetal development, such as sometimes occurs when the mother has German measles during the first trimester of pregnancy.

Congenital defects in one system are frequently accompanied by congenital defects in other systems. Patients with infantile glaucoma occasionally also have congenital cataracts. Pyloric stenosis, deafness, mental deficiency, cardiac anom-alies, etc. may be associated. In the care of these babies such associated defects must be borne in mind.

Signs

Early signs

It is important to make the diagnosis of the glaucoma as early as possible. Symptoms as described below are often more significant than findings at anesthetic examination.

Epiphora, photophobia, and blepharospasm. Epiphora, photophobia, and blepharospasm may be present weeks before corneal hazing or enlargement be-comes obvious to the parent or the pediatrician. Although tear duct occlusion is the usual cause of tearing in a newborn infant, the addition of photophobia should demand careful investigation including a tension determination under anesthesia.

It is probable that the symptoms are related to the irritation of slight corneal edema caused by the increased intraocular pressure. Later in the disease the photophobia may become so intense that the baby will keep its head buried in the pillow. Successful normalization of pressure is usually accompanied by a prompt decrease in these signs.

Corneal edema. Corneal haziness from edema is the sign that brings most of these babies to the physician. In 25% of the cases the edema is present at birth, and in over 60% by the sixth month. The later this sign appears, the better the prognosis. At first, most of the edema is in the corneal epithelium, increasing and decreasing with changes in tension. Removal of the epithelium down to Bowman's membrane frequently permits accurate ophthalmoscopy, gonioscopy, and goniotomy. With progression of the disease, the stretching and edema of the corneal stroma result in irregular opacities, and these are more or less permanent. Corneal edema due to glaucoma must be differentiated from the cloudy cornea secondary to keratitis or trauma. The haze produced by the latter two involves the stroma and has little tendency to clear significantly when the epithelium is removed.

Corneal enlargement. Under the influence of increased intraocular pressure there is progressive enlargement of the infant cornea. This can result in such huge eyes that picturesque terminology such as *buphthalmos,* or *ox eye,* has been used. If pressure does not become elevated until after the age of 3 years, the eyes usually

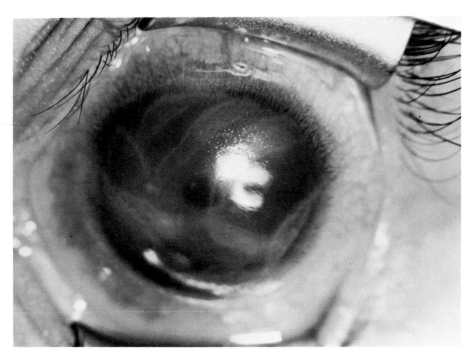

Fig. 17-2. Corneal enlargement with tears in Descemet's membrane in congenital glaucoma.

resist distention. In infants, an increasing corneal diameter is as significant a sign of uncontrolled glaucoma as is a progressing field defect in adult glaucoma. Most infant corneas measure under 10.5 mm in horizontal diameter. A measurement over 12 mm is diagnostic when coupled with tears in Descemet's membrane. The stretching results in irregular corneal astigmatism. The myopia induced by the enlargement of the eye is partially neutralized by the flattening of the cornea.

Tears in Descemet's membrane (Fig. 17-2). The major part of the enlargement of the infant eye occurs at the corneoscleral junction. This places Descemet's membrane under stretch. Since it is less elastic than the corneal stroma, splits in the membrane eventually form. These splits are single or multiple, appearing as an elliptical glassy ridge on the posterior cornea. At first they can be seen in the peripheral cornea, running parallel to the limbus. Later the horizontal meridian is involved, above and below the visual axis. When a tear forms, it is frequently accompanied by sudden clouding of the cornea. This may be total or limited to the area of the tear. The defect is repaired by the endothelium, which produces a new glassy membrane and forms a ridge visible biomicroscopically. Over this area the corneal stroma is usually slightly hazy.

Deep anterior chamber. Since the stretching of the cornea occurs at the limbus in eyes with infantile glaucoma, the anterior chambers are deep. Fortunately

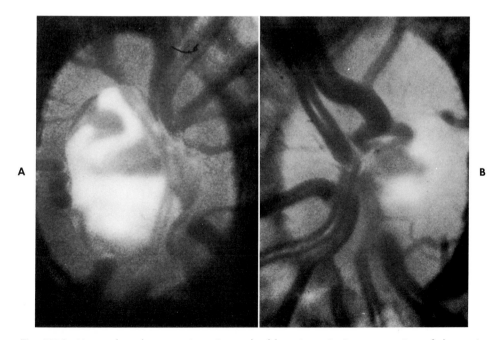

A B

Fig. 17-3. Monocular glaucoma in a 9-month-old patient. **A,** Severe cupping of the optic disc compared with the opposite normotensive eye, **B.** As seen, cupping appears early in infants. Asymmetry is important diagnostically.

this provides the surgeon more space for a better view of the angle and for manipulation of the goniotomy knife.

Cupping and atrophy of optic discs. The part of the examination concerning cupping and atrophy of the optic disc usually requires general anesthesia. Glaucomatous cupping appears early and progresses rapidly with uncontrolled pressures. Asymmetry in cupping of the optic discs is an important early sign of glaucoma (Fig. 17-3).

Late signs

Late changes are the result of progression of the earlier signs. The enlarging cornea becomes hazier and more protuberant; the anterior chamber deepens. Limbal enlargement weakens the zonular ligaments, resulting in iridodonesis and even in subluxation of the lens. These large eyes are easily traumatized, and corneal ulcers, hyphemas, and rupture of the globe are not uncommon. Phthisis bulbi is the eventual fate of many eyes with infantile glaucoma and uncontrolled intraocular pressure.

In most eyes with controlled pressures no further glaucoma damage occurs. In spite of early glaucomatous disc cupping, these eyes may have no detectable field defect in late follow-up. Unfortunately many of these patients will have poor vision due to corneal scarring and anisometropia, which causes amblyopia ex anopsia if there is marked disparity between the two eyes. Patching of the better eye may avoid this complication.

Some patients who as children had a successful operation for monocular glaucoma twenty years previously can have increases in pressure in the apparently normal eye. This means that all these patients must be followed periodically for life. A few others have evidently had endothelial damage and develop corneal edema at relatively low tension levels when they are 20 to 40 years of age.

Differential diagnosis
Megalocornea (Fig. 17-4)

Megalocornea is a condition of abnormal corneal enlargement, usually to 14 to 16 mm in diameter, often with iridodonesis but without such other signs of congenital glaucoma as tears in Descemet's membrane, increased intraocular pressure, or cupping of the nerve head. A sex-linked, recessive inheritance is the rule, 90% of cases occurring in males. Corneal mosaic dystrophy and cataracts have been described in this condition. Gonioscopically, some have normal angles. Some have an area of intense pigmentation that is broader than the usual trabecular pigment band. Others have unusually prominent iris processes.

Megalocornea is by definition a normal eye with a large anterior segment. However, there is good evidence that many of them are formes frustes or cured forms of true infantile glaucoma. Families have been reported with apparent megalocornea in some children and typical infantile glaucoma in others of the sibship. Any case of megalocornea should therefore be followed carefully and not be dismissed as a benign anomaly.

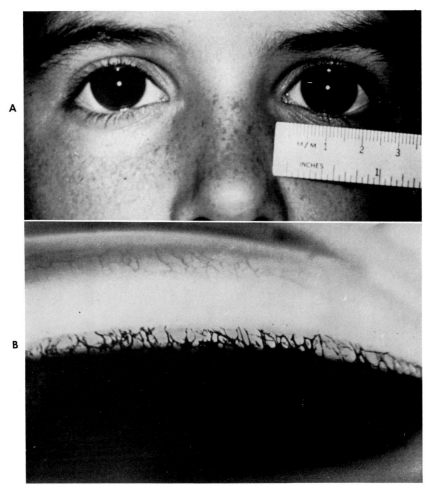

Fig. 17-4. A, Megalocornea. A similar ocular picture is found in three boys, 6, 10, and 12 years of age, and in their father. The cornea is 15 mm in diameter. **B,** Goniophotograph of melgalocornea demonstrating unusually prominent iris processes.

Trauma resulting in corneal haze (Fig. 17-28)

Occasionally, during a difficult delivery, a forceps injury may rupture Descemet's membrane, causing corneal edema that may last for a month or more. The condition is usually unilateral, there is no corneal enlargement, and the tension of the eye is low. Periorbital tissues commonly exhibit signs of trauma if the globe is injured.

Tear duct stenosis

Increased tearing is more commonly caused by obstruction of the nasolacrimal duct. Anesthetic examination may be required to rule out glaucoma. Prolonged use of topical corticosteriods, frequently prescribed with antibiotics for lacrimal obstruction, may induce glaucoma almost indistinguishable from primary infantile glaucoma. Several such cases have been reported. Recognition of this factor may allow return of intraocular pressure to normal without surgery when the steroids are discontinued.

Inflammatory conditions

Rubella keratitis, a viral invasion of the cornea, produces a disciform or diffuse keratitis sometimes without glaucoma. Iridocyclitis or keratoconjunctivitis in infants may lead to misdiagnosis.

Metabolic diseases causing corneal haze

Hurler's disease or gargoylism, corneal lipoidosis, and cystinosis produce diffuse corneal haze.

Other conditions

Idiopathic corneal edema, high myopia with its deep anterior chamber, congenital hereditary corneal dystrophy, and conical cornea can all be confusing if they are not kept in mind.

Examination under anesthesia

Office measurement of the intraocular pressure is usually quite unreliable. Estimations can be made, however, using a topical anesthetic and an oral pacifier if the infant is not struggling. The portable applanation tonometers are more accurate and easier to use than the Schiøtz tonometer. Heavy sedation is not recommended, since it lowers intraocular pressure and has the risks inherent in any form of general anesthesia. Infants should be favored by the best of techniques and anesthetists in well-equipped operating rooms. The surgeon should be prepared to proceed with the operation if it is indicated.

Intraocular pressure and facility of outflow

All general anesthetics tend to lower intraocular pressure, with the possible exception of the dissociative drug ketamine. The high intraocular pressures commonly found in infantile glaucoma can be decreased 15 to 20 mm Hg by the time surgical-depth anesthesia is reached. Since normal infants sometimes have intraocular pressures in the midtwenties, the unwary surgeon may easily be misled. Intraocular pressure should be determined as soon as the child is sufficiently anesthetized to obtain pressure measurements. Intubation is not necessary. Unmistakable signs of infantile glaucoma should be observed before a definite diagnosis is made. If such signs are present, a normal intraocular pressure may not preclude surgical intervention.

Frequently the initial high tension will be reduced when a tear in Descemet's membrane forms. This is sometimes confusing when the ophthalmologist finds the tension lower in the seemingly bad eye than in the eye that has no corneal edema.

Some lowering of tension can be expected if the baby has been dehydrated by the withholding of fluids preoperatively. Because of flattening, edema, and enlargement of the cornea, Schiøtz measurements of intraocular pressure cannot be considered entirely accurate. Horizontal applanation tonometry is superior to that done by the Schiøtz instrument and should be used if it is available.

The facility of outflow in eyes with congenital glaucoma is usually decreased below 0.15, although falsely high measurements may be found when corneal edema permits the tonometer plunger to sink more rapidly into the boggy corneal tissue. In general, tonography has been of little use in evaluating these young patients.

Corneal measurement

The horizontal diameter of the cornea from limbus to limbus is taken by calipers. A measurement over 11.5 mm is suspect. Diameters exceeding 14 mm are typical of advanced glaucoma, and stretching of the cornea to 17 mm is seen occasionally.

Gonioscopic anatomy and microscopic interpretation

A thorough knowledge of gonioscopic and microscopic anatomy is essential for the proper diagnosis and treatment of congenital glaucoma.

Gonioscopy (Fig. 17-5 and Reel II-7). Unless the cornea is perfectly clear, thorough removal of the epithelium down to Bowman's membrane by a curet or No.

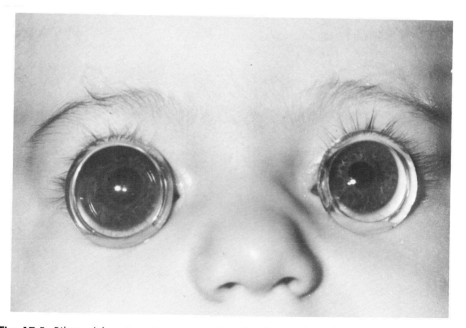

Fig. 17-5. Bilateral lens insertion to reveal angle abnormalities better seen by comparing both eyes.

15 Bard-Parker blade greatly aids clarity of the cornea. Epithelium is also easily removed with a cotton-tipped applicator soaked in 70% alcohol. This method reduces the risk of accidental lacerations to Bowman's membrane and limbal vessels but increases postoperative discomfort. The deep anterior chamber and the flat iris plane are like those of an aphakic eye. The anterior iris mesoderm tends to be hypoplastic and the radial iris vessels prominent, especially if the pressure is elevated. The angle is usually wider than 45°.

Gonioscopically, the flat insertion of iris into the trabecular meshwork is the most characteristic finding. The angle recess, which is beginning to form in most normal newborn eyes, is not seen in the eye with infantile glaucoma. In the less pronounced anomalies, there may be only 0.1 mm difference between normal and abnormal iris insertion. Unfortunately this may be smaller than the resolving power of standard gonioscopic equipment. The peripheral iris and its radial blood vessels lift slightly at their juncture with the trabecular meshwork, producing a scalloped border. The blood vessels then arch backward toward the ciliary body (Fig. 17-6). The iris surface is often covered by a wispy, cottony-like tissue that continues into the angle, extending toward Schwalbe's line.

The trabecular surface glistens like stippled cellophane. Trabecular sheets are much more transparent than the adult tissues with which the examiner is so familiar. In the normal infant eye there is little angle recess, but the anterior ciliary body and its insertion on the scleral spur are directly visible. In the eye with infantile glaucoma the trabecular sheets seem to be thicker. The gray ciliary body band and the white of an apparent scleral spur are visible but are seen through an appreciable bulk of trabecular sheets. Scheie has shown that blood influx into Schlemm's canal can be produced in almost all cases by using jugular compression or by paracentesis if the intraocular pressure is increased. The red streak of blood in Schlemm's canal may seem to be well in front of the iris insertion. This is in part an optical artifact due to the parallax of the gonioscopic view, but is largely a result of the transparency of the tissues as they insert on the trabecular meshwork. There is no abnormal pigmentation of the trabecular surfaces, and Schwalbe's line is in its usual location.

Microscopic interpretation. The microscopic angle anomaly of infantile glaucoma is a specific one. The findings reported are as follows:

1. The scleral spur is poorly developed and can often be located only by the anterior termination of the meridional muscles of the ciliary body.

2. Schlemm's canal is present and patent in most early cases; it is compressed or absent in advanced cases.

3. Trabecular sheets sweep past the scleral spur and are continuous with the longitudinal muscle of the ciliary body. A thin membrane covering the trabecular sheets has been observed by some with the scanning electron microscope (Fig. 17-7), but its presence has been denied by others. This membrane, although described in 1938 by Barkan, had not been well visualized by earlier methods of microscopy. It is possible that the impaired facility of outflow in infantile glaucoma

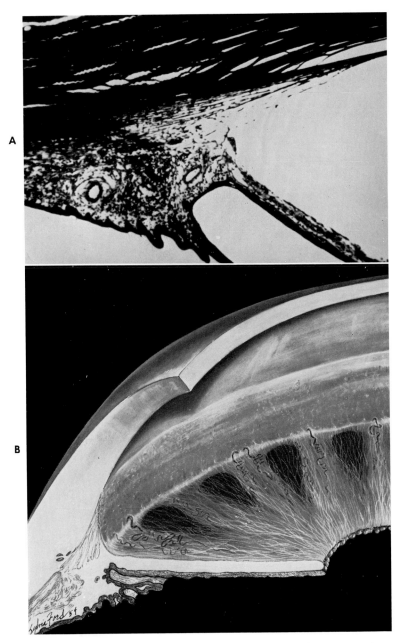

Fig. 17-6. A, Photomicrograph of infantile glaucoma angle. **B,** Composite microscopic and gonioscopic drawing of infantile glaucoma. (**A** courtesy Dr. A. E. Maumenee, Baltimore.)

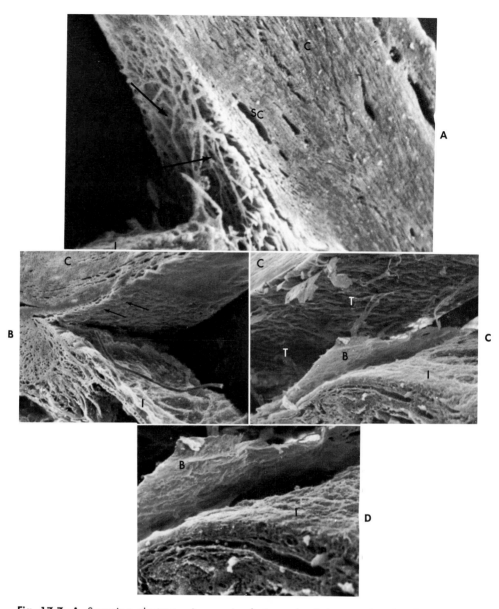

Fig. 17-7. A, Scanning electron microscopic photograph of the anterior chamber angle of the eye of a normal child—fixed, embedded, retrieved, and studied in the same way as the infantile glaucoma eye in **B** to **D.** The uveal meshwork (arrows) of the trabeculum has its usual loosely meshed texture. (×100.) **B,** Scanning electron microscopic photograph of the anterior chamber angle of a 10-month-old infant with infantile glaucoma. A thread from a gauze square lies on the anterior surface of the iris. Beyond it the angle wall can be seen, but no perforations can be seen. The trabecular sheets are compressed. Schlemm's canal is not visible. The arrows point to compressed trabecular meshwork. (×100.) **C,** Under higher magnification an area of the angle wall is shown where the innermost trabecular surface has been torn from the underlying tissues and is lying down on the anterior surface of the iris. The underlying exposed trabecular tissues look more typical of the uveal trabecular meshwork. **D,** The trabecular surface layer, or Barkan's membrane, seems to be imperforate except for small artifactual tears. (×300.) *I,* Iris; *SC,* Schlemm's canal; *C,* cornea; *B,* inner trabecular surface, or Barkan's membrane; *T,* trabecular meshwork behind Barkan's membrane. (**B** to **D** courtesy Dr. D. Anderson and Dr. A. E. Maumenee, Baltimore.)

is due to the impermeable Barkan's membrane. Goniotomy incision through this membrane would permit free outflow of aqueous.

4. The peripheral iris never inserts on the ciliary body but instead runs directly into the inner trabecular meshwork in front of the spur. Embryologically this represents failure of cleavage of the iris from the cornea. The peripheral iris covers one tenth to one half of the trabecular surface and may be partially responsible for the decrease in facility of outflow. Maumenee has suggested that the abnormal pull of the meridional fibers of the ciliary body closes the trabecular sheets.

Ophthalmoscopy

Renewed interest in the pathogenesis of optic nerve damage in glaucoma has led to a reevaluation of previous studies on congenital glaucoma patients. As a result, many old concepts have been abandoned. It is now apparent that glaucomatous cupping appears early in infants with elevated ocular pressure. Changes occur rapidly, often within four to six weeks. Early pathologic cupping is commonly central and deep, with steep margins and a pink-appearing rim of nerve tissue. As cupping progresses, the narrowing rim will remain pink until late in this process (Fig. 17-8).

Pathologic cupping in congenital glaucoma infants may also disappear rapidly after intraocular pressure is controlled (Fig. 17-9). Improvement may be noted within a few days or weeks after surgery and is an excellent indicator of the success of therapy.

Fluorescein studies, as with adult uncontrolled glaucoma, show a marked delay

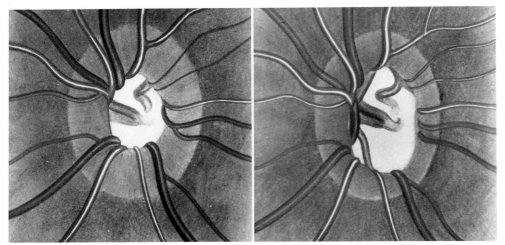

A

B

Fig. 17-8. A, A 4-month-old infant with intraocular pressure 35 and cornea measuring 12 mm in diameter and slightly cloudy. The cup measured 0.3 C/D. **B,** Same infant, disc at 8-week follow-up examination. Intraocular pressure 30 and cornea 12.5 mm and slightly hazy, with a marked increase in cupping to 0.6 C/D.

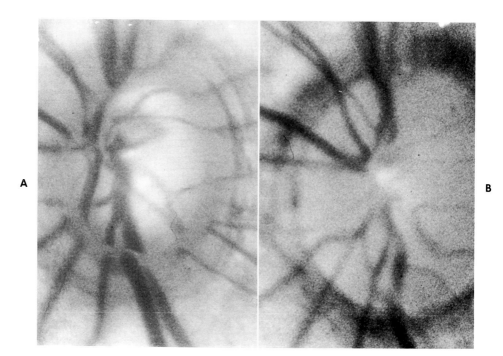

Fig. 17-9. A, Markedly cupped disc of 6-month-old patient with infantile glaucoma, seen through edematous cornea. **B,** Same disc two months after successful goniotomy, with almost complete disappearance of the cup. A slight temporal slope is indicated by lower temporal vessel.

in appearance of the dye (Fig. 17-10). The choroid and optic nerve head supplied by the short posterior ciliary arteries fill later than the central retinal vessels. Although interpretation of these fluorescein findings is speculative, vascular supply to the optic nerve head appears to be decreased during intraocular pressure elevation. It is possible, too, that a relatively low blood pressure in the young permits shunting of blood away from the disc more easily.

Indications of glaucomatous visual damage at an early age come primarily from examination of the optic disc. Marked to moderate cupping would appear to prognosticate a poor visual future, but fortunately this is not necessarily true. After pressure is controlled and the optic disc cup shows improvement, there will be no detectable field defect in a majority of patients later examined (Fig. 17-11).

The sequence of pathologic glaucomatous changes in the infant is probably different from that in the adult. The earliest changes may be due to a loss of intercellular and intracellular fluid and to stretching of the cribriform fascia and scleral canal. Later changes include loss of glial tissue and then atrophy of neurons. Supporting evidence for these changes comes from pathologic specimens (Fig. 17-12), which show early bowing of the cribriform plate while neuronal and glial tissue are still present. The fact that later field examinations are normal despite

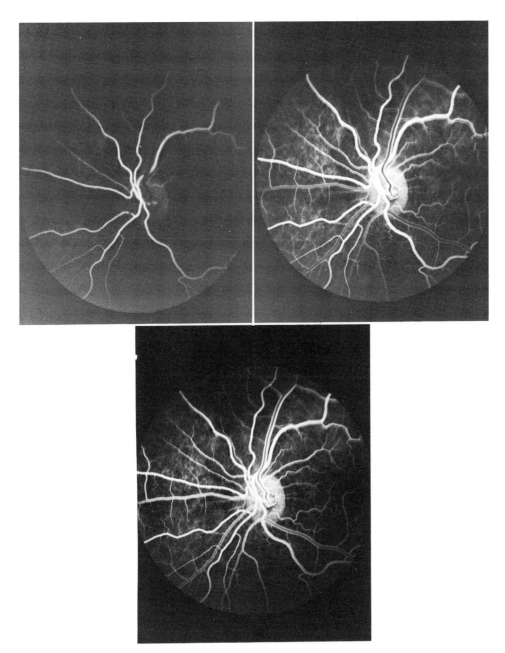

Fig. 17-10. Pattern of fluorescein angiography in infant with increased pressure and glaucomatous cup, showing filling of the central vessels before appearance of the choroidal flush.

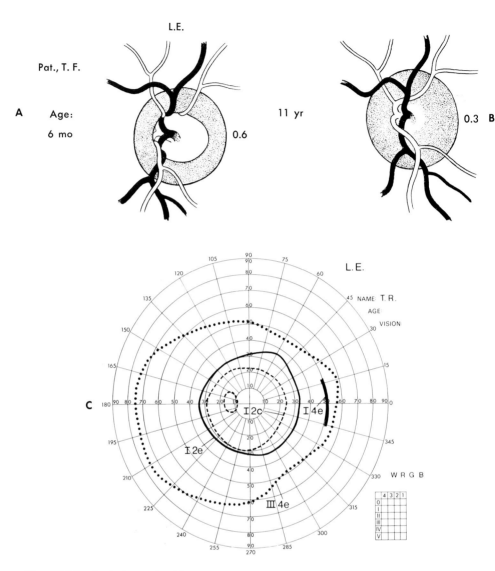

Fig. 17-11. A, A 6-month-old infant with corneal enlargement; intraocular pressure is 35, and cupping 0.6 to 0.7 C/D in the left eye. **B** and **C,** Same patient at 11 years of age. **B,** Intraocular pressure of 15, corneal striae, and 0.3 C/D are seen. **C,** Goldmann field has failed to show a glaucoma defect.

previous extensive glaucomatous cupping supports the findings that nerve fibers had not been destroyed. Changes are reversible in earlier stages when fluids, fibrous supportive tissue, and glial tissue are capable of returning to their normal state. Neurons are incapable of regeneration, and in the late phase the process of cupping is irreversible.

Corneal haze and irregular astigmatism may make fundus examination difficult. After removal of the corneal epithelium, a surprisingly clear look at the disc is possible through the smooth dome of the diagnostic contact lens. If phenyl-

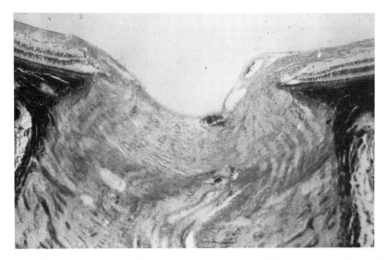

Fig. 17-12. Pathologic specimen shows marked bowing of the lamina cribrosa in a congenital glaucoma patient with moderate cupping and little, if any, nerve fiber damage. (Courtesy Dr. Richard Green and Dr. A. E. Maumenee, Baltimore.)

ephrine (Neo-Synephrine) has been needed to dilate the pupil, it is usually possible to regain miosis promptly for the surgery if 1% pilocarpine solution is used instead of isotonic sodium chloride solution to fill the diagnostic contact lens while doing ophthalmoscopy and gonioscopy.

Treatment
Medical

Miotics are of limited value in the therapy of infantile glaucoma. They are used preoperatively to hold the pupil small for goniotomy, as interval therapy between operations, and terminally to prolong vision in eyes in which surgery has failed. Generally, 2% pilocarpine solution is used every 6 to 8 hours, but stronger miotics are permissible, since they seldom produce the irritation seen in adult eyes. Occasionally miotics can result in troublesome diarrhea. Epinephrine has also been found to be of value in the treatment of these patients.

The carbonic anhydrase inhibitors, like acetazolamide (Diamox), are similarly useful preoperatively. Five to 10 mg of acetazolamide per kilogram of body weight every 6 hours is a safe dose for infants. It will lower the pressure and help reduce corneal edema. In patients without definite diagnosis, carbonic anhydrase inhibitors may lower intraocular pressure, and normal measurements may result in misdiagnosis under anesthesia. Medical therapy is also recommended for the transient elevation of pressure that often accompanies congenital rubella.

Surgical (see also Chapter 26)

Infantile glaucoma is essentially a surgical problem. However, it is not uncommon in normal infant eyes to find intraocular pressures measuring between 20 and

30 mm Hg. Therefore finding such a pressure is not in itself sufficient reason to proceed with surgery. There must be other stigmas of glaucoma, such as corneal edema, corneal enlargement, tears in Descemet's membrane or glaucomatous disc cupping.

Goniotomy. Goniotomy is by far the best procedure for infantile glaucoma if the disease is not too far advanced. When the operation is performed by a competent surgeon with contact lens visualization, the risks are small and the result is gratifying. In three out of four cases the glaucoma can be arrested. Success seems to be the result of opening a route for aqueous flow into Schlemm's canal. It is not yet known whether this is due to incising an impermeable membrane, lowering the point of iris insertion on the trabecular meshwork, or, as suggested by Maumenee, interrupting an abnormal pull of the ciliary muscle on the trabecular fibers. A successful goniotomy increases the facility of aqueous outflow and normalizes intraocular pressure. The improvement in outflow facility tends to be maintained.

Goniopuncture. This procedure is used occasionally, mainly for eyes in which repeated goniotomies have failed or to clear the cornea for definitive surgery by a temporary reduction in pressure. Since it is advisable to maintain a deep chamber after goniotomy, combined goniotomy-goniopuncture is not advocated.

Trabeculotomy. Reports in the European literature indicate a high success rate with trabeculotomy in congenital glaucoma patients (Chapter 25). However, it must be understood that even in experienced hands, identification and probing of Schlemm's canal are difficult, particularly in the infant. Therefore internal goniotomy remains the procedure of choice, with its high success rate, ease of operation, and relatively low risk. Yet when a cloudy cornea prevents adequate visualization of the angle, trabeculotomy may be considered an effective alternative.

Trabeculectomy. The effectiveness of trabeculectomy in the young is fair. There is success in some congenital glaucomas uncontrolled with three or four goniotomies. The technique is the same as in adults (Chapter 25).

Fistulizing procedures. Any of the fistulizing operations for glaucoma can claim an occasional cure but are usually most disappointing. Incisions should be kept small, since ectasias and staphylomas frequently occur when the eye is again subjected to increased intraocular pressure. Thermal sclerostomy and trephination are also logical procedures to try. Iridencleisis is said to carry a higher risk of sympathetic ophthalmia than the same operation in adults.

Cyclocryotherapy. The success of cyclocryotherapy in prolonging visual life of the eye leaves much to be desired. However, it often decreases discomfort and reduces intraocular pressure for several weeks to months. Since connective tissue is less damaged by cold than by heat, staphyloma formation is unlikely to occur with cryotherapy. The incidence of phthisis is extremely low. The procedure may be easily repeated to obtain adequate control.

Prognosis in infantile glaucoma

The earlier any glaucoma is diagnosed and brought under control, the better the prognosis. This is especially true of infantile glaucoma. Although occasionally a spontaneous remission or cure may occur, most of these infants go blind unless successful surgery is performed. If pressure is elevated and the cornea is hazy at birth, there is much less chance of cure than when the symptoms appear after the second month. With the use of goniotomy, less than half of those with signs present at birth can be salvaged, whereas over 80% can be arrested when the disease becomes manifest between the second and ninth months. Of 67 infant eyes followed one to ten years, 85% (57 eyes) were controlled. Of these 57 eyes, 44 (77%) required one goniotomy, 10 (18%) required two goniotomies, and 3 (5%) required three goniotomies.

A series of successfully treated congenital glaucoma patients were subjected to Goldmann field examination at age 5 to 20. Over 80% of these were normal in spite of early pressure, cornea, and disc abnormalities.

Unfortunately, when patients were old enough to obtain reliable visual acuities, 40% had vision below 20/200. An equal percentage had 20/20 to 20/50 vision. Poor visual results have been attributed to corneal opacities, optic nerve damage, and amblyopia ex anopsia with anisometropia and strabismus. Patching the better eye before the age of 5 will sometimes improve visual acuity.

Delay in treatment leads to corneal enlargement and decreases the probability of success. Because of the safety of goniotomy, it is well worth while, even in cases with a relatively poor prognosis, such as corneal diameters over 14 mm or in children more than 1 years of age.

In those unfortunate patients for whom therapy has been unsuccessful, the eyes can be kept free of pain by cyclocryotherapy or retrobulbar alcohol injections. Parents should be encouraged to seek the help of local groups interested in aiding the visually handicapped. Skillful handling of the child and the parents can avoid the psychiatric problems that are sometimes worse than the visual loss.

Patients operated on by Otto Barkan are over 35 years of age. A few who were thought to have been cured are now having recurrence of increased tension, and some have glaucoma in the second eye, which was formerly thought to be normal. Since tonography was not available for these patients in the early postoperative period, it is not possible to say whether the eyes have suffered a decrease in facility of outflow or whether aqueous production has increased to normal values, causing the pressure elevation. In any event, such findings point up the necessity for periodic checkup on all cases of congenital glaucoma if unsuspected loss of sight is to be avoided.

GLAUCOMA ASSOCIATED WITH CONGENITAL ANOMALIES

In the following congenital conditions, the anomaly is present at birth. It is of great importance that pediatricians be alerted to the frequency of glaucoma in these conditions and the need for early ophthalmologic care. Too often the elevated pressure is not noted until irreparable harm has been done to the eye. Sometimes elevations of intraocular pressure are not found until early adulthood. Whether this represents further decrease in an already impaired outflow system or alteration or restoration of aqueous production is not known.

Late-developing infantile glaucoma

There are a few cases of infantile glaucoma in which the pressure elevation is so slight or appears so late that only moderate or no corneal enlargement is found. If there is corneal enlargement with tears of Descemet's membrane, the diagnosis is definite, but it can only be presumptive in their absence. The angle anomaly may be indefinite, since there is a tendency for formation of an angle recess with continuing development. It may be impossible to distinguish this type of glaucoma from open-angle glaucoma.

Aniridia (Fig. 17-13 and Reel III-1)

Aniridia is a bilateral congenital anomaly due to failure of the mesoblast to grow outward over the surface of the lens at the fourth month of fetal life. Numerous associated anomalies of the cornea, lens, anterior chamber angle, retina, central nervous system, and skeletal system have been reported. Wilms' tumor and congenital cataracts are more common with this defect. The prevalence of aniridia in patients with Wilms' tumor is 1:73. More important, about 20% of infants with congenital aniridia have been found to have Wilms' tumors.

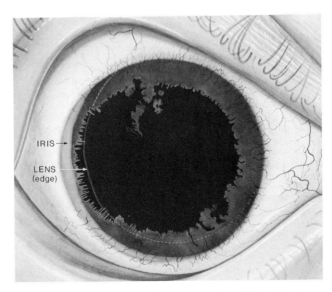

Fig. 17-13. Diagrammatic representation of an eye with aniridia, showing superficial marginal corneal degenerative changes, which are so common. Blood vessel invasion occurs eventually. Eye is turned temporally, showing edge of lens. (Drawing by J. Esperson.)

The condition is genetically determined and is ordinarily dominant, with marked penetrance. A mutant form of the anomaly can appear at a frequency of 1:100,000. Wilms' tumors appear to be more frequently associated with the mutant form of aniridia. As the child grows older, metaplasia of the peripheral corneal epithelium can occur, leading to circumferential degenerative pannus (Fig. 17-13). This can lead, in turn, to complete corneal opacification by the age of 20 to 30 years in some patients. Corneal transplants have been tried in these patients with some success.

There is almost never complete absence of the iris. It may be fairly well developed in some areas, and only a rudimentary stump in others. In some eyes this stump seems to jut directly out from the lower trabecular meshwork. In others it appears to adhere progressively over part of the meshwork, producing a more serious, therapy-resistant form of glaucoma. Abnormal mesodermal tissue is present in the angles of some eyes.

Most of these patients have nystagmus and vision of about 20/100. Poor visual acuity has been attributed to abnormalities of the macula, as seen on pathologic examination, and ophthalmoscopic absence of the foveal reflex. Moderate photophobia may be present even when the eyes are normotensive, and sunglasses or tinted contact lenses are helpful. Attempts have been made to improve nystagmus and visual acuity with painted iris corneal cosmetic contact lenses. The risk of this additional insult in a cornea predisposed to degeneration must be considered.

Early glaucoma occurs in approximately 30% of aniridia patients. In spite of the nystagmus, reasonably valid tonograms can be obtained in patients old enough to cooperate. Decreased outflow facility is the rule in congenital aniridia even before pressure elevations are apparent. Increased intraocular pressure usually appears less dramatically than in the infantile types. Seldom is there severe corneal edema, enlargement, or ruptures of Descemet's membrane. Often pressure elevation is delayed into the early teens, and some eyes remain normotensive. It is important that they be examined periodically.

Reports of operations for glaucoma in patients with aniridia are insufficient for useful statistics as to the proper form of treatment. In general, surgical response has not been gratifying. Therefore medical management is to be employed if possible. If pressures remain elevated, goniotomy (repeated if necessary), trabeculectomy, or external trabeculotomy are at present the advised therapy. Sclerostomy, cyclodialysis, and finally cyclocryotherapy can be used if other measures fail. Grant, during close follow-up, observed increasing peripheral anterior synechia formation of the small iris leaf to trabeculum. This damage may be preventable by early goniotomy. Most of these surgical procedures are complication-prone, particularly to the exposed lens. Cataracts often form in these patients as they get older. Since their vitreous humor is often fluid, lens extraction is hazardous. Patients eventually needing cataract extraction are subjected to further trauma to an already defective cornea. Corneal opacification may result.

Sturge-Weber syndrome (oculofacial angiomatosis) (Figs. 17-14 and 17-15)

The Sturge-Weber syndrome is a cutaneous hemangiomatosis (nevus flammeus) involving the distribution of the fifth cranial nerve and is usually unilateral. Only if it crosses the midline does the attendant glaucoma affect both eyes. Congenital glaucoma is usually associated if there is upper lid involvement. There is almost always concomitant angioma of the choroid and often of the brain. If the brain is involved, x-ray examination may show specks of calcium in the involved areas. Mental deficiency and convulsions are common.

The glaucoma is due to an attendant angle anomaly. In some instances there is increased vascularity of the iris near the angle, but in many cases it is not greater than in infantile glaucoma. The coefficient of aqueous outflow is decreased. Intraocular pressure may be elevated at birth, but more often it is not raised until early childhood or even young adulthood. The adult form is similar to primary open angle glaucoma but associated with dilated conjunctival vessels, heterochromia, choroidal hemangioma, and abnormal retinal vessels.

The same therapy can be advised as in aniridia. Often numerous large vessels

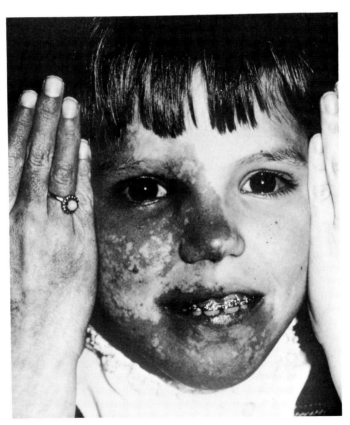

Fig. 17-14. Cutaneous manifestation of Sturge-Weber syndrome.

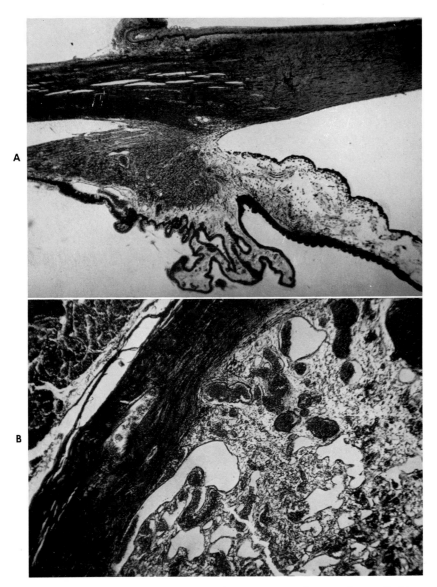

Fig. 17-15. A, Photomicrograph of the angle in Sturge-Weber syndrome. **B,** Photomicrograph of Sturge-Weber choroidal hemangioma. (Courtesy Dr. L. Christensen, Portland, Ore.)

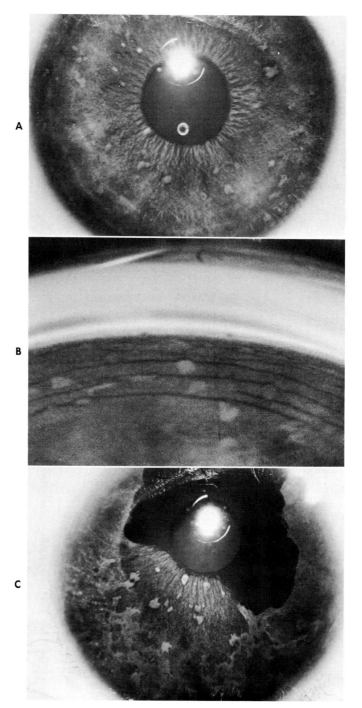

Fig. 17-16. A 22-year-old patient with neurofibromatosis. **A** and **B,** External and gonio-scopic appearance of iris nodules, left eye. **C** and **D,** External and gonioscopic view of abnormally pigmented iris and angle. Note absence of angle recess and high iris inser-tion. **E,** Skin neurofibromas. **F,** *Café au lait* spot.

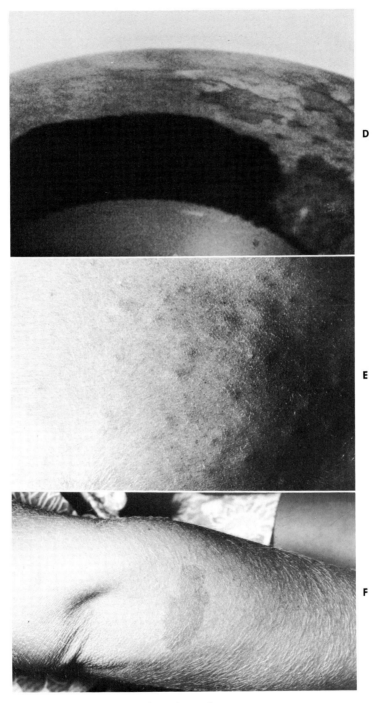

Fig. 17-16, cont'd. For legend see opposite page.

on and in conjunctiva, sclera, and choroid bleed extensively with surgery. More cautery than usual is needed.

Neurofibromatosis (von Recklinghausen's disease)
(Fig. 17-16)

Neurofibromatosis of the skin, particularly of the upper lid, often has an associated glaucoma on the same side. The glaucoma is similar to infantile glaucoma. The syndrome is uncommon but should be recognized readily by pediatricians, ophthalmologists, and plastic surgeons. Too often plastic procedures are performed on the lid without any examination of the underlying eye.

Diagnostic clues may come from examination of the skin for neurofibromas and *café au lait* spots. The iris surface often reveals small, multiple, discrete nodules of neurofibromatous tissue. Large areas of deeply pigmented iris surface can extend into the angle. The angle gonioscopically shows a high, flat insertion of iris tissue, especially at the areas of deep pigmentation. Glaucoma can be due to angle structures that fail to develop normally or from infiltration of the tumor. Optic nerve gliomas and skeletal defects are associated.

The treatment is the same as that for infantile glaucoma, with a much poorer prognosis.

Marfan's syndrome (arachnodactyly)
(Figs. 17-17 and 17-18)

Arachnodactyly, cardiac anomalies, subluxated lenses, and sometimes glaucoma characterize Marfan's syndrome. Sixty percent of patients with this collagen disorder have dislocated lenses, and some of these are associated with microphakia. The lens is spherical and dislocated upward in 80% of cases. Gonioscopically, persistent mesodermal tissue with dense iris processes is commonly seen. The iris surface is usually smooth, and iris processes extend from iris root across the ciliary body face, scleral spur, and trabecular meshwork, possibly to Schwalbe's line. Seventy-five percent of the patients have angle anomalies.

The microscopic anatomy of the angle of such eyes shows a thickened anomalous trabecular meshwork with a large number of the trabecular sheets passing the scleral spur and inserting directly into the ciliary body. The microscopic picture is similar to that in the Sturge-Weber syndrome. In addition to increased intraocular pressure produced by the trabecular anomaly, glaucoma can be caused by the usual complications associated with a dislocated lens. Retinal detachments are also more common among these patients. The syndrome is probably transmitted as a dominant trait. The urine of patients with ectopia lentis and suspected Marfan's syndrome should be examined by the cyanide nitroprusside test for homocystine to rule out possible homocystinuria.

Medical control is preferred as long as possible. Lens removal may become necessary and can be successful though hazardous. Surgical complications occur in 50% of cases. Goniotomy has been effective in a few cases.

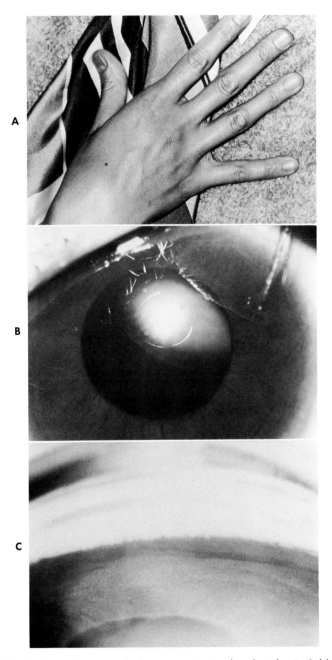

Fig. 17-17. Marfan's syndrome and glaucoma. **A,** Arachnodactyly. **B,** Subluxated lens. **C,** Dense iris processes bridging angle recess on gonioscopy.

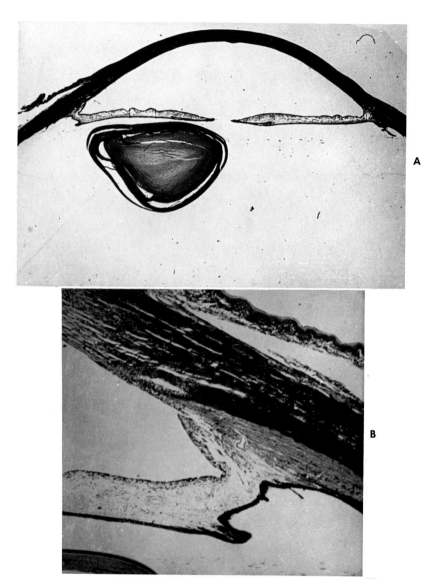

Fig. 17-18. Photomicrographs of an eye from a patient with Marfan's syndrome. **A,** Low power. **B,** High power. (From Reeh, M. J.: Trans. Amer. Acad. Ophthal. Otolaryng. **58:** 212, 1954.)

Pierre Robin syndrome (microgenia and glossoptosis)

Pierre Robin syndrome, which consists of hypoplasia of the mandible, glossoptosis, and usually cleft palate, is occasionally associated with congenital glaucoma. More common ocular complications are high myopia, cataract, retinal detachment, and microphthalmos.

Homocystinuria

Homocystinuria, a recessively inherited metabolic abnormality, consists of mental retardation, convulsions, bilaterally dislocated lenses, fine blond hair, and blue eyes. Kyphoscoliosis, joint laxity, arachnodactyly, and generalized osteoporosis with fractures occur, and the appearance of some patients closely resembles that of those with Marfan's syndrome. There is also a tendency for vascular thrombosis and occlusion of medium-sized veins and arteries.

A deficiency or absence of the enzyme cystathionine synthetase is the probable inborn error of metabolism. Elevated plasma homocystine leads to excretion of this amino acid in the urine. The symptoms and signs may relate to deficiency of cystathionine or cysteine or to the abnormal accumulation of homocysteine, homocystine, or methionine. Pathologically, the zonular fibers are coiled close to the ciliary body, and the nonpigmented epithelium shows patchy atrophy with thickening of the basement membrane. In many individuals only partial expression of the syndrome is apparent. This may be limited to lens dislocation and homocystinuria. Although most of these lenses are displaced posteriorly, pupillary block by a partially dislocated lens is more common than with Marfan's syndrome. The secondary glaucoma so induced is treated much as are other lens subluxations. General anesthesia increases the danger of thromboembolism in patients with homocystinuria.

Goniodysgenesis (iridocorneal mesodermal dysgenesis; Rieger's syndrome; Axenfeld's anomaly; Peter's anomaly)
(Fig. 17-19 and Reel III-2)

Rieger's syndrome and Axenfeld's anomaly are spectacular anomalies inherited dominantly and representing mesodermal dysplasia of the anterior ocular segment. The overlapping descriptions of these defects given by Axenfeld and Rieger create confusion over the appropriate eponym to apply. Goniodysgenesis or mesodermal dysgenesis is suggested as a more useful term.

Posterior embryotoxon is the term applied to an unusual prominence of Schwalbe's line, which stands out like an encircling glass rod inside the limbus. The anteriorly displaced Schwalbe's ring can easily be seen by external inspection or slit-lamp examination. It is estimated to be present to some degree in 15% of individuals, depending on the criteria used for evaluation. Posterior embryotoxon is believed to be a hyperplasia of mesodermal tissue on the posterior cornea near the angle. When dense bands of iris tissue extend and attach to the posterior embryotoxon, the condition is known as *Axenfeld's anomaly,* an incomplete form of the anterior chamber defect described by Rieger. Gonioscopically and to some extent by slit lamp, large, ropy strands of peripheral iris remain attached or semi-attached to Schwalbe's line. Sometimes it looks as if the strands had broken, leaving part attached to the cornea and the rest to the iris. Schwalbe's line itself can occasionally be detached from the cornea in some areas. In some eyes only a few small areas of iris may be involved. In others the entire circumference of the tra-

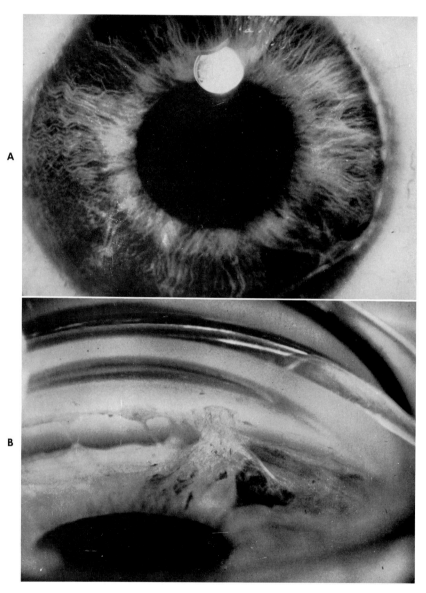

Fig. 17-19. A, Goniodysgenesis (Axenfeld's syndrome) showing posterior embryotoxon. **B,** Goniophotograph of Axenfeld's syndrome, showing iris adhesion to Schwalbe's line. **C,** Goniophotograph of syndrome in brown eye, showing prominent Schwalbe's line with tentlike iris adhesions. **D,** Goniophotograph of syndrome, showing extensive iris adhesions to Schwalbe's line. (**A** and **B** from Wuest, F. C., and Erdbrink, W. L.: Amer. J. Ophthal. **51:**148, 1961.)

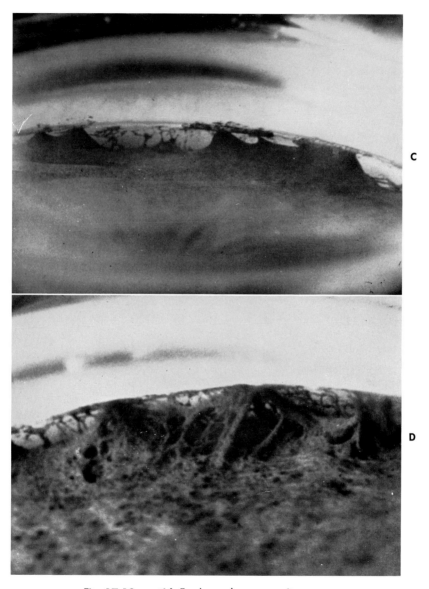

Fig. 17-19, cont'd. For legend see opposite page.

becular meshwork is concealed by the iris curtain. The syndrome sometimes occurs in eyes with microcornea.

Rieger's syndrome refers to a dysgenesis that features bilateral hypoplasia of the iris stroma, posterior embryotoxon and the associated angle anomalies, plus pupillary distortion, polycoria, and a high likelihood of glaucoma. In addition to glaucoma, other defects, usually dental, may be present in Rieger's syndrome. When glaucoma occurs, it usually develops during the first to the third decades, but infrequently presents in infancy.

Peter's anomaly (Fig. 17-20) involves the central portion of the cornea and iris collarette. The adherent iris froms a ring of stroma extending forward to adhere at a defect in Descemet's membrane. Adjacent to the adhesion is a central corneal opacity. These findings are present with or without iridocorneal angle anomalies and glaucoma.

Frequently mesodermal dysgenesis accompanies ectopia of the pupil and polycoria. In these syndromes no new synechias are formed, such as occur in essential iris atrophy. Cataracts are occasionally part of the picture. The syndrome is extremely variable in its expression, with the full-blown disease in one member of a family and only minimal signs in another.

Treatment for goniodysgenesis is the same as that for open-angle glaucoma. If surgery becomes necessary, external filtering operations are needed. Goniotomy can cut off the iris adhesions but does not often permanently lower pressure. Many such eyes do not develop glaucoma.

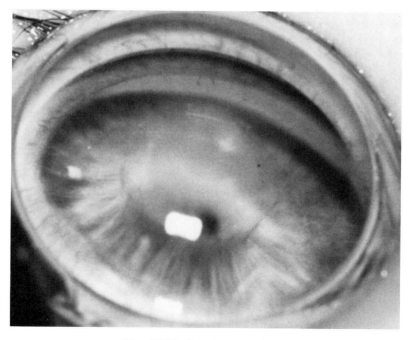

Fig. 17-20. Peter's anomaly.

Lowe's syndrome (oculocerebrorenal syndrome) (Fig. 17-21)

Lowe's syndrome, a rare type of congenital glaucoma. is genetically determined and probably sex linked, since it is seen predominantly in males. The inborn error in metabolism produces children who are mentally retarded, often to the idiot level. They have a disturbance of amino acid metabolism, resulting in aminoaciduria. The ocular signs include cataracts in 50% to 90% and glaucoma that resembles infantile glaucoma. Fine lens opacities are frequently found in the mother. Most investigators believe that the glaucoma is due to an incomplete angle cleavage. Pathologically, the iris may extend onto the trabecular meshwork. Microphakia is a common associated finding.

Some eyes have been cured by goniotomy, and from the results obtained in the few patients studied, this appears to be the procedure of choice at present. It should be remembered that aminoaciduria may be normally present in infants up to the age of 3 to 4 months.

Microcornea

In microcornea (Fig. 17-22) the eye is usually hyperopic and has a cornea whose horizontal diameter is usually less than 10 mm, with such shallow chambers and narrow angles that an attack of acute glaucoma can occur at any time. Symptoms, signs, and treatment are the same as for angle-closure glaucoma. Iridencleisis, trabeculectomy, or a guarded thermal sclerostomy should be considered when filtering surgery is needed in these narrow-angled eyes. The incarcerated

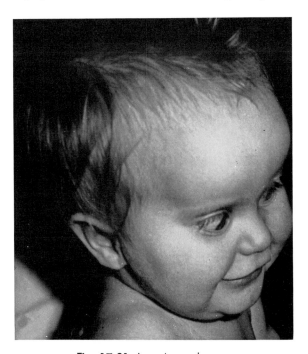

Fig. 17-21. Lowe's syndrome.

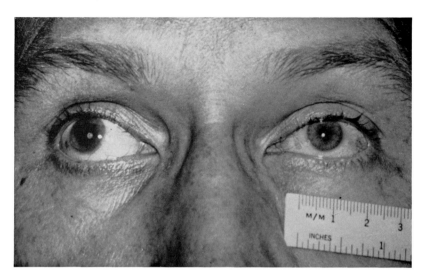

Fig. 17-22. Microcornea.

and retracted iris with iridenclesis will widen the angle area opposite the surgical incision. There are some eyes with microcornea whose angles are definitely open, sometimes to Grade 3, but that have decreased facility of outflow, increased tension, and clinical course similar to open-angle glaucoma. A few of such eyes also show the classic features of Axenfeld's syndrome.

Spherophakia (Marchesani's syndrome)
(Fig. 17-23)

Marchesani described a syndrome that includes microspherophakia, brachycephaly, brachydactyly, flexure deformities, a short pyknic build, and mental retardation. The lens is so reduced in diameter that its edges can often be seen through a mid-dilated pupil. High degrees of myopia are usually present and should alert one to this diagnosis, especially in young persons. The high myopia and iridodonesis caused by the spherical lens become worse when the lens subluxates, usually downwards. Such lenses tend to dislocate when patients are in the teens or early twenties (Fig. 17-23). The lens causes pupillary block and angle-closure glaucoma that is increased by miotics. An acute attack can be broken by intense mydriasis, iridectomy, or lens extraction. Iridectomy permits the use of miotics. The long-term prognosis is not good, in part because most cases are not diagnosed until permanent synechias have closed the angle and marked visual loss has occurred.

Mesodermal dysgenesis of the anterior chamber angle can be associated with the syndrome. A recessive genetic pattern is the rule, but the condition may appear as a dominant trait.

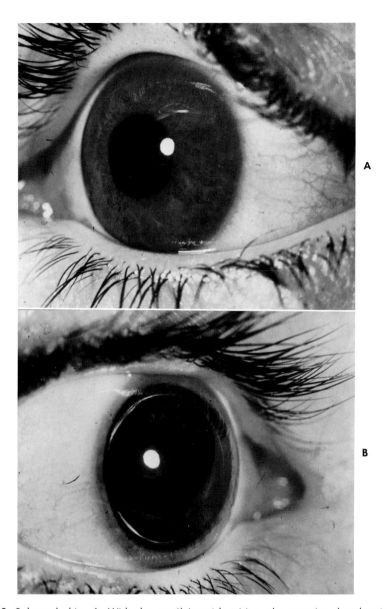

Fig. 17-23. Spherophakia. **A,** With the pupil in midposition, the anterior chamber is shallow, pupillary block and angle closure are present, and the intraocular pressure is elevated. **B,** In the other eye the pupil is widely dilated, the pupillary block is broken, and the anterior chamber angle has opened. Note the reflex of the spherical lens just inside the pupillary border.

Rubella (Fig. 17-24)

Glaucoma occurs in 10% to 25% of infants with proved rubella syndrome. This is much lower than the incidence of congenital cataracts, mental retardation, deafness, and cardiac anomalies concurrent with rubella. These cases present a very special problem in diagnosis and management.

Rubella keratitis, often of relatively short duration, causes corneal clouding with or without pressure elevation. When present, the corneal haze is deep, diffuse, or disciform, resisting attempts at clearing by removal of epithelium. Care must be taken not to confuse keratitis with the corneal edema of glaucoma.

Rubella glaucoma can be permanent or transient. Proved rubella with increased pressure, corneal edema, and disc changes may subside completely in a few weeks without therapy. An inflammatory reaction is probably responsible for this transient condition that is best managed medically. However, developmental defects of the angle do occur in some rubella patients. This group of cases represents the percentage developing a permanent pressure rise and responds best to goniotomy. Gonioscopically and pathologically, the anterior chamber appears not unlike that of typical congenital glaucoma.

Confusion caused by inconsistencies in rubella cases calls for conservative management until a diagnosis of true congenital glaucoma can be established. When management is questionable, it is advisable to use carbonic anhydrase inhibi-

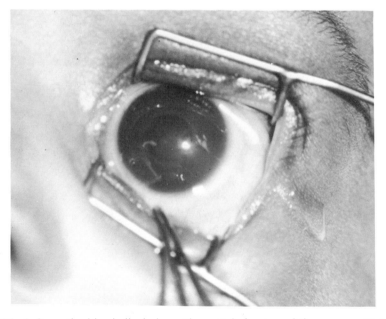

Fig. 17-24. A 3-month-old rubella baby with partial clearing of the cornea. At 1 month, pressure was 32 mm Hg in both eyes, with marked corneal clouding. Pressure gradually normalized without surgery, and the corneas cleared completely by 6 months of age.

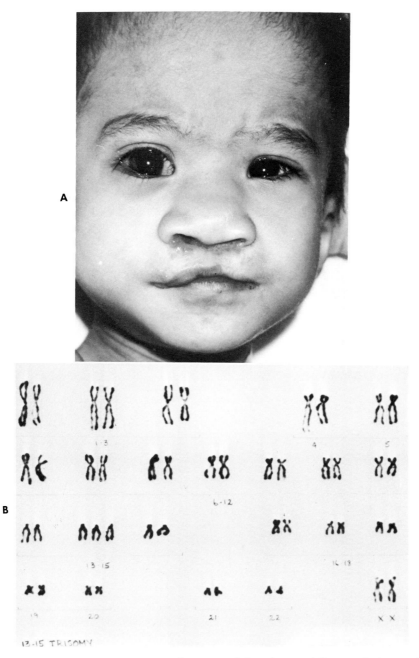

Fig. 17-25. A, Child with unilateral glaucoma, cleft palate and lip, renal abnormalities, and mental retardation caused by a trisomy 13-15 (D) pattern. **B,** Example of trisomy pattern.

tors to control pressure for a few weeks to see if the abnormal findings clear spontaneously.

Chromosome abnormalities (trisomy 13-15 [D]; trisomy 17-18 [F]) (Fig. 17-25)

In some infants with multiple congenital anomalies, chromosome analysis of leukocytes or dermal cells in mitosis reveals chromosome abnormalities of trisomy 13-15 (D) or 17-18 (F). Congenital glaucoma occurs, caused by incomplete cleavage of mesoderm in the anterior chamber angle. Other ocular defects include microphthalmos, colobomas, optic atrophy, retinal dysplasia, and cataracts. A variety of general deformities such as deafness, cleft lip and palate, microcephaly, and maldevelopment of the hands and feet, kidneys, and heart occur. These infants are mentally retarded and usually die very early in life.

Broad thumb syndrome (Rubinstein-Taybi syndrome) (Fig. 17-26)

Congenital glaucoma has been discovered in patients with broad thumbs and great toes. Radiologic evidence of these abnormalities of the phalanges are reported in various combinations with mental and motor retardation, highly arched palate, lid colobomas, unusual facial features, strabismus, and cataract. Chromosome patterns have been normal.

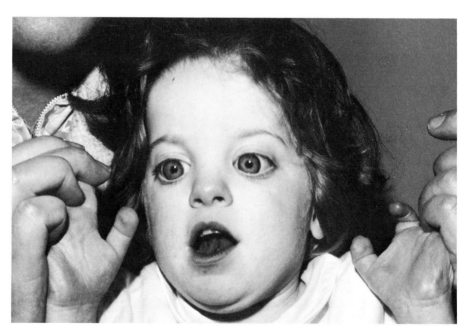

Fig. 17-26. Broad thumb syndrome and congenital glaucoma. (Courtesy Dr. R. J. Keefe, San Francisco.)

Persistent hyperplastic primary vitreous

Typically, persistent hyperplastic primary vitreous occurs unilaterally in a microphthalmic eye. The white retrolental mass is made up of the primary vitreous plus the remains of the hyaloid arterial system. Many eyes have been enucleated with the mistaken diagnosis of retinoblastoma. The clinical course is varied, but there tends to be progressive extension of the opacification into the lens, which becomes cataractous. Swelling of the lens or iris bombé can produce angle-closure glaucoma. More frequently, after the fourth month of life, massive and repeated hemorrhages into the eye occur, with secondary glaucoma. No definitive treatment can be suggested.

SECONDARY GLAUCOMA IN INFANTS

It is theoretically possible for infants to develop any of the secondary glaucomas to which adults are susceptible. Only a few of the more common types can be mentioned.

Retrolental fibroplasia

Since premature infants have been receiving only the absolute minimum amount of oxygen consistent with survival, the dread disease retrolental fibroplasia has become very rare. Some reports, however, suggest that the disease again may become more frequent. When it occurs, the combination of retinal edema and the contraction of the retrolental fibrous tissue forces the lens forward, causing a very shallow anterior chamber and angle closure in some cases. Ciliary processes can be seen peripherally, made visible by the pull of the contracting connective tissue or the ciliary body. Pressure levels are usually not very high, and surgical intervention is usually not helpful. Occasionally, if an acute attack occurs, a peripheral iridectomy may be helpful.

Tumors

Glaucoma in infants may result from intraocular tumors.

Retinoblastoma

Retinoblastoma is the commonest tumor of infancy that can produce glaucoma. In the late stages, pain and enlargement of the globe occur. It is diagnosed by the ophthalmoscopic demonstration of the intraocular tumor. Occasionally the finding of calcifications in the tumor by x-ray examination proves helpful.

Juvenile xanthogranuloma (nevoxanthoendothelioma) (Fig. 17-27)

Juvenile xanthogranuloma, an uncommon benign xanthomatous skin disease, has its onset in infancy and slowly subsides spontaneously over a period of years. It is characterized by widespread yellow to orange skin nodules, which are present at or shortly after birth in most cases. Skin lesions appear in crops and regress spontaneously. Some authors regard this as a form of Hand-Schüller-Christian

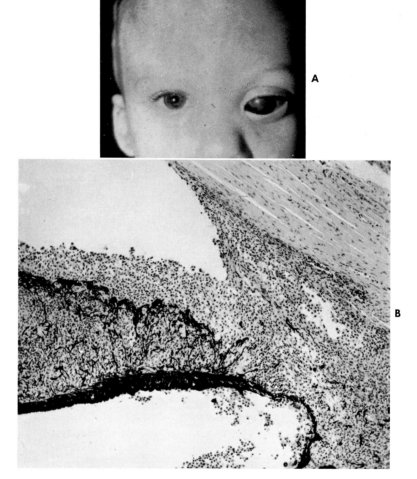

Fig. 17-27. A, Child with unilateral glaucoma secondary to xanthogranuloma of the iris. **B,** Xanthogranuloma of the iris with obstruction of the trabecular meshwork. (**A** courtesy Dr. T. E. Sanders, St. Louis; **B** from AFIP collection.)

disease. Histologically, these tumors consist of lipid-filled histiocytes. Fever and proptosis are rarely encountered, and there may be radiologic evidence of bone destruction. Glaucoma results when there is an anterior chamber hemorrhage or the angle is involved with the neoplastic tissue.

Ocular involvement described includes vascularized lesions in the iris and ciliary body as well as one report of an epibulbar mass. A salmon-colored or yellowish thickening of the iris or angle is seen, and anterior chamber hemorrhages occur. Any infant seen with a spontaneous anterior chamber hemorrhage and secondary glaucoma should be suspected of having this disease. A biopsy of one of the skin lesions establishes the diagnosis, but such skin nodules are not always present.

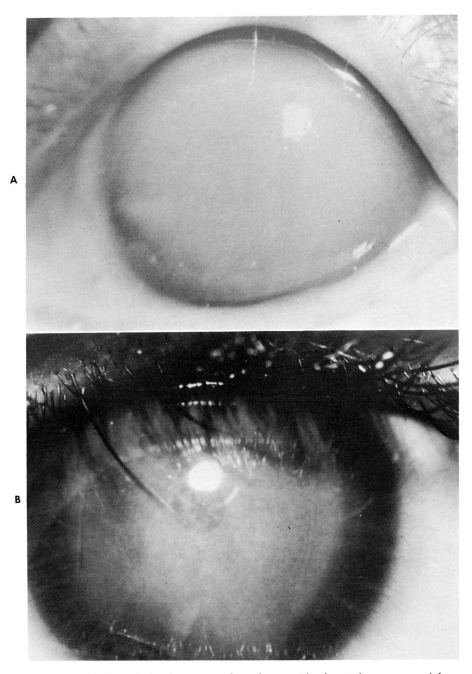

Fig. 17-28. A, Unilateral cloudy cornea of newborn, with elevated pressure and forceps injury to face. **B,** One year later, tension was normal, with gradual corneal clearing. (Courtesy Dr. D. Loeb, San Francisco.)

Since the skin lesions subside spontaneously, if the glaucoma can be controlled with acetazolamide (Diamox), the ocular lesions may also disappear. Systemic and subconjunctival steroids sometimes result in a regression of this lesion. Rapid regression has also been reported after x-ray therapy. Small doses (200 R) should be used. Larger or repeated doses risk production of cataract but may be necessary to save the eye.

Inflammation

Keratitis and uveitis in utero or in infancy can result in damage to the outflow mechanism and increased tension. The glaucoma can be caused by angle closure or it may be open angle in type. It differs from the adult forms only by the capacity of the infant eye to stretch when subjected to increased pressure. Therapy is the same as that for adult secondary glaucoma of similar etiology.

Trauma (Fig. 17-28)

Infants and children are unhappily prone to suffer blunt and penetrating injuries. The glaucoma resulting from such injuries depends on the nature and extent of the direct damage as well as on the consequences of hemorrhages and the surgical repair.

Treatment of penetrating injuries consists of prompt repair. Hemorrhages require bed rest, sedation, and a regimen much as for adults (Chapter 14).

Birth injuries, especially those due to forceps damage, can present a very difficult problem in the differential diagnosis of congenital glaucoma. Skin evidence of trauma to the periorbal area should be helpful when the glaucoma is unilateral. Injury may produce a transient elevation of pressure in which surgery is contraindicated. Conservative management with acetazolamide for a few weeks is recommended. Breaks in Descemet's membrane with corneal edema are the typical findings; usually the eye will be hypotonic. Edema usually disappears in a few weeks when Descemet's membrane has healed.

PROBLEMS FOR CONSIDERATION

It is generally agreed that the developmental anomalies of the anterior chamber angle of the eye are responsible for infantile glaucoma. The exact nature of these anomalies and especially the manner in which obstruction to aqueous outflow occurs are uncertain. Additional histologic studies and careful electron microscopic studies are required. An impermeable endothelial layer lying over the trabecular meshwork has been described by some observers. Careful electron microscopic studies should be able to verify the existence of such a membrane or offer new explanations for the mechanism of this disease. Histochemical techniques for identification of the angle abnormality and better in vivo methods should be sought. Few electron microscopic descriptions of the angle structures in normal infant eyes are available, and additional studies are needed to verify this finding.

Reports suggest that rubella may be much more important than previously thought in many ocular developmental diseases. The roles of this and other viruses as etiologic factors in infantile glaucoma should be investigated. Rubella keratitis has been described as a cause of corneal cloudiness even when not associated with infantile glaucoma. The differential diagnosis of these conditions can be quite difficult, and better diagnostic criteria are needed.

Few studies have been performed to establish values for intraocular pressure and outflow facility in normal infant eyes. If these parameters are to be intelligently used in the management of eyes with infantile glaucoma, better information on normal eyes must be obtained. This will require rigid standardization of depth of anesthesia and the use of applanation tonometers in the horizontal position. Reliable hand applanation tonometers should permit accurate pressure determinations even in the unanesthetized infant. New, controlled studies of the effects of various anesthetic agents on intraocular pressure and outflow facility are needed. Since deep anesthesia is required to obtain pressure-outflow values in infants, the effects of anesthetic agents may be of considerable importance in the management of children with the disease.

Whereas the delineation of the anatomic abnormalities of infantile glaucoma requires additional histologic study, the mechanism of action of the surgery used to correct these abnormalities is in equal need of such study. Goniotomy has been used for about thirty-five years and has proved to be an effective surgical procedure. However, few follow-up studies have been made of eyes that have had successful goniotomies. Careful tonographic, gonioscopic, and histologic evaluation of these eyes would be of considerable value in determining the mechanism of action of goniotomy.

Although presently used surgical methods are successful in most eyes with infantile glaucoma, many eyes are not controlled and continue to show progressive damage. There is good reason to suggest that the failure of some surgical procedure may be as much related to the scarring and damage produced by the surgery as to the disease itself. Present surgical techniques may be too gross to perform accurately a procedure that may be so delicate it requires the incision of a membrane one cell layer thick. Carefully controlled microsurgery with visualization of the angle structures under high magnification and perhaps even with motor-driven stereotactic instruments that can be accurately positioned may be used to help define the mechanism of action of surgical procedures.

Certain congenital metabolic diseases are often associated with anomalies of the chamber angle and infantile glaucoma. Increased knowledge of the metabolic defects in such diseases as homocystinuria, Lowe's syndrome, and Marfan's syndrome may provide valuable clues to the biochemical regulation of cleavage and development of the angle structures.

References—Section V

Abbassi, V., Lowe, C. U., and Calcagno, P. L.: Oculo-cerebro-renal syndrome; a review, Amer. J. Dis. Child. **115**:145, 1968.

Alkemade, P. P. H.: Dysgenesis mesodermalis of the iris and the cornea, Springfield, Ill., 1969, Charles C Thomas, Publisher.

Allen, R. A., Straatsma, B. R., Apt, L., and Hall, M. O.: Ocular manifestations of Marfan's syndrome, Trans. Amer. Acad. Ophthal. Otolaryng. **71**:1, 1967.

Anderson, J. R.: Hydrophthalmia or congenital glaucoma, London, 1939, Cambridge University Press.

Armaly, M. F.: Effect of corticosteroids on intraocular pressure and fluid dynamics. I. The effect of dexamethasone in the normal eye, Arch. Ophthal. **70**:482, 1963.

Armaly, M. F.: Effect of corticosteroids on intraocular pressure and fluid dynamics. II. The effect of dexamethasone in the glaucomatous eye, Arch. Ophthal. **70**:492, 1963.

Armaly, M. F.: The heritable nature of dexamethasone-induced ocular hypertension, Arch. Ophthal. **75**:32, 1966.

Ashton, N., Shakib, M., Collyer, R., and Blach, R.: Electron microscopic study of pseudoexfoliation of the lens capsule. I. Lens capsule and zonular fibers, Invest. Ophthal. **4**:141, 1965.

Ballintine, E. J.: Clinical tonography, Cleveland, 1954, American Academy of Ophthalmology and Otolaryngology.

Barkan, O., and others: Symposium: The infantile form of congenital glaucoma, Trans. Amer. Acad. Ophthal. Otolaryng. **59**:322, 1955.

Becker, B.: Intraocular pressure response to topical corticosteroids, Invest. Ophthal. **4**:198, 1965.

Becker, B., and Hahn, K. A.: Topical cortico-steroids and heredity in primary open-angle glaucoma, Amer. J. Ophthal. **57**:543, 1964.

Becker, B., Keskey, G. R., and Christensen, R. E.: Hypersecretion glaucoma, Arch. Ophthal. **56**:180, 1956.

Becker, B., and Kolker, A. E.: Topical steroid testing in conditions related to glaucoma. In Schwartz, B., editor: Corticosteroids and the eye, vol. 6, Boston, 1966, Little, Brown & Co.

Becker, B., Kolker, A. E., and Roth, F. D.: Glaucoma family study, Amer. J. Ophthal. **50**:557, 1960.

Becker, B., and Mills, D. W.: Corticosteroids and intraocular pressure, Arch. Ophthal. **70**:500, 1963.

Becker, B., and Morton, W. R.: Phenylthiourea taste testing and glaucoma, Arch. Ophthal. **72**:323, 1964.

Becker, B., and Ramsey, C. K.: Plasma cortisol and the intraocular pressure response to topical corticosteroids, Amer. J. Ophthal. **69**:999, 1970.

Becker, B., and Shin, D. H.: Response to topical epinephrine—a practical prognostic test in patients with ocular hypertension, Arch. Ophthal. (To be published.)

Bertelsen, T. I., Drablös, P. A., and Flood, P. R.: The so-called senile exfoliation (pseudoexfoliation) of the anterior lens capsule, a product of the lens epithelium. Fibrillopathia epitheliocapsularis. A microscopic, histochemic, and electron microscopic investigation, Acta Ophthal. **42**:1096, 1964.

Bito, L. Z., and Salvador, E. V.: Intraocular fluid dynamics. III. The site and mechanism of prostaglandin transfer across the blood intraocular fluid barriers, Exp. Eye Res. **14**:233, 1972.

Blanton, F. M.: Anterior chamber angle re-

318

cession and secondary glaucoma, Arch. Ophthal. **72:**39, 1964.

Burian, H. M., and Allen, L.: Histologic study of the chamber angle of patients with Marfan's syndrome, Arch. Ophthal. **65:**323, 1961.

Burian, H. M., Braley, A. E., and Allen, L.: External and gonioscopic visibility of the ring of Schwalbe, Trans. Amer. Ophthal. Soc. **52:**389, 1954.

Buxton, J. N., and Preston, R. W.: Tonography in cornea guttata, Arch. Ophthal. **77:**602, 1967.

Chandler, P. A.: Narrow-angle glaucoma, Arch. Ophthal. **47:**695, 1952.

Chandler, P. A., Simmons, R. J., and Grant, W. M.: Malignant glaucoma; medical and surgical treatment, Amer. J. Ophthal. **66:**495, 1968.

Clark, W. B., editor: Symposium on glaucoma, St. Louis, 1959, The C. V. Mosby Co.

Cross, H. E., and Jensen, A. D.: Ocular manifestations in Marfan's syndrome and homocystinuria, Amer. J. Ophthal. **75:**405, 1973.

Crouch, E. R., and Frenkel, M.: Amino caproic acid in the treatment of traumatic hyphema, Amer. J. Ophthal. **81:**355, 1976.

Curran, E. J.: A new operation for glaucoma involving a new principle in etiology and treatment of chronic primary glaucoma, Arch. Ophthal. **49:**131, 1920.

Curtin, V. T., Joyce, E. E., and Ballin, N.: Ocular pathology in oculo-cerebro-renal syndrome of Lowe, Amer. J. Ophthal. **64:**533, 1967.

Dickson, D. H., and Ramsay, M. S.: Fibrillopathia epitheliocapsularis (pseudoexfoliation): a clinical and electron microscopic study, Canad. J. Ophthal. **10:**149, 1975.

Duke-Elder, S., editor: System of ophthalmology. Vol. III. Normal and abnormal development, Part 2: Congenital deformities, St. Louis, 1963, The C. V. Mosby Co.

Duke-Elder, E., editor: System of ophthalmology. Vol. XI. Diseases of the lens and vitreous; glaucoma and hypotony, St. Louis, 1969, The C. V. Mosby Co.

Duque-Estrada, M. W.: L'hypertension oculaire dans le syndrome de Weill-Marchesani, Bull. Soc. Franc. Ophtal. **64:**729, 1961.

Eakins, K. E., Whitelocke, R. A. F., Bennett, A., and Martenet, A. C.: Prostaglandin-like activity in ocular inflammation, Brit. Med. J. **3:**454, 1972.

Feibel, R. M., and Bigger, J. F.: Rubeosis iridis and neovascular glaucoma; evaluation of cyclocryotherapy, Amer. J. Ophthal. **74:**5, 1972.

Fralick, F. B.: Symposium: Office management of the primary glaucomas, Trans. Amer. Acad. Ophthal. Otolaryng. **64:**105, 1960.

Goldmann, H.: Some basic problems of simple glaucoma, Amer. J. Ophthal. **48:**213, 1959.

Grant, W. M., and Walton, D. S.: Distinctive gonioscopic findings in glaucoma due to neurofibromatosis, Arch. Ophthal. **79:**127, 1968.

Hansen, E., and Sellevold, O. J.: Pseudoexfoliation of the lens capsule. I. Clinical evaluation with special regard to the presence of glaucoma, Acta Ophthal. **45:**1095, 1968.

Haut, J., and Joannides, Z.: A propos de 55 cas de syndrome de Lowe, Arch. Ophthal. **26:**21, 1966.

Henkind, P., and Ashton, N.: Ocular pathology in homocystinuria, Trans. Ophthal. Soc. U.K. **85:**21, 1965.

Henkind, P., Siegel, I. M., and Carr, R. E.: Mesodermal dysgenesis of the anterior segment: Rieger's anomaly, Arch. Ophthal. **73:**810, 1965.

Hoskins, H. D., Jr.: Neovascular glaucoma: current concepts, Trans. Amer. Acad. Ophthal. Otolaryng. **78:**330, 1974.

Hyams, S. W., Friedman, Z., and Neumann, E.: Elevated intraocular pressure in the prone position, Amer. J. Ophthal. **66:**661, 1968.

Jensen, A. D., Cross, H. E., and Paton, D.: Ocular complications in the Weill-Marchesani syndrome, Amer. J. Ophthal. **77:**261, 1974.

Jerndal, T.: Goniodysgenesis and hereditary juvenile glaucoma, Goteborg, 1970, Elanders Boktryckeri Aktiebolag.

Kass, M. A., Kolker, A. E., and Becker, B.: Chronic topical corticosteroid use simulating congenital glaucoma, J. Pediat. **81:**1175, 1972.

Kass, M. A., Kolker, A. E., and Becker, B.: Glaucomatocyclitic crisis and primary openangle glaucoma, Amer. J. Ophthal. **75:**668, 1973.

Kayes, J., and Becker, B.: The human trabecular meshwork in corticosteroid-induced glaucoma, Trans. Amer. Ophthal. Soc. **67:**339, 1969.

Keith, C. G.: The ocular manifestations of trisomy 13-15, Trans. Ophthal. Soc. U.K. **86:**435, 1966.

Kirsch, R. E.: Glaucoma following cataract extraction associated with use of alpha-chymotrypsin, Arch. Ophthal. **72:**612, 1964.

Kirsch, R. E.: A study of provocative tests for angle closure glaucoma, Arch. Ophthal. **74:**770, 1965.

Kwitko, M. L.: Glaucoma in infants and children, New York, 1973, Appleton-Century-Crofts.

Larsen, J. S.: Senile exfoliation (pseudo-exfoliation, fibrillopathia epithelio-capsularis) of the lens capsule in a postmortem material, Acta Ophthal. **47:**679, 1969.

Layden, W. M., and Shaffer, R. N.: Exfoliation syndrome, Trans. Amer. Ophthal. Soc. **71:**128, 1973.

Levene, R. Z., and Schwartz, B.: Depression of plasma cortisol and the steroid ocular pressure response, Arch. Ophthal. **80:**461, 1968.

Leydhecker, W.: Glaukom, ein Handbuch, Berlin, 1959, Springer-Verlag.

Lieberman, T. W., Podos, S. M., and Hartstein, J.: Acute glaucoma, ectopia lentis and homocystinuria, Amer. J. Ophthal. **61:**252, 1966.

Lowe, C. U., Terrey, M., and MacLachlan, E. A.: Organic-aciduria, decreased renal ammonia production, hydrophthalmos, and mental retardation; a clinical entity, Amer. J. Dis. Child. **83:**164, 1952.

Lowe, R. F.: Acute angle-closure glaucoma: the second eye; an analysis of 200 cases, Brit. J. Ophthal. **46:**641, 1962.

Lowe, R. F.: Primary angle-closure glaucoma; a review of provocative tests, Brit. J. Ophthal. **51:**727, 1967.

Mann, I.: Development of the human eye, ed. 3, New York, 1964, Grune & Stratton, Inc.

Marchesani, O.: Brachydaktylie und angeborene Kugellinse als Systemerkrankung, Klin. Mbl. Augenheilk. **103:**1392, 1939.

Maumenee, A. E.: The pathogenesis of congenital glaucoma: a new theory, Trans. Amer. Ophthal. Soc. **56:** 507, 1958.

Maumenee, A. E., Paton, D., Morse, P. H., and Butner, R.: Review of 40 histologically proven cases of epithelial downgrowth following cataract extraction and suggested surgical management, Amer. J. Ophthal. **69:**598, 1970.

Minas, T. F., and Podos, S. M.: Familial glaucoma associated with elevated episcleral venous pressure, Arch. Ophthal. **80:**202, 1968.

Neufeld, A. H., and Sears, M. L.: The site of action of prostaglandin E$_2$ on the disruption of the blood-aqueous barrier in the rabbit eye, Exp. Eye Res. **17:**445, 1973.

Podos, S. M., Becker, B., and Kass, M. A.: Prostaglandin synthesis, inhibition, and intraocular pressure, Invest. Ophthal. **12:**426, 1973.

Podos, S. M., Joffe, B. M., and Becker, B.: Prostaglandins and glaucoma, Brit. Med. J. **4:**232, 1972.

Reese, A. B., and Ellsworth, R. M.: The anterior chamber cleavage syndrome, Arch. Ophthal. **75:**307, 1966.

Richardson, K. T., and Shaffer, R. N.: Optic-nerve cupping in congenital glaucoma, Amer. J. Ophthal. **62:**507, 1966.

Rieger, H.: Beiträge zur Kenntnis seltener Missbildungen der Iris, Arch. Ophthal. **133:**602, 1935.

Rohen, J. W., Linner, E., and Witmer, R.: Electron microscopic studies on the trabecular meshwork in two cases of corticosteroid-glaucoma, Exp. Eye Res. **17:**19, 1973.

Roy, F. H., Summit, R. L., Hiatt, R. L., and Hughes, J. G.: Ocular manifestations of the Rubinstein-Taybi syndrome, Arch. Ophthal. **79:**272, 1968.

Schwartz, A.: Chronic open-angle glaucoma secondary to rhegmatogenous retinal detachment, Amer. J. Ophthal. **75:**205, 1973.

Schwartz, J. T., Reuling, F. H., Feinleib, M., Garrison, R. J., and Collie, D. J.: Twin study on ocular pressure following topically applied dexamethasone. II. Inheritance of variation in pressure response, Arch. Ophthal. **90:**281, 1973.

Sears, D., and Sears, M.: Blood-aqueous barrier and alpha-chymotrypsin glaucoma in rabbits, Amer. J. Ophthal. **77:**378, 1974.

Sears, M. L., Neufeld, A. H., and Jampol, L. M.: Prostaglandins, Invest. Ophthal. **12:**161, 1973.

Shaffer, R. N.: The role of vitreous detachment in aphakic and malignant glaucoma, Trans. Amer. Acad. Ophthal. Otolaryng. **58:**217, 1954.

Shaffer, R. N.: A review of angle-closure glaucoma. In Newell, F. W., editor: Glaucoma: Transactions of the First Conference, New York, 1956, Josiah Macy, Jr., Foundation.

Shaffer, R. N : New concepts in infantile glaucoma, Trans. Ophthal. Soc. U.K. **87:**581, 1967.

Shaffer, R. N.: The role of the astroglial cells in glaucomatous disc cupping, Docum. Ophthal. **26:**516, 1969.

Shaffer, R. N., and Hetherington, J., Jr.: The glaucomatous disc in infants, Trans. Amer. Acad. Ophthal. Otolaryng. **73:**929, 1969.

Shaffer, R. N., and Weiss, D. I.: Congenital and pediatric glaucomas, St. Louis, 1970, The C. V. Mosby Co.

Shin, D. H., Kolker, A. E., Kass, M. A., and Becker, B.: Long-term epinephrine therapy for ocular hypertension, Arch. Ophthal. (To be published.)

Shin, D. H., Waltman, S. R., Palmberg, P. F., and Becker, B.: HLA-B12 and HLA-B7 in primary open-angle glaucoma. (To be published.)

Sugar, H. S.: Pigmentary glaucoma; a 25 year review, Amer. J. Ophthal. **62:**499, 1966.

Sunde, O. A.: On the so-called senile exfoliation of the anterior lens capsule: a clinical and anatomical study, Acta Ophthal., supp. 45, p. 1, 1956.

Tarkkanen, A.: Pseudoexfoliation of the lens capsule, Acta Ophthal., supp. 71, 1962.

Theobold, G. D.: Pseudo-exfoliation of the lens capsule: relation to "true" exfoliation of the lens capsule as reported in the literature and role in production of glaucoma capsulocuticulare, Amer. J. Ophthal. 37:1, 1954.

Tonjum, A. M.: Intraocular pressure disturbances early after ocular contusion, Acta Ophthal. **46:**874, 1968.

Tonjum, A. M.: Intraocular pressure and facility of outflow late after ocular contusion, Acta Ophthal. **46:**886, 1968.

Van Herick, W., Shaffer, R. N., and Schwartz, A.: Width of chamber angle, Amer. J. Ophthal. **68:**626, 1969.

Vannas, A.: Fluorescein angiography of the vessels of the iris in pseudoexfoliations of the lens capsule, Acta Ophthal. **105**(supp.):1, 1969.

Waardenburg, P. J., and others: Genetics and ophthalmology, vol. 2, Springfield, Ill., Charles C Thomas, Publisher.

Wachtel, J. G.: The ocular pathology of Marfan's syndrome, Arch. Ophthal. **76:**512, 1966.

Winter, F.: The second eye in acute, primary, shallow-chamber angle glaucoma, Amer. J. Ophthal. **40:**557, 1955.

Wolff, S. M., and Zimmerman, L. E.: Chronic secondary glaucoma associated with retro-displacement of iris root and deepening of the anterior chamber angle secondary to contusion, Amer. J. Ophthal. **54:**547, 1962.

Worst, J. G. F.: The pathogenesis of congenital glaucoma, Springfield, Ill., 1966, Charles C Thomas, Publisher.

Wyllie, A. M., and Wyllie, J. H.: Prostaglandins and glaucoma, Brit. Med. J. **3:**615, 1971.

Zink, H. A., Palmberg, P. F., and Bigger, J. F.: Increased sensitivity to theophylline associated with primary open-angle glaucoma, Invest. Ophthal. **12:**603, 1973.

Zink, H. A., Palmberg, P. F., Sugar, A., Sugar, H. S., Cantrill, H. L., Becker, B., and Bigger, J. F.: Comparison of in vitro corticosteroid response in pigmentary glaucoma and primary open-angle glaucoma, Amer. J. Ophthal. **80:**478, 1975.

Zink, H. A., Podos, S. M., and Becker, B.: Inhibition by imidazole of the increase in intraocular pressure induced by topical prostaglandin E_1, Nature [New Biol.] **245:**140, 1973.

SECTION **VI**

MEDICAL TECHNIQUES

In most large clinics the number of patients discovered to have open-angle glaucoma has increased dramatically, largely as a result of greater awareness of the disease and better methods for its detection. In spite of the increased number of patients, there has been a drastic decline in glaucoma surgery, with the sole exception of peripheral iridectomies for angle-closure glaucoma. The reduction in surgery for open-angle glaucoma does not reflect the lack of effective surgical procedures but rather is a consequence of better medical therapy. Moreover, surgery for angle-closure glaucoma is now more frequently successful, thanks to the newer medical agents that have made possible more adequate preparation for the surgery and a more leisurely evaluation of the decongested eye.

CHAPTER **20**   **HYPEROSMOTIC AGENTS AND OTHER MEDICATIONS**

CHAPTER **18**

Medications that increase the
facility of outflow

MIOTICS
Mechanism of action of miotics
Angle-closure glaucoma

In angle-closure glaucoma, agents that constrict the pupil are capable of relieving the obstructive effects of peripheral iris blocking the trabecular meshwork. This is a consequence of the pull of the pupillary sphincter, which reduces the volume of iris in the angle and tightens the iris periphery. However, constriction of the pupil increases the area of contact between the iris and lens, thus increasing the resistance between the posterior and anterior chambers and resulting in a greater tendency to iris bombè. This is particularly true in eyes with "flabby" peripheral irides. In most instances the milder miotics, for example, pilocarpine, carbachol, and neostigmine (Prostigmin), will permit greater access of aqueous humor to trabecular structures. The risk of inducing angle occlusion is greater with stronger miotics, for example, isoflurophate (DFP), demecarium bromide (Humorsol), and echothiophate (Phospholine), which produce more intense miosis, greater vascular congestion, and an initial pressure rise. Such anticholinesterase agents are difficult to reverse and are rarely indicated in the unoperated angle-closure glaucomas. After peripheral iridectomy these drugs may be used if necessary and are often most effective.

Open-angle glaucoma

In the open-angle glaucomas various miotics improve outflow facility. This is true of both normal eyes and those suffering from glaucoma. The mechanism here remains obscure. It does not appear to depend on the effects of the various agents on the sphincter of the pupil, for one may dilate the pupil with phenylephrine (Neo-Synephrine) without affecting the improved outflow facility. Their effectiveness may relate to the stimulation of ciliary musculature, resulting in a pull on the scleral spur or trabecular meshwork, or perhaps to direct cholinergic effects on those parts

325

of the trabecular meshwork bordering Schlemm's canal, which may constitute the major resistance site. Miotics in open-angle glaucoma do not constitute a cure of the basic outflow disorder. They merely relieve the obstructed outflow, thus lowering intraocular pressure and avoiding optic nerve damage.

Classification (Figs. 18-1 and 18-2)

The medications that act predominantly in increasing outflow facility may be classified as parasympathomimetic (cholinergic) agents, which presumably act on the motor end plate, and anticholinesterase drugs, which reversibly or irreversibly inhibit cholinesterase, permitting local accumulation of acetylcholine.

Parasympathomimetics

Parasympathomimetic agents act in the same way as acetylcholine. Acetylcholine itself may be used in the anterior chamber as a means of stimulating parasympathetic end organs in the iris, ciliary body, and trabecular meshwork. Unfortunately for the therapy of glaucoma, it penetrates the cornea poorly and is too evanescent because of its rapid destruction by cholinesterase.

Pilocarpine. Pilocarpine is the most important and useful miotic available. It has been in use since 1877 (Weber). It is an alkaloid obtained by extraction from *Pilocarpus microphyllus.* It is used as water-soluble hydrochloride or nitrate in

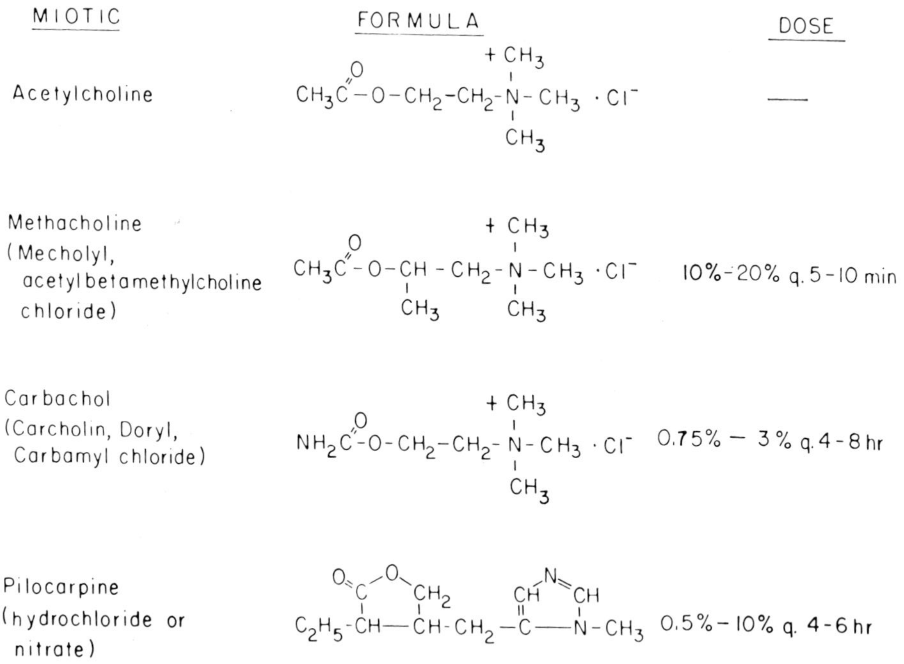

Fig. 18-1. Parasympathomimetic (cholinergic) agents.

solutions varying from 0.5% to 10%. It acts directly on parasympathetic organs. Miosis begins in 10 to 15 minutes and lasts 4 to 8 hours. The aqueous solutions are stable, they penetrate the cornea well and consistently, and there is a very low incidence of allergic reactions. It is wise to administer pilocarpine at least twice a day. It may be used chronically as often as every 4 hours or acutely as frequently as every minute. For prolonged administration there seems to be little advantage in using concentrations in excess of 4% or in applying more frequently than every 4 hours.

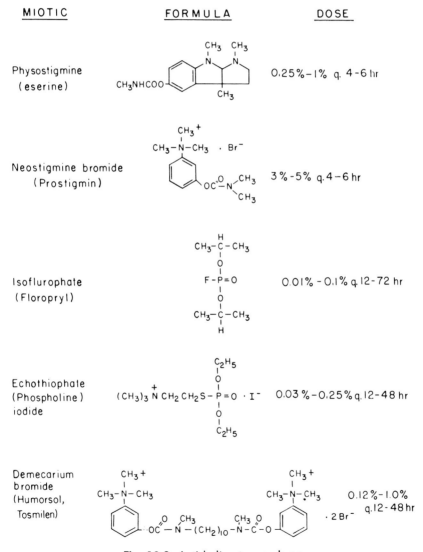

Fig. 18-2. Anticholinesterase drugs.

Methacholine chloride (acetyl-β-methylcholine; Mecholyl). Methacholine chloride is a synthetic, substituted acetylcholine, which is very short acting (less than 1 hour). It penetrates the cornea poorly and is used only in freshly prepared solutions. Concentrations of 10% to 20% are applied every 5 to 10 minutes in angle-closure glaucoma. Under these circumstances it is wise to precede its administration by a topical anesthetic to improve penetration. This drug is rarely used for long-term administration (2% to 3% solutions). It is contraindicated in asthmatic patients and is dangerous to use subconjunctivally or by retrobulbar injection. Systemic reactions are not infrequent and include sweating, flushing, an increase in pulse rate, and a fall in blood pressure.

Carbachol (carbamylcholine chloride; Carcholin; Doryl). Since carbachol is more resistant to splitting by cholinesterase, it is a longer-acting synthetic derivative of choline than is methacholine. It is somewhat stronger than pilocarpine but unfortunately does not penetrate as well. It is used for chronic administration in aqueous solutions of 0.75% to 3% every 4 to 8 hours. Better penetration may be obtained by its use in a petrolatum base ointment or with a wetting agent such as benzalkonium chloride (1:5000). Carbachol is an excellent replacement or alternate drug for pilocarpine or other miotics when resistance or intolerance has developed. This often permits carrying the patient along under good control with later possibility of returning to the original medication.

Anticholinesterase agents

By their inhibition of cholinesterase, anticholinesterase agents potentiate the action of acetylcholine on the parasympathetic end organs. In general, these agents are less well tolerated and produce more orbicularis, ciliary, and iris muscle spasm, irritation, hyperemia, and congestion of the globe than do the parasympathomimetics.

Physostigmine (eserine). Physostigmine was the first medical therapy used in the treatment of glaucoma (Laqueur, 1876). It is an alkaloid obtained from Calabar (or "ordeal") beans, the seeds of the vine *Physostigma venenosum.* Physostigmine temporarily inactivates cholinesterase. It is used in aqueous solution as a salicylate in concentration of 0.25% to 1% every 4 to 6 hours. It may also be used in ointment or as an alkaloid in oily vehicles. The drug is sensitive to light and heat and should not be used when it has turned red. It produces miosis in 30 minutes, persisting for many hours (12 to 36 hours). Eserine can rarely be used for long periods of time because of irritation and follicular hypertrophy of the palpebral conjunctiva.

Neostigmine (Prostigmin). Neostigmine is used as the bromide in concentrations of 3% to 5% every 4 to 6 hours. It is a synthetic anticholinesterase similar in action to physostigmine. It is more stable than eserine and causes less vascular congestion and folliculosis. A number of patients can tolerate it for long periods of time.

Isoflurophate (Floropryl; DFP). Isoflurophate is an extremely potent anticholinesterase agent. It has its major action against the nonspecific or pseudocholinesterases. It produces intense miosis associated with ciliary spasm and headache. Until such agents as pyridine-2-aldoxime methiodide (P_2AM) became available (p. 334), isoflurophate was considered an irreversible inhibitor of cholinesterase. Its greatest usefulness is in the open-angle glaucomas, particularly in aphakic glaucoma. Unfortunately it is rapidly hydrolyzed and inactivated by water. Touching the lids during application may get tears on the dropper and inactivate the solution. Isoflurophate was previously available as a 0.01% to 0.1% solution in anhydrous peanut oil. At present only a 0.025% ointment is marketed. Its side effects, uses, and contraindications are much the same as those of demecarium bromide and echothiophate.

Echothiophate iodide (Phospholine iodide). Echothiophate iodide is a white crystalline solid and a long-acting, potent cholinesterase inhibitor. It has much the same action as isoflurophate but is water soluble and more stable. It should be kept under refrigeration when in solution. It may be made up in concentrations of 0.03% to 0.25% and is used once every 12 to 48 hours. In the initial therapy of open-angle glaucoma, use of 0.06% echothiophate permits somewhat easier administration and better round-the-clock pressure control than is obtained with pilocarpine and with fewer side effects than with the 0.25% concentration of echothiophate. This has some additional advantages in young people, for the miosis and induced myopia are more constant. However the systemic and ocular side effects of echothiophate have led most ophthalmologists to start with pilocarpine and to reserve anticholinesterase agents for the patient who fails to respond to the parasympathomimetic agents.

Echothiophate iodide, 0.25%, induces miosis in about 30 minutes, lasting several days to three weeks. It improves outflow facility and reduces intraocular pressure in both normal and most glaucomatous eyes. Fortunately this agent is able to improve outflow facility even in some glaucomatous eyes not controlled by other miotics and carbonic anhydrase inhibitors (Fig. 29-15). Intraocular pressure can be normalized with echothiophate iodide for long periods in about 30% to 40% of eyes uncontrolled on other agents. Maximum effect is usually produced with the 0.125% concentration; only rarely is the 0.25% solution necessary.

Demecarium bromide (Humorsol; Tosmilen). Demecarium bromide is a long-acting, water-soluble cholinesterase inhibitor with considerable specificity for acetylcholinesterase. It is stable in solution and does not require refrigeration. It may be administered in concentrations of 0.12% to 1% at time intervals of 12 to 48 hours. The 0.12% solution is used much as is 0.06% echothiophate iodide. With the use of 0.25% demecarium bromide, some 30% to 55% of patients with uncontrolled glaucoma can be brought under reasonable control. If 1% solutions are used, the results are somewhat better than those with 0.25% echothiophate iodide. The 1% solution was clinically evaluated but never commercially marketed. Demecarium bromide was withdrawn from the market by the manufacturer several years ago, ostensibly because of packaging difficulties, but has been reintroduced and is now readily available.

Use

In the use of miotic agents it is wise to start with the weaker ones and lower concentrations and to work up to the higher concentrations and stronger anticholinesterase agents. Although opinions differ, there appears to be no special advantage to the use of mixtures of miotics. Rare instances of potentiation can be found, but more commonly the maximum effect of the combination can be obtained with one or the other of the agents when given in adequate concentration. Occasionally the use of more than one agent results in a decreased total effect. The use of combinations of miotics leads to the development of resistance to both agents and does not allow time for responsiveness of the eye to the original miotic to return. Frequently, after the use of an anticholinesterase and the avoidance of pilocarpine for a period of time, the patient responds again dramatically to the reinstitution of pilocarpine (Fig. 29-17).

In open-angle glaucomas there appear to be no contraindications to the use of topical epinephrine or carbonic anhydrase inhibitors with miotics. In fact, there is every indication that miotic therapy should be continued when secretory suppressants are used. It is important to reemphasize that the patient should know what medication he is taking and that the name and concentration of the agent should be on the label.

When the more potent miotic agents are to be used, especially in stronger concentrations, it has been found advisable to see the patient within the first few days of use. This permits better evaluation of response and side effects such as severe ocular reactions (iritis, acute angle closure, etc.). It is most important to repeat visual field studies within a short time after starting these drugs, to establish a new base line with the smaller pupils. The more intense miosis produced by these agents may reduce sensitivity and produce artifactual depression of the visual field. If this is not discovered for several months, progression of field loss is suspected.

If filtering surgery becomes necessary because of failure of medical control, it is wise to discontinue the administration of the ineffective anticholinesterase agent two to four weeks prior to the operation. Its continued use to the time of surgery leads to a greater inflammatory response in the eye, with increased chance for the formation of synechias and scarring. Pilocarpine may be substituted for the anticholinesterase drops during this interval.

Side effects

Ocular side effects

The side effects of all miotics are qualitatively similar but differ markedly in magnitude. They are much more common and severe with anticholinesterase drugs than with the parasympathomimetics. Ciliary and conjunctival congestion, ocular and periorbital pain, twitching lids, headaches, and accommodative myopia are frequent when any miotic is started. Pain is usually relieved by salicylates, and other side effects rarely persist beyond the first week of administration. Some patients are relieved of such side effects by starting with lower concentrations and gradually increasing to the desired strength. Most patients on miotic therapy have poor vision in dim light, making driving at night hazardous and best avoided if possible. Proliferation of pigment epithelium and nodular excrescences or cysts at the pupillary margin, frequently seen with the anticholinesterases, may further reduce the pupillary opening. The use of phenylephrine may inhibit such proliferations or make them less apparent. Rarely, pigmented cysts or proliferations of the epithelium of the ciliary body narrow the chamber angle. This and the increased pupillary block caused by the intense miosis may lead to angle closure. Occasionally vitreous hemorrhages and retinal detachments are seen, and rarely fibrinous iritis may occur. Allergic conjunctivitis and dermatitis are seen, and occasional instances of stenosis of the lacrimal canaliculi have been noted.

It is important to appreciate that many eyes subjected to anticholinesterase agents such as echothiophate iodide develop posterior synechias even in the absence of overt iritis. There is also considerable clinical evidence that cataracts occur

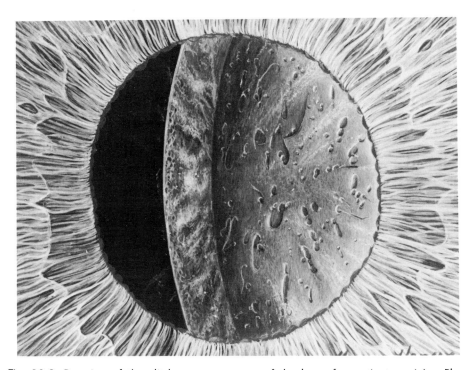

Fig. 18-3. Drawing of the slit-lamp appearance of the lens of a patient receiving Phospholine iodide. The patchy superficial opacification is seen in the direct beam. The vacuoles and irregular streaks are better visualized by retroillumination. (From Shaffer, R.N., and Hetherington, J., Jr.: Amer. J. Ophthal. **62:**613, 1966.)

more frequently and progress more rapidly in patients over 50 years of age treated with echothiophate iodide. The initial changes consist of collections of small vacuoles located in the anterior subcapsular region and arranged in clusters, giving a characteristic mossy appearance (Fig. 18-3). Such changes may occur in 8% to 10% of nonglaucomatous eyes and in a similar percentage of eyes treated with pilocarpine or carbachol, but they are seen in up to 60% of eyes treated with echothiophate iodide for over six months. Similar changes are noted in patients treated with demecarium bromide or insoflurophate. Visual acuity may not be affected by these changes initially, and most cases do not progress when the medication is stopped at this stage. On continuous therapy for three years about 50% of eyes demonstrate loss of visual acuity of two lines or more due to lens changes. When cataract surgery becomes necessary, one should omit strong miotics for two to four weeks preoperatively to avoid marked postoperative inflammatory reaction. It is also necessary to sweep the posterior synechias free with a spatula.

The accommodative spasm is usually most marked and most intolerable in younger patients. Clip-on minus lens corrections may provide some relief from the induced myopia. The symptoms are most marked with agents required several times daily because of the great fluctuation in induced ciliary spasm. Topical epinephrine is an excellent alternative if adequate control can be maintained. Many younger patients tolerate the strong anticholinesterase drugs used as a single dose at bedtime. This results in excellent control and a fairly constant accommodative status that can be corrected with glasses.

When the stronger anticholinesterase agents are used, ocular side effects, particularly headaches and ache about the eye, are noted by many patients. In approximately 20% of patients these side effects prevent use of the drug. Tolerance of the side effects depends greatly on the enthusiasm of the physician. Since most side effects are markedly reduced after 5 to 10 days of use of a miotic agent, encouragement by the ophthalmologist often makes the difference between success and failure.

It is important to reemphasize that stronger miotics are contraindicated or should be used only with the greatest caution in the treatment of patients with narrow angles. In susceptible eyes, physiologic iris bombè may increase to partial or complete angle closure because of the increased resistance between the posterior and anterior chambers produced by the intense miosis. Vascular congestion may intensify this effect. Similar paradoxical pressure reactions to even the weaker miotics may be seen. This is particularly common in spherophakia because of the pupillary block induced by miosis. Some eyes with hemorrhagic glaucoma also demonstrate pressure rises after miotics, perhaps on the basis of increased vascular congestion.

Dilation of the pupil becomes necessary to evaluate the status of the retina, avoid adhesions to the lens, evaluate the visual field, and improve visual acuity, particularly in those patients with lens changes. From this point of view, it is most interesting and practical that 10% phenylephrine hydrochloride can overcome the

Table 18-1. Effect of 10% phenylephrine (Neo-Synephrine) on demecarium-treated open-angle glaucoma (mean values for 16 patients)

	Applanation pressure (mm Hg)	Outflow facility (μl/min/mm Hg)	Pupillary size (mm)
Before demecarium bromide	29.8	0.09	3.2
After demecarium bromide	17.6	0.22	1.6
After demecarium bromide and 10% phenylephrine	15.8	0.22	4.1

miosis induced by even such agents as isoflurophate, echothiophate iodide, and demecarium bromide without altering the effects of these agents on outflow facility and intraocular pressure. This is true for normal eyes as well as for those with open-angle glaucoma. Thus, as demonstrated in Table 18-1, patients under reasonable control with demecarium bromide can have their pupils dilated from an average of 1.6 to 4.1 mm without detracting from their control. After prolonged use of anticholinesterase agents, however, fibrosis of the iris sphincter muscle occurs, and pupillary dilatation is not possible with any agent.

It is important to emphasize that in some glaucomatous eyes echothiophate iodide and demecarium bromide induce significant decreases in ocular rigidity for various periods of time. This results in underestimation of intraocular pressure by Schiøtz tonometry if one weight only is used and leads to false optimism as to status of control. It is wise to confirm routine intraocular pressure measurements with several Schiøtz weights or to use applanation tonometry in the follow-up of patients with glaucoma, particularly those recently started on the stronger miotics.

Systemic side effects

Systemic side effects, especially of anticholinesterase agents, include nausea, vomiting, diarrhea, bradycardia, salivation, sweating, and central nervous system reactions such as vivid dreams, depression, and delusions. Such symptoms are particularly likely in farm workers exposed to organophosphorus insecticides in addition to their eye medication. They are a consequence of systemic absorption of the drug and reduction of serum and red cell cholinesterase and are usually rapidly relieved by administration of systemic propantheline (Pro-Banthine) or atropine and by stopping the anticholinesterase drug. Although rare, the systemic side effects of these drugs must be appreciated not only by the ophthalmologist but also by the internist and surgeon treating the patient. Failure to recognize the systemic anticholinesterase effects of such medications applied topically to the eye has resulted in unnecessary extensive medical and x-ray studies. Exploratory laparotomies have been done while maintaining the patient faithfully on his glaucoma drops! It behooves the ophthalmologist using these potent cholinesterase inhibitors to inquire about the presence of systemic side effects and to inform a patient's other physicians as to the potential toxicity of these drugs. The low levels of serum pseudocholinesterase in patients using echothiophate eye drops may risk protracted apnea if succinylcholine is used during general anesthesia. The dangers of added exposure to anticholinesterase agents used in insect sprays have not received sufficient attention. The use of P_2AM (Protopam) or related compounds permits reversal of all ocular effects of the anticholinesterase agents. When administered in doses of 0.2 ml of a 4% solution of P_2AM subconjunctivally, the effects of pupillary size, outflow facility, and intraocular pressure are all reversed.

Alternative drug delivery systems

Topically effective drugs for glaucoma are usually combined with preservatives and wetting agents and administered as eye drops. Two recent alternatives to this method of administration may prove useful for some patients, especially in resistant cases.

Soft contact lenses. Hydrophilic soft contact lenses, particularly the Bionite lens, have the property of taking up drugs when soaked in solution and eluting the medication when worn. Wearing a soft contact lens for 30 minutes that had previously been soaked for 2 minutes in 1% pilocarpine reduces intraocular pressure for 24 hours. Some patients uncontrolled on drops were successfully treated in this fashion. The soft contact lens appears to enhance corneal penetration of the pilocarpine.

Membrane-controlled delivery (Ocusert). A drug delivery system has recently been developed in which the active drug, usually as free base, is sealed within a multilayered polymer envelope about 13 x 5 mm in size. Construction of the membrane envelope permits continuous diffusion of active drug into the cul-de-sac at a predetermined rate. Pilocarpine Ocuserts have been prepared, which release pilocarpine continuously for one week at the rate of 20 to 40 μg/hr. The lower rate gives an intraocular pressure response comparable to 1% pilocarpine drops every 6 hours, and the higher rate is approximately comparable to 2% to 4% pilocarpine every 6 hours. The Ocusert is worn in the cul-de-sac and changed weekly. Advantages of the system include less miosis, less induced myopia, and, theoretically, better diurnal pressure control compared to drops. Some patients have difficulty in retaining the Ocusert in the cul-de-sac, especially during the early months of use. Often the level of pressure reduction has not equalled that from a comparable dose of pilocarpine.

EPINEPHRINE

Although the effects of topical epinephrine were originally thought to be predominantly on aqueous flow (Chapter 19), increases in outflow facility are noted. These may be seen very soon after the start of epinephrine therapy and are very common after prolonged daily or twice daily administration. In one series of patients with open-angle glaucoma studied for periods of six months to more than two years, 55% to 65% had a greater than 50% increase in outflow facility on prolonged epinephrine therapy without change in the miotic used. Furthermore, 50% to 60% of eyes with initial facility below 0.13 demonstrated outflow facilities persistently over 0.18 on prolonged epinephrine therapy. The increase in outflow facility is found to be particularly characteristic of early cases of open-angle glaucoma. In a second series, patients with symmetrical open-angle glaucoma were used, and only one eye was treated with 2% epinephrine hydrochloride, the opposite eye constituting the control. A most significant increase in outflow facility occurred in the treated eyes at both three and six months, and no change was noted in the contralateral control eyes. Epinephrine therapy alone has proved useful in the treatment of early open-angle glaucomas, but its side effects must be taken into consideration (Chapter 19).

The mechanism of this action of epinephrine remains unknown. No changes in accommodation have been noted, and the pupils are somewhat dilated. The possible explanations include (1) direct or indirect effects of epinephrine on the outflow channels, blood vessels, and autonomic nerve supply to the eye, (2) effects of lowered intraocular pressure or reduced secretion of aqueous humor or its constituents on the function of the trabecular meshwork, and (3) spontaneous variations characteristic of the early disease process.

SUMMARY

Agents that improve the outflow facility of the glaucomatous eye remain the mainstay of present-day therapy of open-angle glaucomas. Newer, more potent agents make it possible to control the intraocular pressure effectively and avoid further loss of visual function, even in eyes with advanced glaucoma. It is important for the ophthalmologist to appreciate that the use of these powerful drugs may produce ocular and even systemic side effects. With increased understanding of the anatomy, physiology, and enzymatic biochemistry of the outflow channels and the single or multiple defects of this mechanism that characterize the various glaucomas, one may expect the discovery and introduction of a wide variety of medications with increased specificity and reduced side effects.

CHAPTER **19**

Medications that decrease the rate of aqueous formation

Intraocular pressure is dependent on a balance between the rate of aqueous secretion and the facility of outflow. In fact, in glaucomatous eyes with impaired outflow facility it is the spontaneous decrease in the rate of aqueous formation that often normalizes pressure. In his Proctor Lecture, Friedenwald raised the question as to "whether more effort might not profitably be directed toward a reduction in the formation of aqueous in cases of glaucoma, in addition to the present approach, which concerns largely an effort to increase the outflow of fluid from the eye." With the availability of such potent carbonic anhydrase inhibitors as acetazolamide, this prediction became a reality less than five years later. This chapter describes briefly the principal secretory suppressants that are useful for lowering intraocular pressure in glaucomatous eyes. In addition, the present status of the use of carbonic anhydrase inhibitors in therapy for glaucoma is outlined.

CARBONIC ANHYDRASE INHIBITORS

Carbonic anhydrase was first described in rabbit ciliary body–iris preparations by Wistrand. This finding and the excess of bicarbonate noted in the rabbit aqueous humor, as well as the need for bicarbonate buffering in the ciliary body as postulated in the theory of Friedenwald, suggested one or more roles for carbonic anhydrase in the formation of aqueous humor. When sulfanilamide was reported to inhibit carbonic anhydrase, unsuccessful attempts were made to alter intraocular pressure with this drug. Successful inhibition of aqueous secretion became possible only when sulfonamide derivatives, which were more potent carbonic anhydrase inhibitors, were synthesized. Almost all potent carbonic anhydrase inhibitors tested have been found to lower intraocular pressure in similar fashion in rabbits, guinea pigs, dogs, cats, and man. Acetazolamide was selected for clinical trial because it was the first potent agent available and because it had had a most extensive pharmacologic investigation as a diuretic. The large clinical experience with acetazolamide, its remarkable effectiveness, and our knowledge of its side effects still make it the drug of choice for systemic carbonic anhydrase inhibition. Newer agents have proved no more effective except in isolated instances in which they are better tolerated.

Research

The usefulness of carbonic anhydrase inhibitors in ophthalmology has not been limited to the therapy of the glaucomas. The application of such agents as research tools has contributed greatly to our knowledge of aqueous humor dynamics. The availability of means for altering the rate of secretion of aqueous humor has resulted in extensive observations of the effects of such alteration on its chemical composition as well as on the turnover of various substances. In addition, it has been possible to quantitate their effects on secretion by such physical methods as tonography and perfusion and compare the results with the various chemical methods. There is now almost complete agreement among investigators that systemic carbonic anhydrase inhibition results in some 40% to 60% suppression of aqueous flow in both human and experimental animal eyes. Similar values are obtained by independent methods such as repeated tonography, study of alterations in composition of the aqueous humor, and interpretation of induced changes in turnover measurements. As indicated in Chapter 8, the agreement obtained by such completely independent methods, each with its own assumptions and errors, strongly suggests the basic validity of current concepts of aqueous humor dynamics and rate of formation of aqueous humor.

Unfortunately the knowledge that carbonic anhydrase is necessary for the formation of normal amounts of aqueous humor has not resolved the details of the mechanism of aqueous secretion. In fact it has raised more questions than it has answered. As in other secretory sites where carbonic anhydrase has proved necessary, the intimate mechanism of the role of the enzyme remains speculative. Most theories fall into two categories, attributing either a direct or indirect role to the enzyme. Those who believe that carbonic anhydrase enters *directly* in the secretory processes consider it a means of providing the hydrogen ion or bicarbonate ion needed for secretion. These ions may then be transferred by specific ion carriers or exchanged for the cations or anions to be transported. The advocates of an *indirect* role of carbonic anhydrase believe it to provide buffering capacity for the cell. Thus cells secreting acid will themselves become alkaline and need a supply of hydrogen ion to maintain a pH permitting continued secretory function. Other cells secreting fluids of high pH or exchanging sodium for hydrogen ions might need a supply of bicarbonate to avoid excessive fall in pH.

It is of considerable practical as well as theoretic interest that even with massive doses of effective carbonic anhydrase inhibitors, some 40% to 50% of the normal rate of secretion persists. This may be attributed to the adequacy for residual secretion of the uncatalyzed rate of hydration and dehydration of carbon dioxide or to aspects of the secretory process that are independent of the enzyme carbonic anhydrase. Although limiting the therapeutic efficacy of carbonic anhy-

Carbonic Anhydrase Inhibitors	Formula	Dose
Acetazolamide (Diamox)	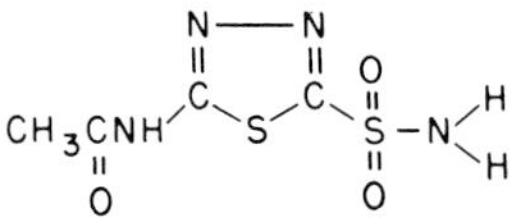	125-500 mg q. 4-12 hr 5-10 mg/Kg q. 4-6 hr (for infants) 250 mg in 2.5 ml distilled H_2O I.V. or I.M.
Methazolamide (Neptazane)	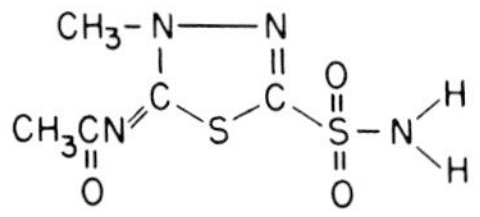	50-100 mg q. 8 hr
Dichlorphenamide (Daranide)	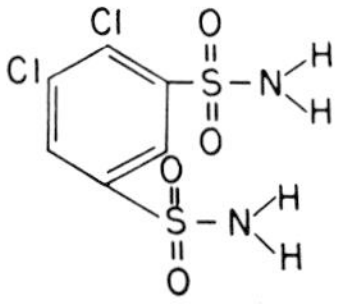	50-200 mg q. 6-8 hr
Ethoxzolamide (Cardrase)	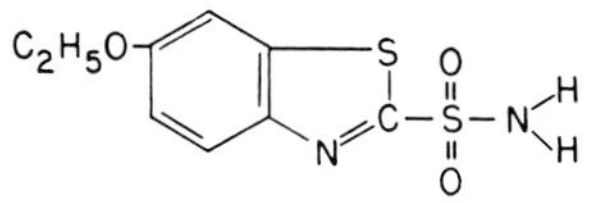	50-250 mg q. 4-8 hr

Fig. 19-1. Carbonic anhydrase inhibitors.

drase inhibitors, the remaining flow may well explain the absence of ocular toxicity, providing a built-in safety factor for maintaining nutritional supply to lens, cornea, and other intraocular structures as well as to many other organs of the body.

Agents available (Fig. 19-1)

The most effective carbonic anhydrase inhibitors available are the sulfonamides, RSO_2NH_2. As Roblin has postulated, the structure of the enzyme substrate H_2CO_3 and the sulfonamide portion of the inhibitor closely resemble one another. Thus the inhibitor may occupy the active site on the enzyme surface, making it unavailable to the substrate.

Various carbonic anhydrase inhibitors with differing in vitro and in vivo potency require different doses when used clinically. However, when they are given in adequate amounts, their effectiveness in lowering intraocular pressure and their side effects are very much the same. Thus the so-called more potent inhibitors are not more effective but merely accomplish the same decrease in intraocular pressure and induce essentially the same unpleasant side effects but at lower dose levels.

Acetazolamide (Diamox). Of the inhibitors, acetazolamide has had the most extensive study and largest clinical trials. For emergency use it is supplied in ampules containing 500 mg to be dissolved in 5 to 10 ml of distilled water and used by intravenous or intramuscular injection. For oral administration 250 mg tablets are available. The dose varies from 125 mg every 12 hours to 500 mg every 4 hours and must be individualized for the particular patient, his needs, and his side effects. The most common dose is 250 mg every 6 hours. Newer long-acting preparations (Diamox Sequels) make it possible to give 500 mg every 12 hours. Aside from the important convenience of less frequent administration, no significant differences are noted in responsiveness or side effects of the two preparations. In practice it is usually best to begin with 250 mg of regular acetazolamide every 12 hours or 500 mg of sustained release acetazolamide once daily and to modify the dose as to needs and tolerance. Although 1 Gm per day is the most frequent dose, many patients are controlled with less than this amount. Although higher doses may have slightly greater effect, it is rare to use acetazolamide in doses over 1 Gm per day, mainly because of increased side effects. The use of 1 tablet (250 mg) per day, as suggested for diuresis, is rarely effective in normalizing intraocular pressure around the clock. Infants tolerate acetazolamide well and with minimal side effects in doses of 5 to 10 mg/kg body weight every 4 to 6 hours.

After intravenous administration of acetazolamide to adults, pressure begins to fall within the first few minutes, reaching a minimum in approximately ½ to 4 hours. After oral administration, intraocular pressure begins to fall in 1 to 2 hours, reaching a low in 3 to 5 hours, with recovery in 6 to 12 hours.

Ethoxzolamide (Cardrase; Ethamide). Ethoxzolamide is another carbonic anhydrase inhibitor that is extremely potent in vitro. In vivo it has much the same action as acetazolamide but may be administered in smaller milligram doses. It is supplied in 125 mg tablets. It is administered orally in doses of 50 to 250 mg every 4 to 8 hours. The most frequently used dose is 125 mg every 6 to 8 hours.

Dichlorphenamide (Daranide; Oratrol). Dichlorphenamide is a useful substitute for acetazolamide. It is administered in doses of 50 to 200 mg every 6 to 8 hours. It is said to produce less metabolic acidosis but may induce more pronounced renal loss of potassium.

Methazolamide (Neptazane). Methazolamide has only slightly greater in vitro activity than acetazolamide. However, this agent penetrates the aqueous humor and spinal fluid some three to five times as readily as does acetazolamide. This may account for its effectiveness in lowering intraocular pressure at lower doses than are required of acetazolamide. It is available in 50 mg tablets and is administered orally in doses of 50 to 100 mg every 8 hours. Methazolamide is used most frequently in patients unable to tolerate acetazolamide because of renal calculi or other side effects.

Clinical use
Angle-closure glaucoma

The short-term use of carbonic anhydrase inhibitors in acute angle-closure glaucoma has received widespread acceptance. If the patient is vomiting, it is necessary to use parenteral medication. The only drug available at the present time that can be given parenterally is acetazolamide. It is best to give one half of the ampule (250 mg in 5 ml of distilled water) intravenously and the remainder intramuscularly. It may be necessary to repeat the parenteral injection in 2 to 4 hours.

Oral medication should be begun as soon as it can be retained. Lowering of the intraocular pressure results in clearing of corneal edema and time for more adequate examination and evaluation of the eye by gonioscopy, ophthalmoscopy, and tonography. It also permits surgery to be delayed so that the operation may be done on a less inflamed eye.

It is important to emphasize that carbonic anhydrase inhibitors are only a temporary preoperative medication in eyes with unoperated angle-closure glaucoma. Undue reassurance and procrastination in lieu of surgery result in failure to recognize intermittent mild episodes of recurrent angle closure. Eventually the angle is sufficiently compromised that simple peripheral iridectomy is no longer curative. It then becomes necessary to perform filtering procedures with their attendant increased hazards and complications. This misuse of carbonic anhydrase inhibitors must be reemphasized, for it is still prevalent and is causing much unnecessary visual loss.

Carbonic anhydrase inhibitors have also proved useful in the postoperative management of angle-closure glaucoma. It is often necessary to use these agents in those eyes with unsuccessful filtering procedures or in those in which the outflow facility is so impaired after peripheral iridectomy that the intraocular pressure is elevated even with maximum miotic therapy. In these eyes, one is essentially treating a secondary glaucoma.

Open-angle glaucoma (Fig. 29-18)

Carbonic anhydrase inhibitors have proved of greatest value in the long-term therapy of primary open-angle glaucoma. It is now quite clear that some patients with otherwise uncontrolled open-angle glaucoma can be maintained normotensive and without further field loss for periods of up to twenty years. It must be emphasized that the effects of carbonic anhydrase inhibitors are reversible at any time, necessitating continuous round-the-clock medication. Before the undertaking of long-term administration it has proved ideal to hospitalize patients for establishment of base-line tension curves, urinalysis, and blood counts. In this fashion the best carbonic anhydrase inhibitors as well as its dose, frequency of administration, and side effects can be determined for an individual patient. In clinical practice, it is more practical to arrive at these decisions slowly by trial and error. Miotic therapy should be continued when carbonic anhydrase inhibitors have been added to the regimen of the patient. In some instances dramatic improvement in outflow facility is seen after the addition of a carbonic anhydrase inhibitor. This improvement remains unexplained but may relate to the greater effectiveness of miotics when intraocular pressure is reduced or to possible unknown effects of carbonic anhydrase inhibitors on outflow channels.

Secondary glaucoma

Short-term administration of carbonic anhydrase inhibitors is of use in the self-limited secondary glaucomas (e.g., trauma, glaucomatocyclitic crisis, and uveitis). In these patients carbonic anhydrase inhibition should be maintained only as long as the impaired outflow facility requires. Long-term administration is required in some cases of chronic secondary glaucoma, with effectiveness equal to that in primary open-angle glaucoma.

Congenital glaucoma

In congenital glaucoma, carbonic anhydrase inhibitors are very useful pre-operatively. By lowering intraocular pressure, they permit surgery to be delayed and at the same time afford some clearing of the cornea. It then becomes possible to evaluate ophthalmoscopic, gonioscopic, and tonographic findings and to per-form goniotomy on a softer eye under direct visualization of the angle.

Results

Short-term therapy

A decrease in aqueous secretion of over 40% was observed in 83% of one series of 440 glaucomatous eyes treated with acetazolamide. Only 27 eyes (6%) failed to obtain 20% inhibition of secretion. Results from other clinics are very similar. The short-term administration of methazolamide and other agents that cannot be given parenterally results in suppression of aqueous secretion of more than 40% in only some 60% of eyes.

Long-term therapy

Five out of 6 patients with primary open-angle glaucoma respond initially to carbonic anhydrase inhibition with satisfactory falls in pressure if adequate doses are used. However, less than half the responders can be maintained at pressure levels of 24 mm Hg or less on such medication for periods of more than two to three years. When acetazolamide is used, more than two thirds of the failures are due to intolerable side effects. The remainder are attributed to inadequate pressure control because of poor drug absorption, development of tolerance to the carbonic anhydrase inhibitor, or further impairment of outflow facility. With the use of methazolamide in those patients who fail to tolerate acetazolamide, it has been possible to increase the number of patients successfully controlled for over three years to approximate more closely the 50% figure.

In the review of such statistics, however, it must be pointed out that the selec-tion of patients largely determines the outcome. If one chooses those out of control on all miotic therapy and with far-advanced glaucoma, even 50% inhibition of secretion may fail to normalize pressure. There is also evidence in all reported series that during the long-term follow-up some of the failures after initial success can be attributed to progression of the outflow disorder. Failures in everyday prac-tice also include inability to continue medication because of expense, lack of under-standing, and failure to return for follow-up visits. At any rate, with the round-the-clock use of carbonic anhydrase inhibitors available at present, almost 50% of consecutive patients with open-angle glaucoma referred because of failure to re-spond satisfactorily to miotics can be successfully controlled without field loss for periods of at least three years.

Side effects

Ocular side effects

It is most important to emphasize that no ocular damage has been reported as a consequence of reduction of aqueous formation, lowering of intraocular pressure, or inhibition of carbonic anhydrase (present in lens, vitreous humor, retina, and uveal tract). Thus after acetazolamide no functional or anatomic alterations have been detected in ocular circulation, appearance or metabolism of the lens, function of the macula, dark adaptation, flicker fusion, etc. However, several instances of transient myopia have been reported similar to that which occasionally follows the use of other sulfonamides.

Systemic side effects

Almost all patients who are started on carbonic anhydrase inhibitors experience paresthesia, but it is rarely incapacitating. The side effects that necessitate discontinuance of carbonic anhydrase inhibitors are predominantly gastrointestinal (loss of appetite) and urinary (ureteral colic). With methazolamide there are more complaints of generalized malaise and excessive fatigue. Other carbonic anhydrase inhibitors present much the same side effects as acetazolamide. The patient's tolerance to most of the side effects depends to a large extent on the enthusiasm and encouragement of the physician as well as on the understanding and convictions of the patient. The physician, however, must be aware of the side effects and discontinue the drug when they become intense. Severe mental depression and confusion have occasionally been seen with use of carbonic anhydrase inhibitors. Such symptoms may incorrectly be considered the result of cerebral arteriosclerosis, especially in elderly patients. The symptoms are reversible with withdrawal of the drug.

The rare instances of repeated ureteral colic constitute a contraindication to the use of carbonic anhydrase inhibitors. The formation of ureteral calculi may be related to the marked reduction in urinary citrate excretion that follows carbonic anhydrase inhibition. However, several patients who have experienced ureteral colic after acetazolamide have been able to tolerate the smaller doses needed of methazolamide without further stone formation.

The occurrence of sulfonamide sensitivity manifested by a skin rash requires stopping the particular drug used. Fortunately some of these patients can be maintained on other carbonic anhydrase inhibitors. Bone marrow depression is a rare side effect of sulfonamide therapy and has been reported with use of acetazolamide. Grant states that this is an idiosyncratic reaction. Repeated blood studies are not indicated. Elevation of blood uric acid with development of acute gouty arthritis has been reported in a patient taking acetazolamide. The mechanism of the hyperuricemia is unknown. Since some patients who fail to tolerate one of these agents can be controlled on another, it is essential that ophthalmologists familiarize themselves with the use and side effects of all available carbonic anhydrase inhibitors.

SYMPATHOMIMETIC AGENTS

Epinephrine, phenylephrine (Neo-Synephrine) hydrochloride, naphazoline (Privine), and other related compounds have been known for many years to decrease intraocular pressure when applied topically to the eye. Tonographic and fluorescein turnover studies have demonstrated that these agents decrease the rate of aqueous formation in human eyes. The mechanism of action on the secretory process remains speculative but is most likely a beta-adrenergic effect. Vasoconstriction does not appear to be essential for the suppression of secretion. Thus isoproterenol (Isuprel), which has very little vasoconstrictor activity, is effective in reducing aqueous flow.

Epinephrine hydrochloride, bitartrate, or *borate* is the most popular and useful of the sympathomimetic agents. It is used topically as a 0.5% to 2% solution that contains an antioxidant and is administered once every 12 to 24 hours. Commercial preparations are usually described as concentration of epinephrine salt rather than as concentration of available free epinephrine. This is particularly important in the case of epinephrine bitartrate, where a 2% solution contains approximately 1.1% epinephrine. Fortunately evidence indicates that 0.5% epinephrine is about equally effective as the 2% concentration.

Epinephrine reduces the rate of aqueous formation by approximately 30% to 35%. It is of considerable practical significance that this reduction of flow is independent of and in addition to the effects of carbonic anhydrase inhibitors. Thus one may induce some 50% suppression of flow by acetazolamide and obtain an additional 30% effect on the residual flow with topical epinephrine, resulting in some 65% to 70% suppression of aqueous formation. Furthermore, in the management of glaucoma treated with miotics, topical epinephrine provides an excellent means of further lowering intraocular pressure, often without the need for the addition of carbonic anhydrase inhibitors. It must be emphasized that even when miotics are used, topical epinephrine will produce some pupillary dilation. This dilation may improve vision in patients with lens changes but may also induce acute angle closure in eyes with narrow angles. Therefore, in eyes that are capable of angle closure, it is unwise to use topical epinephrine until after peripheral iridectomy has been done.

As indicated in Chapter 18, evidence has been accumulated to indicate that epinephrine improves outflow facility in glaucomatous eyes. This effect is in addition to the depressed aqueous secretion. It is noted particularly in eyes with early primary open-angle glaucoma, and is thought to be an alpha adrenergic effect.

Side effects

Too little attention has been directed to the side effects of topical epinephrine therapy. These include not only such common ocular complaints as reactive hyperemia (which the patient claims is "relieved" by the use of the epinephrine drops) and brow ache but also hypersensitivity reactions of the conjunctiva and lids. These are probably allergic reactions to phenolic breakdown products or oxidized polymers of epinephrine, for often the reaction can be alleviated in spite of the continued use of epinephrine if one changes to a different salt or even obtains a fresh bottle of the same preparation. Discolored solutions should be discarded. In some 20% of patients epinephrine is not tolerated because of hyperemic and sensitivity reactions. The allergic reaction can be controlled with topical corticosteroids, but even weak steroids induce pressure elevations in primary open-angle glaucoma when continued for long periods. Two new steroid preparations have become available that alleviate the sensitivity without causing increased intraocular pressure. Medrysone (HMS), 1%, is a progesterone-related steroid that does not produce elevated intraocular pressure and yet has significant anti-inflammatory activity. Tetrahydrotriamcinolone, 0.25%, is a more potent corticosteroid still classified as investigational that does not increase pressure. Both drugs have been used two to four times daily for up to five years in glaucoma patients to control allergic epinephrine reactions without adversely affecting the glaucoma. In addition to the local hypersensitivity to epinephrine, melanin-like pigment deposits are seen on the lids, encysted in the conjunctiva and even in the cornea. Pigmented lacrimal stones may also occur and cause epiphora due to obstruction.

Of much greater significance are the complaints of visual haze and the rare occurrence of documented central scotoma after the use of topical epinephrine. Dramatic decreases in visual acuity have been noted occasionally after repeated use of epinephrine preparations, particularly in aphakic patients. The decrease is usually associated with vascular spasm, edema, and occasionally fine hemorrhages about the macula. When use of topical epinephrine is stopped, visual acuity recovers in most instances. Although the pathogenesis of these vascular changes is not known and the causative role of epinephrine has not been proved, the vasospastic nature of the process forces one to consider it as a possible iatrogenic process. Unfortunately these macular findings are not usually blamed on epinephrine, and so most patients are continued on epinephrine, with unexplained visual loss. Present evidence suggests that this maculopathy may occur in up to 20% of aphakic patients treated with topical epinephrine.

In a few persons corneal haze and edema occur after topical epinephrine. Halos or blurred vision is noted by the patient despite excellent control of intraocular pressure. Prompt improvement follows discontinuation of epinephrine.

In the reading of repeat tonograms, it is a common occurrence to note irregularities of the transmitted pulse after topical epinephrine therapy is begun. Electrocardiograms demonstrate some of these to be premature ventricular contractions (Fig. 29-19). In some patients palpitations are noted but are usually reported to the internist rather than to the ophthalmologist. Blood pressure elevations have also been noted. It is easy to prove the topical epinephrine to be causative, and it is important to inform the internist that the drug is being used.

CARDIAC GLYCOSIDES

In experimental animals cardiac glycosides such as ouabain and digoxin inhibit sodium and potassium–activated adenosinetriphosphatase of the ciliary epithelium and suppress secretion of aqueous humor. This effect is additive to that of carbonic anhydrase inhibitors. Unfortunately, at reasonable dose levels, digoxin has failed to prove of value in the management of glaucoma uncontrolled on other medications. The topical application of cardiac glycosides has been attempted, but the inhibition of transport induced in the cornea results in corneal edema, which precludes the use of the cardiac glycosides that are available at the present time.

VASOPRESSIN

The antiduretic vasopressin (beta-hypophamine) lowers intraocular pressure in rabbits and in patients. After topical administration of 1 to 2 units of vasopressin, aqueous humor secretion may be decreased by as much as 60%. Unfortunately the rapid development of a state of resistance to the drug limits its use to short-term application.

ADRENOLYTIC AGENTS

Such drugs as phentolamine methanesulfonate (Regitine), *N, N*-dibenzyl-beta-chloroethylamine (Dibenamine), ergotamine, phenoxybenzamine (Dibenzyline), and guanethidine (Ismelin) are found to lower intraocular pressure in experimental animals. Unfortunately these agents are either too toxic for human use or not effective in lowering intraocular pressure in patients with glaucoma.

Topical use of some of these drugs has been proposed for therapy of open-angle glaucoma. In some patients with glaucoma uncontrolled on miotics and epinephrine, the addition of topical 10% guanethidine results in a dramatic fall in intraocular pressure. Most often this occurs without change in outflow facility, but an early transient increase in outflow facility may be observed. Ptosis and miosis are usually seen after occasional initial mydriasis following 10% guanethidine. The picture is that of peripheral chemical sympathectomy (Chapter 6). The transient increase in outflow facility and mydriasis may represent release of norepinephrine preceding its depletion. Guanethidine alone has proved to be of little value in glaucoma therapy, but its use with topical epinephrine is reported to produce an additive effect. It is not available in the United States but is used in Europe.

6-Hydroxydopamine. Recently Holland reported that subconjunctival 6-hydroxydopamine produces a chemical sympathectomy of the anterior segment of the eye and results in a hypersensitivity to topical epinephrine in lowering intraocular pressure. Some glaucoma patients appear particularly sensitive to this effect. The sympathectomy is not permanent, and repeated administration of 6-hydroxydopamine may be required at two- to four-month intervals.

Thymoxamine. When applied topically to the eye, the alpha-adrenergic blocker thymoxamine hydrochloride, 0.5%, induces rapid miosis. The dilator muscle of the iris is inhibited, permitting the iris sphincter to constrict unopposed. In the normal eye this occurs without effect on intraocular pressure or outflow facility. In acute angle-closure glaucoma, however, miosis may open the angle and terminate the attack. Thymoxamine has been shown to be of value in acute angle-closure glaucoma, often relieving the attack without other miotic or hyperosmotic therapy. The drug is available in Europe but classified as investigational in the United States.

RETROBULBAR ANESTHETICS

Retrobulbar injection of procaine and epinephrine lowers intraocular pressure in glaucomatous and normal eyes, probably as a consequence of a decrease in aqueous secretion. This method of lowering intraocular pressure has proved useful as a preoperative procedure or to break the cycle in a few instances of angle-closure or secondary glaucoma with markedly elevated intraocular pressure. With newer agents such as intravenous hyperosmotics available, it is rarely necessary to utilize retrobulbar injection, particularly because of the hazard of retrobulbar hemorrhage.

INFLAMMATORY AGENTS

Radiation, trauma, surgical procedures, histamine, and other inflammatory agents reduce aqueous secretion and lower intraocular pressure. The effects are usually explainable on the basis of the inflammation they induce in the anterior segment of the eye, and these agents are not practical methods of treatment.

SUMMARY

Secretory suppression by means of systemic carbonic anhydrase inhibitors or topical epinephrine provides a most valuable adjunct to miotics in therapy for glaucoma. As greater knowledge of the intimate detailed mechanism of aqueous production is acquired, it can be anticipated that newer and more effective secretory inhibitors will become available for use by the research worker and the clinician.

20

Hyperosmotic agents and other medications

HYPEROSMOTIC AGENTS

Hyperosmotic agents have become an important part of the therapeutic armamentarium for the management of glaucoma. They have proved most useful in the therapy of acute glaucoma and have all but eliminated the necessity to operate on an eye with markedly elevated intraocular pressure.

Mechanism of action

Hyperosmotic agents lower intraocular pressure by producing a rapid increase in blood osmolality. This induces an osmotic gradient between the blood and ocular fluids, resulting in loss of water from the eye to the hyperosmotic plasma. Evidence indicates that sudden small changes in blood osmolality can also alter intraocular pressure by affecting osmoreceptors in the hypothalamus. The response appears to be mediated via the optic nerve, since transection of the nerve eliminates the effect. For clinical use, most agents produce effective lowering of intraocular pressure when blood osmolality is increased by some 20 to 30 mOsmol/L.

The osmotic gradient

Various factors are important in determining the osmotic gradient induced between the blood and ocular fluids. Since the change in blood osmolality depends on the number of milliosmols of substance administered, agents with low molecular weight have potentially greater effect than large molecular weight compounds at the same dosage. Agents confined to the extracellular fluid space (e.g., mannitol) produce a greater effect on blood osmolality at the same dosage than do agents distributed in total body water (e.g., urea). Some drugs rapidly enter the eye (e.g., alcohol), thereby producing less of an osmotic gradient than those which penetrate slowly or not at all (e.g., glycerol). Agents administered intravenously bypass gastrointestinal absorption and produce a more rapid and somewhat greater effect. Other factors such as rate of elimination from the circulation and production of hypo-osmotic diuresis (alcohol) also affect the osmotic change that these agents produce.

It is a happy coincidence that the above factors balance each other sufficiently that most hyperosmotic drugs currently used are effective at a dose in the range of 1 to 2 Gm/kg.

Agents available

Intravenous agents (Table 20-1)

All the intravenous hyperosmotic agents have the advantage of more rapid onset of action compared to the orally administered drugs. They are administered at a rate of approximately 60 drops per minute, with the total dose usually given within 45 to 60 minutes.

Mannitol. Intravenous mannitol is a very effective hyperosmotic drug that is presently the agent of choice for intravenous administration. The usual dose is 2.5 to 10 ml/kg of the 20% solution. It penetrates the eye very poorly, is not metabolized, and is rapidly excreted in the urine. The 20% solution is stable and is much less irritating than urea if the infusion extravasates. Its major disadvantages are the comparatively larger volume required because of limited solubility and the greater likelihood of cellular dehydration due its confinement to extracellular water.

Urea. Urea is administered as a 30% solution in 10% invert sugar in a dose of 2 to 7 ml/kg. It produces a rapid lowering of pressure, is not metabolized, and is rapidly excreted in the urine. Its major disadvantage is that it penetrates the eye reasonably well, especially when the eye is inflamed. As the urea is cleared from the circulation, the blood osmolality may fall below that of the vitreous, resulting in a rebound phenomenon. The solution tends to be unstable and must

Table 20-1. Intravenous hyperosmotic agents

Agent	Molecular weight	Distribution	Ocular penetration	Usual dose
Urea	60	Total water	Good	1-2 Gm/kg (30% solution)
Mannitol	182	Extracellular	Very poor	1-2 Gm/kg (20% solution)
Ascorbate	198*	Total water	Good	0.5-1 Gm/kg (20% solution)

*1 mOsmol = 99 mg.

Table 20-2. Oral hyperosmotic agents

Agent	Molecular weight	Distribution	Ocular penetration	Usual dose*
Glycerol	92	Extracellular	Poor	1-1.5 Gm/kg
Isosorbide	146	Total water	Good	1-2 Gm/kg
Alcohol	46	Total water	Good	0.8-1.5 Gm/kg

*Usually given in 50% solutions.

be mixed just before use. If the solution extravasates, slough and phlebitis may occur.

Sodium ascorbate. Intravenous sodium ascorbate is used as a 20% solution in doses of 2 to 5 ml/kg. Since the compound is ionized in solution, each milliosmol given provides two milliosmols. Although ascorbate is normally found in relatively high concentration in the eye, when the concentration in plasma exceeds that of the vitreous an osmotic gradient is produced. Solutions of ascorbate are unstable and must be prepared fresh before use.

Oral agents (Table 20-2)

Orally administered agents tend to act more slowly than those given intravenously, although the difference is not great. Compensating for this, however, is the greater safety of these drugs, particularly from overloading the circulation in patients with borderline cardiac status.

Glycerol. Glycerol is used as a 50% solution in fruit juice or cola drink in a dose of 1.5 to 3 ml/kg solution (0.7 to 1.5 ml/kg of glycerol) and is presently the most widely used hyperosmotic agent. It is very effective in lowering intraocular pressure, penetrates the eye poorly and is confined to extracellular water. Its major disadvantage is the frequency with which it induces nausea and vomiting. Another disadvantage is its caloric value, particularly when repeated administration is necessary or for use in diabetics.

Isosorbide (Hydronol). Isosorbide is an effective oral hyperosmotic agent that is presently available only on an investigational basis. It is absorbed rapidly and quantitatively from the gastrointestinal tract and excreted unchanged in the urine. Rapid decrease in intraocular pressure is produced when it is given as a 50% solution in doses of 2 to 4 ml/kg. It produces less nausea than glycerol, is stable in solution, and can be stored in a soda-type bottle for emergency office use.

Ethyl alcohol. Oral ethyl alcohol has been evaluated as a hyperosomotic agent and found to be very effective. It is used as a 50% solution in fruit juice or as straight bourbon or Scotch whiskey in doses of 2 to 3 ml/kg (1 to 1.8 ml/kg of absolute alcohol). Alcohol inhibits antidiuretic hormone (ADH) production, inducing a hypotonic diuresis and thereby prolonging and increasing the hyperosmolality of the blood. It penetrates the eye rapidly, but vitreous penetration is sufficiently delayed so that an osmotic gradient is created. Ethyl alcohol is rarely employed therapeutically but certainly can be used in an emergency situation as straight whiskey.

Clinical use
Angle-closure glaucoma (Fig. 29-11)

Hyperosmotic agents have their greatest value in the management of acute angle-closure glaucoma. Many ophthalmologists keep oral glycerol in their offices for use in such cases. Pure glycerol, 1 ml/kg in an equal volume of fruit juice or cola drink, along with topical miotics will terminate most attacks of acute angle-closure glaucoma. Isosorbide can also be used. If the patient is vomiting, intravenous mannitol should be administered as soon as he arrives at the hospital. A dose of 1 Gm/kg given over 30 to 60 minutes will lower intraocular pressure in almost all patients. Lower doses are frequently sufficient, and the administration should be stopped when the pressure has fallen and the pupil has become miotic. Once the acute attack has terminated, iridectomy becomes a much safer and often a curative procedure.

Secondary glaucoma

In the secondary glaucomas, hyperosmotic agents are valuable preoperatively or as a means of controlling pressure and preventing damage until the underlying disease process is controlled. Surgery for lens-induced glaucoma becomes much safer when performed at normal pressures after osmotic therapy. The acute glaucoma after blunt trauma will frequently subside spontaneously after several days but may be uncontrollable until then. Oral hyperosmotic agents can be given daily, or even several times a day, for up to several weeks without complications. Isosorbide avoids the caloric value of glycerol and alcohol in these instances. In markedly inflamed eyes and in hemorrhagic glaucoma, oral glycerol or intravenous mannitol are preferable because they penetrate the eye poorly. Surgery for traumatic hyphema with secondary glaucoma is often avoided when hyperosmotic agents are given. Clearing of the hyphema and normalization of pressure are frequently seen after oral glycerol or intravenous mannitol.

Malignant glaucoma (ciliary-block glaucoma)

Hyperosmotic agents are particularly useful in malignant glaucoma. As water is transferred from the vitreous to the circulation, vitreous volume is decreased, and the vitreous face moves posteriorly. Strong mydriatics (3% atropine, 10% phenylephrine [Neo-Synephrine]) will usually break posterior synechias and dilate the pupil, establishing communication between the anterior and posterior chambers. In the phakic eye, atropine also tightens the zonules and pulls the iris-lens diaphragm posteriorly. Most cases of malignant glaucoma are terminated in this fashion.

Open-angle glaucoma

Hyperosmotic agents are most useful in open-angle glaucoma as a means of lowering intraocular pressure prior to surgery. Oral ascorbic acid, 0.5 Gm/kg per day in four doses, has recently been used in the treatment of primary open-angle glaucoma. The drug appears effective when given in this fashion but requires the administration of 70 to 80 tablets of ascorbic acid per day. In addition, many patients develop gastrointestinal irritation and diarrhea with this amount of medication. It is doubtful that hyperosmotic drugs will be useful for long-term therapy of primary open-angle glaucoma.

Side effects

Side effects from use of hyperosmotic agents are frequent. Some of these are serious and even potentially fatal. Fortunately the more serious side effects are uncommon.

Headaches, nausea, and vomiting are the most frequent side effects and are seen to some degree with all the agents. Oral glycerol is particularly prone to induce nausea. Intense diuresis after osmotic therapy may lead to urinary retention, requiring catheterization. Pulmonary edema and congestive heart failure may be precipitated in elderly patients with borderline cardiac and renal status. This is especially true of mannitol. Being confined to the extracellular fluid space, mannitol greatly increases blood volume and may overload the circulation. Cellular dehydration, including cerebral dehydration with resultant disorientation, may also occur more often with mannitol than with the other agents.

CENTRAL NERVOUS SYSTEM DEPRESSANTS

Sedatives and tranquilizers produce inconsistent effects on intraocular pressure in normal and glaucomatous patients. Drinking of alcoholic beverages tends to lower intraocular pressure. There are repeated reports in the literature of the use of chlorpromazine, barbiturates, meprobamate, etc. for long-term administration to patients with glaucoma. There is evidence that these agents may alter the patient's emotional response to his disease process, but there is very little evidence that they alter the disease process itself or its control. Some of these agents may affect osmoreceptors in the hypothalamus.

MYDRIATIC AGENTS

In the secondary glaucomas associated with inflammatory diseases, use of a mydriatic (parasympatholytic agent) dilates the pupil, relieves ciliary and pupillary spasm, and avoids posterior synechias. Although these agents can induce angle-closure glaucoma in susceptible eyes and may raise intraocular pressure in primary open-angle glaucoma, they still find considerable use in eyes with active inflammation and glaucoma. When intraocular pressure is elevated, it is often wise to use a weaker mydriatic such as 2% to 5% homatropine, for these agents are more readily reversed by miotics if this becomes necessary (e.g., in the event of a sharp pressure rise). With the availability of carbonic anhydrase inhibitors and stronger miotics, many ophthalmologists now prefer 1% to 2% atropine or 0.2% scopolamine.

Phenylephrine hydrochloride, 10%, is an excellent agent for pupillary dilation. As do other sympathomimetic agents, it also tends to lower intraocular pressure in glaucomatous eyes. As indicated in Chapter 18, phenylephrine proves useful in the ophthalmoscopic examination of eyes with open-angle glaucoma on prolonged miotic therapy. This is particularly valuable, for the pupillary dilation induced does not impair the improved outflow facility. In many instances of glaucoma, central lens opacities may be of sufficient magnitude to decrease vision when miotics are used. In these eyes phenylephrine may improve visual acuity sufficiently to warrant its use along with the miotic agents. It must be stressed that the mydriatic effects of phenylephrine can overcome even the most potent miotics available. This serves to reemphasize the need for caution in the use of this agent in eyes with angle-closure glaucoma before iridectomy. Phenylephrine should be used with suitable precautions such as applying pressure over the tear ducts after administrations. Systemic effects can be of danger to hypertensive patients.

ANTI-INFLAMMATORY AGENTS

The adrenal steroids have proved of enormous value in decreasing the inflammatory response of the eye. In eyes with glaucoma secondary to active inflammation, the topical or systemic use of these agents may decrease reaction sufficiently to normalize outflow facility. Although it is rarely seen after systemic steroid therapy, the prolonged topical use of potent corticosteroids may produce elevations of intraocular pressure in susceptible eyes (Chapters 14 and 15). Some 30% to 40% of patients with secondary glaucomas fall into the susceptible category. For these patients, steroids can be used if needed, but with due caution. Steroid testing of the fellow normal eye may help to differentiate disease-caused outflow impairment from that induced by corticosteroids.

In many eyes with inflammation, hyposecretion of aqueous humor results in hypotony in spite of obstructed outflow channels. In some of these eyes the decrease in inflammation that follows steroid therapy may improve function of the ciliary body and restore the blood-aqueous barrier, so that effective secretory activity is restored and intraocular pressure rises abruptly. The pressure rise may be to glaucomatous levels if outflow facility is decreased or insufficiently normalized by the anti-inflammatory agents.

References—Section VI

Abraham, S. V.: Miotic iridocyclitis, Amer. J. Ophthal. **43**:298, 1957.

Armaly, M. F., and Rao, K. R.: The effect of pilocarpine Ocusert with different release rates on ocular pressure, Invest. Ophthal. **12**:491, 1973.

Axelsson, U.: Glaucoma, miotic therapy, and cataract, Acta Ophthal., supp. 102, 1969.

Ballin, N., Becker, B., and Goldman, M.: Systemic effects of epinephrine applied topically to the eye, Invest. Ophthal. **5**:125, 1966.

Becker, B.: Use of methazolamide (Neptazane) in the therapy of glaucoma: comparison with acetazolamide (Diamox), Amer. J. Ophthal. **49**:1307, 1960.

Becker, B., Kolker, A. E., and Krupin, T.: Hyperosmotic agents. In Leopold, I. H., editor: Symposium on ocular therapy, vol. 3, St. Louis, 1968, The C. V. Mosby Co.

Becker, B., and Ley, A. P.: Epinephrine and acetazolamide in the therapy of the chronic glaucomas, Amer. J. Ophthal. **45**:639, 1958.

Fralick, F. B.: Symposium: Office management of the primary glaucomas, Trans. Amer. Acad. Ophthal. Otolaryng. **64**:105, 1960.

Grant, W. M.: Physiological and pharmacological influences upon intraocular pressure, Pharmacol. Rev. **7**:143, 1955.

Grant, W. M.: Ocular complications of drugs: glaucoma, J.A.M.A. **207**:2089, 1969.

Halasa, A. H., and others: Thymoxamine therapy for angle-closure glaucoma, Arch. Ophthal. **90**:177, 1973.

Holland, M. G.: Treatment of glaucoma by chemical sympathectomy with 6-hydroxy-dopamine, Trans. Amer. Acad. Ophthal. Otolaryng. **76**:437, 1972.

Kolker, A. E., and Becker, B.: Epinephrine maculopathy, Arch. Ophthal. **79**:552, 1968.

Kronfeld, P. C., and others: Tonography Symposium, Trans. Amer. Acad. Ophthal. Otolaryng. **65**:133, 1961.

Leopold, I. H.: Ocular cholinesterase and cholinesterase inhibitors, Amer. J. Ophthal. **51**:855, 1961.

Leydhecker, W.: Glaukom, ein Handbuch, Berlin, 1959, Springer-Verlag.

Maren, T. H., Mayer, E., and Wadsworth, B. C.: Carbonic anhydrase inhibition. I. The pharmacology of Diamox 2-acetylamino-1,3,4-thiadiazole-5-sulfonamide, Bull. Johns Hopkins Hosp. **95**:199, 1954.

Paterson, G. D., and Paterson, G.: Drug therapy of glaucoma, Brit. J. Ophthal. **56**:288, 1972.

Podos, S. M., Becker, B., Asseff, C., and Hartstein, J.: Pilocarpine therapy with soft contact lenses, Amer. J. Ophthal. **73**:336, 1972.

Sears, M. L., and Neufeld, A. H.: Adrenergic modulation of the outflow of aqueous humor, Invest. Ophthal. **14**:83, 1975.

Shaffer, R. N., and Hetherington, J., Jr.: Anticholinesterase drugs and cataracts, Amer. J. Ophthal. **62**:613, 1966.

21

General care of the surgical patient

There is nothing more reassuring to the surgical patient than to feel complete confidence in his physician. The preparation of a patient for surgery is really begun by the care and thoroughness with which the ophthalmologist conducts the history-taking and physical examination. He must be interested in the past medical history and in the present physical status of the patient. If possible, the family physician should have examined the patient recently.

PREOPERATIVE CARE
Instructions to the patient

The patient should be told in a general way what to expect during his hospital stay. An explanation of likely complications is necessary. Physicians are now in fact legally required to provide this information in order to obtain the patient's agreement (informed consent) to operate. Patients must be told they may develop, for example, cataracts or infection. The probability of success of a procedure should also be stated so that patients are not disappointed. The surgery itself can be explained reassuringly. It is important to tell the patient that the local anesthesia is momentarily painful but that the surgery itself is painless. A patient thus prepared is quieter, less apprehensive, and more cooperative. Preoperative sedation is more effective, and the surgery will go more smoothly for patient and surgeon alike. As Atkinson says, "Fear invites complications."

Before the orders are made out, the surgeon should question the patient about possible allergy to medications. He should be told to take with him to the hospital any medications he is routinely using at home. These will include systemic medications as well as glaucoma drops and tablets. He should continue to use these the day of admission on the same schedule as at home. Misplaced orders, closed pharmacies, and the overloaded workday of nurses too often result in delay in obtaining and giving new medications. Patients facing surgery are apprehensive, and their confidence in both the hospital and the surgeon can be shaken by failure to receive promptly medication that they have been told is vital.

357

Use of anticholinesterase agents preoperatively

There is considerable evidence that eyes under treatment with such anticholinesterase drugs as demecarium bromide (Humorsol) or echothiophate iodide (Phospholine iodide) develop a more marked inflammatory response after filtering operative procedures. This consists of fibrin and cells in the anterior chamber, rapid formation of posterior synechias to the lens, and greater chance of developing anterior synechias as well as blocking off the filtration area.

Since failure of the stronger medical agents to control the glaucoma is the reason for surgery, it is logical to change the patient's medication from anticholinesterase drugs to pilocarpine for a period of two to three weeks preceding the operation. Anticholinesterase agents lower blood pseudocholinesterase and prolong apnea if succinylcholine (Anectine) is used during general anesthesia. Pseudocholinesterase levels may be reduced for weeks or months after medication is discontinued. Therefore, if general anesthesia is used, the anesthesiologist should be informed of any anticholinesterase agents used by the patient during the preceding months.

Preoperative orders

Lavatory and chair privileges

There should be as little interference with the patient's routine as possible. He may be permitted to continue the use of his own medications in his room unless there is some physical reason that makes this undesirable.

Secobarbital (Seconal) or pentobarbital (Nembutal)

Secobarbital or pentobarbital, 0.1 Gm by mouth, should be given at bedtime and repeated 2 hours before surgery. Premedication with barbiturates is advisable when local anesthetics are to be used. One of the most common mistakes in preoperative sedation is to give the medication too late to obtain maximal effect. In some elderly patients the barbiturates may act as excitants. An excellent substitute is chloral hydrate, 0.5 to 1 Gm by mouth.

Meperidine (Demerol)

Meperidine, 25 to 75 mg, combined with equal amounts of hydroxyzine hydrochloride (Vistaril) should be given intramuscularly 1 hour before surgery. Hydroxyzine hydrochloride potentiates the sedation of the narcotic and decreases any tendency for nausea. Meperidine as an analgesic is well tolerated and has few toxic reactions. Hydroxyzine hydrochloride is preferable to promethazine (Phenergan) because of its diminished hypotensive action.

Particularly in older patients, excessive doses of the combination of a barbiturate plus meperidine and hydroxyzine hydrochloride can result in sedation that is the equivalent of a light stage of general anesthesia. If this occurs, the patient must be carefully watched during surgery, preferably by an anesthesiologist. Under such circumstances several instances of cardiac arrest have been reported.

OPERATIVE CARE

Every surgeon should be aware of the incidence of cardiac arrest and should be familiar with its emergency management. Cardiac arrest during general anesthesia occurs in 1 in 3000 adults and 1 in 700 infants. The incidence, furthermore, is five times greater in poor-risk patients as compared with healthy patients. These figures point out the occasional need for resuscitation equipment, medications, and personnel in preventing a disaster. Techniques and procedures can be learned with practice sessions and drills.

Neuroleptanalgesia (ataractic)

Neuroleptanalgesia is especially useful when general anesthesia is unnecessary or contraindicated and when the usual mild preoperative sedation is inadequate. There are several advantages to the use of this medication. Ataractics provide comfort to the anxious patient and better control in higher-risk cases. No intubation is required. The patient becomes emotionally detached from his surroundings, often with amnesia for the procedure. Analgesia, hypomobility, antiemesis, and vasomotor stability are attained. Extrapyramidal reactions are rare. The usual local ocular anesthesia is necessary, however, and the patient should be monitored by an experienced anesthesiologist.

The strength of the medication used depends on factors such as the patient's size, age, health, and emotional status. Preoperatively medications for the average adult are as follows: hydroxyzine pamoate, 100 mg by mouth 2 hours before surgery; hydroxyzine hydrochloride, 50 mg, and meperidine, 50 mg, injected intramuscularly 1 hour before surgery. At surgery, meperidine is administered in an intravenous drip in small increments while vital signs and level of conscious response are monitored. A local retrobulbar and periorbital anesthetic is needed.

Ketamine hydrochloride

Ketamine hydrochloride, a phencyclidine compound, produces a dissociative form of anesthesia by depressing corticothalamic pathways. Given intramuscularly or intravenously, it is considered to be safer than other anesthetics and especially useful for short-term procedures in children. Unlike other anesthetic agents, ketamine may produce an increase in blood pressure and intraocular pressure. This effect is minimized with intramuscular administration. Vivid dreams and hallucinations occur in some patients during the recovery period and contraindicate its use except in young children. The recovery period is prolonged, especially with the addition of a general anesthetic, presenting problems with ketamine anesthesia for outpatient examination of children with infantile glaucoma. A period of apnea has been noted in a few infants less than 3 months of age.

Local anesthesia

The technique for local anesthesia is standard. Tetracaine (Pontocaine) drops, 0.5% to 1% in sterile ampules, are given four times at 30-second intervals, an extra drop or two being given after the skin preparation has been completed. Lidocaine (Xylocaine), 2% solution, with hyaluronidase is used for van Lint or O'Brien akinesia and retrobulbar injection. If these are used for subconjunctival injection, a small portion is directed along the superior rectus tendon to prevent pain when the superior rectus fixation suture is placed. Epinephrine drops should not be used if one wants to avoid dilating the pupil. It is difficult to obtain spontaneous iris prolapse for a small peripheral iridectomy if the pupil is too large.

POSTOPERATIVE CARE
Postoperative orders
Position and activity

Usually only one eye is patched. There is no real reason for keeping a patient in bed after an iridectomy if the incision is well closed or after a filtering procedure, unless there is overfiltration with a flat anterior chamber. Sometimes limited activity reduces flow through the filtration area in the early postoperative period. Therefore the usual order is for the patient to be up as soon as the effects of sedation have subsided. In the case of cyclodialysis and goniotomy, the patient is kept in bed with the head turned away from the operative site so that blood will drain away from the incision area. He is permitted activity as soon as the blood is largely absorbed.

Topical medication

All miotic drops should be ordered at specific hours for the unoperated eye. If medications are ordered three times a day, it is the usual practice on general wards to give medicines every 4 hours for 12 hours. The patient then has no medication for 12 hours. This might be disastrous for an eye with glaucoma. The eye operated on is usually dilated daily with 10% phenylephrine (Neo-Synephrine) or with parasympatholytic agents. This is best done by the surgeon when dressing the eye. Topical corticosteroids should be used if there is much postoperative reaction.

Systemic steroids have been used with success in postoperative glaucoma surgery where previous procedures have failed. Contraindications and side effects of systemic steroids must be kept in mind.

Acetazolamide (Diamox) or other carbonic anhydrase inhibitors

After a filtering operation it is wise to stop carbonic anhydrase inhibitors if the condition of the second eye permits. The formation of a functional bleb as well as the re-formation of the anterior chamber may well be dependent on a free flow of aqueous. The depression of aqueous production that follows surgery may negate the effect of stopping carbonic anhydrase inhibitors. Nevertheless, if increased aqueous production aids even slightly in promoting eventual success of the filtering procedure, discontinuing carbonic anhydrase inhibitors would seem desirable.

Other medications

Aspirin or a similar analgesic, 1 or 2 tablets by mouth every 3 hours, is ordered as necessary for pain. Meperidine, 50 to 100 mg every 6 hours subcutaneously, may be used if necessary for pain. Hydroxyzine pamoate or hydrochloride 25 to 50 mg, or prochlorperazine dimaleate (Compazine), 10 mg, by mouth or intramuscularly every 6 hours, may be needed to alleviate nausea. Hydroxyzine pamoate or hydrochloride potentiates the action of meperidine to double its original effectiveness. The dose of meperidine should then be reduced to half when these drugs are combined. Pentobarbital or secobarbital, 100 mg by mouth at bedtime, is ordered if necessary for sleep.

Postoperative instructions

Instructions vary markedly depending on the type of glaucoma procedure performed, the preoperative condition of the eye, the complications during the operation, the patient's general health, and the postoperative appearance of the eye. A patient with a hemorrhage, for example, would require an entirely different management from another patient. For this reason, postoperative patient instructions are governed by the individual surgical situation.

Generally patients leave the hospital on the second postoperative day and are told to limit their activity for one to two weeks. Postoperative office visits are usually every 2 to 5 days, depending on the procedure and time since surgery. Removable sutures are usually taken out 5 to 10 days postoperatively.

It is important that the pupil be dilated daily to prevent posterior synechias. With filtering surgery, 1% to 4% atropine solution or 0.2% scopolamine hydrobromide is usually needed. In iridectomy, 10% phenylephrine is usually sufficient. After trabeculotomies and cyclodialysis procedures, miotics reportedly increase the chances of success. For this, pilocarpine has been suggested.

Topical steroid medications instilled every 2 to every 6 hours may prevent inflammation and reduce fibrosis (scarring) in the postoperative eye. Steroids are especially needed in eyes with a history of inflammatory disease.

Patients will generally ask a number of specific questions. "Can I drive?" "Take a shower?" "Wash my hair?" "When will my vision return?" "When can I go back to work?" Answers to these questions require judgment on the part of the surgeon and can only be in general terms, such as: "You can tentatively plan on returning to work three weeks after surgery, but please understand that this estimate may change markedly according to your response to surgery."

Massage

When a filtering bleb is desired, massage of the eye two or three times daily may be suggested and may be begun as soon as the anterior chamber is re-formed and the pressure is above 10 mm Hg.

The purpose of massage is to help prevent the adherence of subconjunctival tissue to the sclera, with resultant closure of the translimbal channel. Clear instructions should be given to the patient, together with a demonstration of the technique. Two methods are employed. First, direct pressure through the lower lid to the inferior portion of the eyeball is used to force aqueous through the opening and under the conjunctival flap. Second, massage on the superior portion of the globe by alternate pressure of the two index fingers through the upper lid with the patient looking down tends to spread the aqueous and may help promote a more diffuse bleb formation.

Whether much is accomplished by massage is unknown. It may have some beneficial effect in continuing to force aqueous humor through a partly closed incision, thus helping to maintain patency. Strenuous massage is, of course, contraindicated for fear of damage to intraocular structures.

22

Surgical anatomy

There is no more critical millimeter in ophthalmic surgery than the transition zone at the corneoscleral junction known as the limbus. Here are made most of the glaucoma surgical incisions, often with success or disaster dependent on the accuracy of that incision. It is essential that the ophthalmic surgeon visualize the relationship between the external and internal ends of the incision. The plane of this incision must be varied when shifting from an ab externo incision to one with a keratome or when operating on an eye with a crowded anterior segment or an enlarged eye of congenital glaucoma.

CONJUNCTIVA AND TENON'S CAPSULE

The conjunctiva and a very thin subconjunctival fascia extend from the fornices to the limbus. Tenon's capsule is the denser subconjunctival connective tissue that is continuous with the muscle sheaths. Both the fascia and the conjunctiva are more dense and succulent in youth, becoming far thinner in the elderly. Tenon's capsule is thickest in the fornices, becoming thinner as the limbus is approached. Here it is unidentifiable as a separate layer from the wispy subconjunctival connective tissue that continues to lie between conjunctiva and sclera when the flap is turned down over the cornea. Dividing this connective tissue reveals a tiny ridge where the conjunctival epithelium merges with the corneal epithelium at the end of Bowman's membrane. This marks the anterior limit of the limbus.

The necessity of removing a portion of Tenon's tissue during filtering surgery is a controversial point. The fact that conjunctiva and Tenon's capsule combine near the limbus prevents practical manipulation and removal of tissues in a crucial filter area. Additional destruction of Tenon's capsule away from the limbus predisposes the eye to a thin-walled flap and may increase fibrosis and scarring. The indication for removal comes from clinical impressions and needs validation (Chapter 24).

BLOOD SUPPLY TO THE ANTERIOR SEGMENT (Plate 5 and Fig. 22-1)

Conjunctival blood vessels are usually not troublesome unless the eye is congested. Tenon's capsule has no large vessels, and bleeding occurs only when the

363

unwary surgeon incising the fascia cuts into the underlying muscle. This can be avoided by carrying incisions of the conjunctiva and Tenon's capsule down to the sclera in the quadrants between the muscles before completing the incision over the muscle.

There are many tiny surface scleral vessels. When subconjunctival injections are made, the sharp tip of the needle should be kept away from the sclera. In the reflection of the conjunctiva these vessels should be avoided. Procedures that require scleral incisions can be preceded by light cautery to the area.

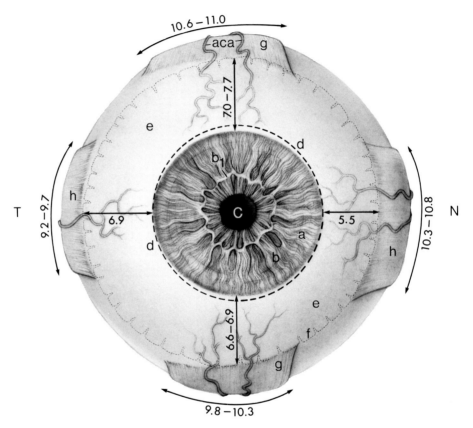

Fig. 22-1. Normal human eye, anterior aspect. *N,* Nasal aspect; *T,* temporal aspect. The cornea *(a)* is anterior to the iris *(b)* and pupil *(c).* The elliptical shape of the anterior corneal margin (arrows) is compared to the round shape of its posterior one (dotted line). The collarette of the iris is evident at b_1. The pupil is displaced slightly to the nasal side of the eye. The limbal area and external scleral sulcus surround the margin of the cornea *(d).* The sclera *(e)* is peripheral to the limbus. The sclera has been made artificially transparent to show the ora serrata *(f),* which are farther posterior on the temporal than on the nasal side. The superior and inferior rectus tendons *(g)* are curved and are inserted obliquely to the axis of the eye. The tendons of the medial and lateral recti muscles *(h)* also have curved insertions that are not oblique to the horizontal meridian. Each rectus muscle has two anterior ciliary arteries *(ACA),* except the lateral rectus, which has one. The measurements of all these structures are given in the illustration. (From Hogan, M. J., et al.: Histology of the human eye, Philadelphia, 1971, W. B. Saunders Co.)

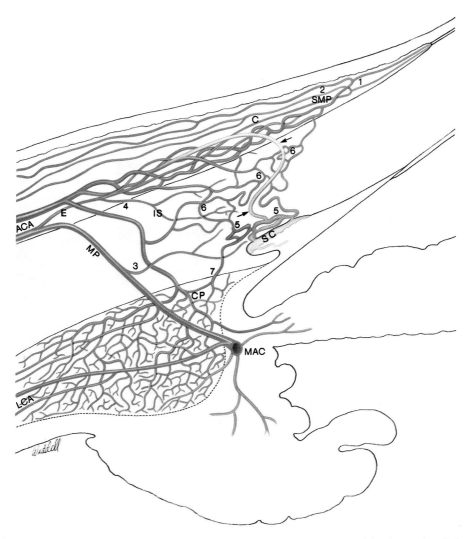

Plate 5. Drawing of a meridional section of the eye to show the blood supply of the limbal area.

Red indicates arterial channels. An anterior ciliary artery *(ACA)* divides to form an episcleral *(E)* and a major perforating *(MP)* branch. The episcleral branches produce episcleral, conjunctival *(C)*, and intrascleral *(IS)* nutrient vessels. The conjunctival vessels form the superficial marginal plexus of the cornea *(SMP)*. Two sets of vessels arise from the superficial marginal plexus: one *(1)* extends forward to form the peripheral corneal arcades; the other forms recurrent vessels *(2)* that run posteriorly to supply 3 to 6 mm of the perilimbal conjunctiva. The latter eventually anastomose with the recurrent conjunctival vessels from the fornices. The major perforating artery passes through the sclera to join the major arterial circle *(MAC)* of the iris. 3, Point at which a branch from the major perforating artery passes forward to form the intrascleral arterial channels of the limbus. This region often is supplied by a vessel that arises directly from the anterior ciliary artery as an episcleral vessel *(4)*.

Venous channels are blue. The major venous drainage from the limbus is into the episcleral veins, which then unite with the ophthalmic veins. The deep scleral venous plexus *(5)* is close to Schlemm's canal *(SC)*. An aqueous vein (arrows) arises from the deep scleral plexus and joins the episcleral veins. The intrascleral venous plexus *(6)* forms an extensive network in the limbal stroma. An important part of the drainage from the ciliary plexus *(CP)* is into the deep and intrascleral venous plexuses *(7)*. (From Hogan, M. J., et al.: Histology of the human eye, Philadelphia, 1971, W. B. Saunders Co.)

The major blood vessels pass through the sclera in relation to the recti muscles. The anterior ciliary vessels run with the muscles, penetrating the sclera to enter the ciliary body 1 to 3 mm in front of the tendinous insertions of the muscles. The long posterior ciliary arteries run in the two horizontal meridians, entering the ciliary body 8 mm behind the limbus. These points of entry need to be kept in mind when one sweeps a cyclodialysis spatula through the suprachoroidal space or does a cyclodiathermy procedure.

LIMBUS OR CORNEOSCLERAL JUNCTION (Fig. 22-2)
Anatomy

The gray transition zone between the white stroma of the sclera and the transparent corneal tissue is known as the limbus. The limbus is wider above, making the cornea oval horizontally. Internally the ring made by Schwalbe's line is almost perfectly circular. With the conjunctiva reflected, the corneoscleral sulcus can often

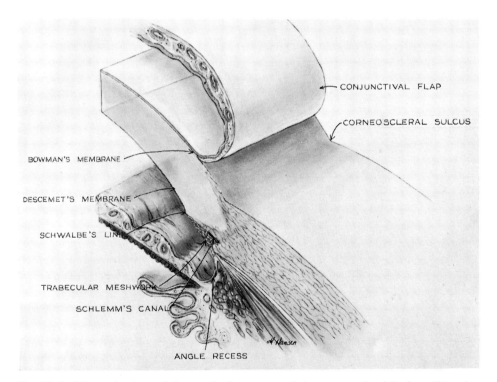

Fig. 22-2. Schematic view of the surgical anatomy of the corneoscleral limbus. This schematic diagram emphasizes the fact that in eyes with wide angles a vertical corneal incision at the conjunctival reflection enters the anterior chamber well in front of Schwalbe's line. A vertical incision at the corneoscleral sulcus tends to enter just behind Schwalbe's line. In a wide-angle eye there are approximately 2 mm of leeway before the angle recess is reached. In a narrow-angle eye an incision over 1 mm posterior to the conjunctival incision may enter the ciliary body.

be seen. This is the point at which the corneal curve merges with the greater radius of curvature of the sclera.

Incisions

How is the ophthalmic surgeon to place a limbal incision safely? The answer lies in complete understanding of the anatomic landmarks and meticulous attention to the direction taken by each incision into the anterior chamber.

The most helpful landmarks are the reflection point of the conjunctiva at the cornea, the corneoscleral sulcus, and the 1.5 mm gray merging zone of the corneal and scleral fibers in this area. This gray transition zone is produced by the two thin triangles of white scleral fibers enclosing the wedge of clear corneal tissue, which ends at the level of the scleral spur. The apex of the external triangle of scleral fibers is at Bowman's membrane; the internal one, composed of corneoscleral trabecular fibers, has its apex at Schwalbe's line.

After the incision of the conjunctiva and connective tissue, the sclera is exposed. The flap can be turned downward over the cornea after it is freed with the help of blunt dissection. The external anterior limbal border is often still concealed by a last wisp of tightly adherent subconjunctival connective tissue, which may have to be incised with a knife. A clean circular ridge is seen where the conjunctiva joins the corneal epithelium at Bowman's membrane. Although the exact width of the limbus varies from eye to eye, this conjunctival insertion marks the anterior limit of the limbus unless previous surgery or inflammation has disturbed the landmarks. An incision at the site of conjunctival insertion directed toward the anterior chamber runs immediately into clear corneal tissue and enters the chamber anterior to Schwalbe's line. Such an incision runs the risk of buttonholing the conjunctiva.

The gray of the limbus merges with the white of the sclera about 1.5 mm posterior to the conjunctival insertion, approximately at the corneoscleral sulcus. An incision exactly perpendicular at this point enters the chamber in the mid-trabecular area of most wide-angled eyes but may be in the area of the angle recess or even in the ciliary body of an eye with a small anterior segment. Therefore it is necessary to bevel or to angle incisions slightly toward the anterior chamber and to start the incision in a narrow-angled eye between the corneoscleral sulcus and the conjunctival reflection. The surgeon should be able to see clear corneal tissue after cutting the external scleral fibers if the incision is truly limbal.

Fewer complications arise if the ab externo or "scratch" incision is used. The same technique can be used for all glaucoma operations at the limbus and also for making the groove for the McLean suture in cataract surgery. Thus even the occasional operator can build up experience and greater knowledge of the anatomy of this critical zone. This results in safer, more accurate, and more successful surgery.

Incisions made by the keratome or Graefe knife are usually parallel to the iris and slant through the limbal tissues. Consequently they can safely begin farther from the limbus than a more nearly perpendicular ab externo incision and still reach the trabecular meshwork in front of Schlemm's canal. This is why many older texts advise incisions 2 mm behind the limbus. A perpendicular ab externo incision in that position can go directly into the ciliary body, particularly in eyes with small anterior segments. The tragic results of this surgical error can be seen in any laboratory of ophthalmic pathology where enucleated eyes show intravitreal hemorrhage, lens dislocations, cataract, intravitreal fibroblastic proliferation with retinal separation, uveitis, and sympathetic ophthalmia.

Trabeculectomy and trabeculotomy procedures require a knowledge of the limbal area as it is approached through a scleral flap incision. Deeper landmarks may be confusing, and an unwary surgeon will miss Schlemm's canal attempting trabeculotomy. Most important is the color change from the white of the sclera to the bluish cast given off by cornea adjoining sclera. At this point, the scleral spur and, just anterior to it, Schlemm's canal are located. Experience, however, is needed to increase the skill of the surgeon in locating small structures in this critical area. Technique can be developed by occasionally performing surgery with the operating microscope on unused eye bank eyes.

DESCEMET'S MEMBRANE

Descemet's membrane does not cut like corneoscleral fibers. When the incision has reached Descemet's membrane, or the inner trabecular fibers, the surgeon no longer feels the grating of the tip of the knife as it slides over collagenous bundles. Like cellophane, these inner tissues resist cutting until an initial perforation has been made; then they split easily. It is important to recognize this point. Otherwise, the surgeon is tempted to push harder and harder in an attempt to enter the anterior chamber, with the danger of damage to iris and lens when the penetration occurs suddenly. The No. 67 Beaver blade may be turned upward so that only the tip is in contact with the membrane to make the last controlled entry into the chamber. A razor-blade knife or a keratome enters even more easily, and the depth of penetration is more readily controlled when cutting upward rather than pressing down toward the iris.

CHAPTER 23

Surgery to break pupillary block

As stated in Chapters 12 and 13, the presence of a pupillary block represents a surgical emergency in almost all cases. The eye cannot return to normal until aqueous humor is free to come forward into the anterior chamber. In the interim, irreparable harm can be done to both the anterior and posterior ocular segments. Preoperative goals are designed to obtain a normotensive, quiet, white eye by medical means just as quickly as possible. This means that treatment with oral hyperosmotic agents, miotics, and acetazolamide (Diamox) is started in the office and the patient is hospitalized immediately for intensive topical and systemic therapy, including intravenous hyperosmotic agents if necessary. Neither the surgeon nor the patient should be misled by an initially normalized pressure into continuation of medical therapy. Iridectomy should be delayed only until the eye is no longer dangerously inflamed. Occasionally it is impossible to lower the intraocular pressure by medical means. In such cases a posterior sclerotomy with vitreous aspiration should precede the iridectomy. If the second eye has a narrow angle also, miotics should be used to avoid angle closure until a prophylactic iridectomy can be performed.

IRIDECTOMIES
Peripheral iridectomy

Peripheral iridectomy is the safest of the glaucoma operations when performed skillfully and is one of the few glaucoma operations that merits genuine enthusiasm for its effectiveness. Iridectomy should always be preferred to a filtering operation if there is any reasonable chance of success (Fig. 23-1).

Local anesthesia is usually used. General anesthesia should be employed if the eye is so painful and congested that local anesthesia may be ineffective or if the patient is nauseated or overly apprehensive. In either case a miotic pupil is essential during the surgery. Pilocarpine, 2%, should be used four times immediately preceding the operation. Added miotics should be given in the second eye if its chamber angle is narrow and it has not been operated on.

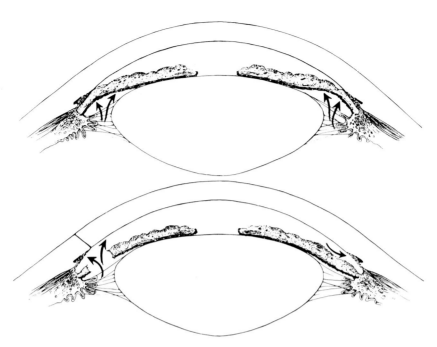

Fig. 23-1. Angle-closure glaucoma showing how iridectomy breaks the pupillary block and results in opening of the entire peripheral angle if no permanent peripheral anterior synechias are present.

Procedure

Incision (Figs. 23-2 to 23-4). A small peritomy is prepared in the upper temporal quadrant. The incision should not extend beyond the 12 o'clock meridian, since the opposite quadrant may be required for future filtering surgery. When only a small peritomy is used (Fig. 23-2), it is usually possible to perform a filtering procedure in the future at the same site, should this be necessary. Because of this, some surgeons prefer to do iridectomies in the upper nasal quadrant, and many confine their initial glaucoma surgery to the 12 o'clock position.

Between the corneoscleral sulcus and the corneoconjunctival junction, an ab externo groove, 4 mm in length, is made halfway through the limbus at right angles to the peripheral corneal surface. It is important to keep this incision far enough anterior that there can be no risk of damaging the ciliary body. If there is any doubt concerning the landmarks, the incision should be beveled anteriorly, and corneal tissue should be identified before the anterior chamber is entered. A keratome incision is contraindicated. A track suture may be placed before the groove is made and replaced across the groove, or a McLean suture may be used. The 7-0 silk or mild chromic suture is pulled out in a loop, which the assistant uses to hold the edges of the incision apart. With the use of the sharp end of the No. 67 Beaver blade, the central 2 mm of the incision is slanted toward the anterior

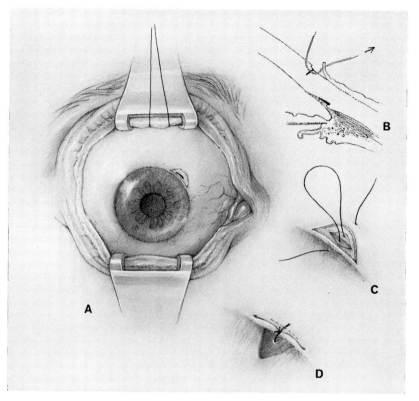

Fig. 23-2. Peripheral iridectomy using peritomy incision. **A,** Conjunctival incision and limbal groove. **B,** Cross section showing placement of McLean suture. **C,** McLean suture pulled out of limbal incision. **D,** Suture tied after completion of iridectomy.

chamber and is deepened to Descemet's membrane. Descemet's membrane is then split with the point of the knife, taking great care to avoid deep penetration into the anterior chamber. Usually a tiny loss of aqueous humor can be seen as the chamber is opened. The peripheral iris drops against the 1 mm inner incision and seals it.

Iridectomy (Fig. 23-5 and Reels I-4 and I-5). If the incision has entered the anterior chamber without damage to intraocular structures, the anterior chamber will still be full. If the pupil is dilated at this stage, acetylcholine (Miochol) is instilled to constrict the pupil rapidly. The surgeon is then able to perform a peripheral rather than an undesired mid-iris or sector iridectomy.

With the assistant pulling the incision apart by the suture, the surgeon presses vertically downward against the back lip of the incision with a small iris forceps. A tiny bubble of iris tissue containing posterior chamber aqueous humor will be forced through the incision. When enough iris has been pushed out to elongate the upper pupillary margin halfway to the limbus, the iris is grasped by toothed forceps, and a piece is excised with de Wecker scissors. The excised tissue should be

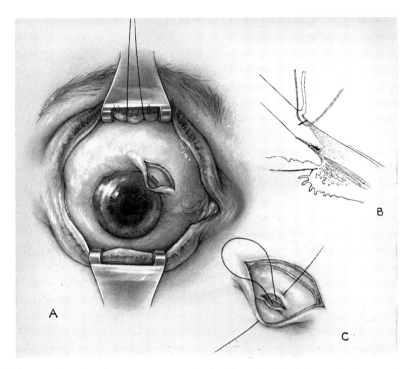

Fig. 23-3. Peripheral iridectomy using a limbus-based scleral flap. **A,** Conjunctival and outer limbal incision. **B,** Cross section of the limbus, showing outer limbal incision and McLean suture. **C,** McLean suture pulled out of limbal incision.

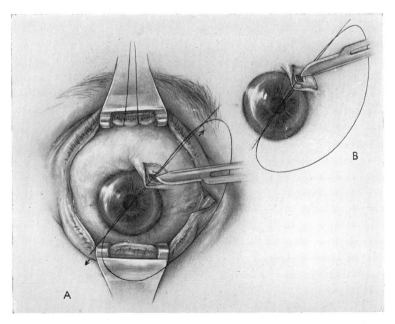

Fig. 23-4. Peripheral iridectomy. **A,** Deepening incision to Descemet's membrane. **B,** 1.5 mm opening through Descemet's membrane made with the tip of the knife.

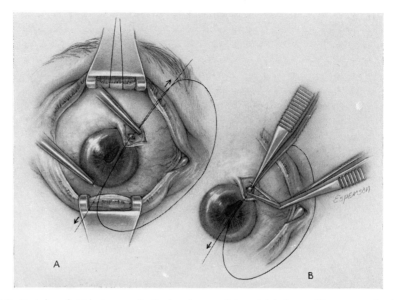

Fig. 23-5. Peripheral iridectomy. **A,** Prolapsing peripheral iris by pulling open the incision with sutures, plus pressure behind the incision and at the opposite limbus. **B,** Peripheral iridectomy.

inspected to be sure that the pigmented epithelium has been included. If smooth forceps are used, there is more risk that the superficial iris tissue will be excised, leaving behind an intact iris pigment layer. If there is no spontaneous prolapse of iris, smooth forceps must be used in the anterior chamber to pick up the iris in order to avoid injury to the lens. Particular care is then needed to be certain that the pigment layer is included and that a through-and-through iridectomy has been accomplished. Such assurance is impossible with an iridotomy.

Failure of the iris to prolapse. The following causes of failure of the iris to prolapse should be investigated.

1. Inaccurate incision. It may have been placed too far back, and the apparent opening into the anterior chamber will be actually on top of the ciliary body. If so, it is best to close the incision by the McLean suture and make a new, properly placed incision in a different quadrant. An incision placed too far into the cornea will not be plugged by the iris dropping against it. Instead, aqueous humor will leak out slowly and make prolapse of the iris difficult.

The incision may not have gone through into the anterior chamber or it may be too small. By keeping in the same incision plane and rigidly controlling the depth of penetration of the knife tip, the incision may be enlarged and deepened. Unless peripheral anterior synechias are present, an opening of approximately 1 mm should be ample.

2. The eye may be too soft because of preoperative medications and the retrobulbar anesthetic. While the back lip of the incision is kept depressed by the for-

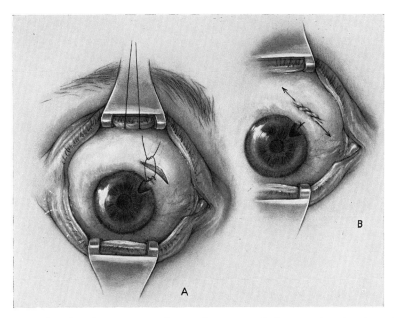

Fig. 23-6. Peripheral iridectomy. **A,** After re-formation of the anterior chamber, the first half of a surgeon's knot can be tightened to permit gonioscopy. **B,** McLean suture tied. Conjunctiva closed with a running black silk suture.

ceps, the intraocular pressure is increased by gentle pressure against the eye at the opposite limbus with the use of the side of the de Wecker scissors or a muscle hook. With a patent incision, this maneuver is almost always successful.

3. Peripheral anterior synechias may be present. A spatula must now be used. Usually the opening will have to be enlarged to 2 mm to accommodate a 1 mm spatula. While the back of the incision is depressed with the spatula, the tip can be moved forward under Descemet's membrane into the anterior chamber. Care is necessary to prevent detaching Descemet's membrane with the spatula (Reel III-7). Efforts should be made to avoid losing aqueous humor when the spatula is inserted or withdrawn. If there is still aqueous humor trapped behind the iris, pressure on the eye produced as before results in iris prolapse.

4. A hole may have been made in the iris, or aqueous humor may have escaped from behind the iris into the anterior chamber. If so, there will not be sufficient aqueous humor behind the iris to produce prolapse. With a knife or scissors the limbal incision must be enlarged sufficiently to permit entry and opening of forceps in the anterior chamber. Using smooth iris forceps to avoid trauma to the lens, the iris is grasped and pulled out, and a piece is excised. Be sure that the pigment layer of the iris has been included.

Completion of surgery (Fig. 23-6). Repositing the iris is easy if the pupil is miotic and the sphincter has not been injured by too large an iridectomy. Massaging through the conjunctiva or tapping the outside edge of the incision with a spatula plus the pull of the sphincter will open up the iridectomy and restore a central pupil. Anterior chamber irrigation may be required occasionally. The edges of a small iridectomy opening may become trapped in the limbal incision, requiring release with a cyclodialysis or iris spatula.

If the anterior chamber has been lost, it should be restored. This is best done by a commerically available plastic irrigator with a half-curved, flattened, silver needle. Normal isotonic sodium chloride solution may be used, but Locke's or Ringer's solution is less irritating. With the use of the back of the flattened needle to depress the posterior lip of the incision, the stream of the solution will flush peripheral iris out of the incision at the same time that the chamber is filled. It may be necessary to have the suture ready to tie if there is a tendency for the incision to leak.

In the past, preplaced paracentesis was used to be sure that the anterior chamber could be re-formed after the iridectomy. This added maneuver has proved unnecessary when the technique just described is used. With the pupillary block broken, the chamber is seldom lost and is easily re-formed. When the surgeon cannot see the iridectomy clearly, acetylcholine instilled in the anterior chamber will constrict the pupil and expose the excision site. Pigment removal does not guarantee a patent iridectomy. The opening can be sealed in prolapsed iris at the wound. If there is any need to examine the anterior chamber angle, the McLean suture can now be tied singly, and gonioscopy can be performed.

Postoperative treatment

It is very important to dilate the pupil daily in order to avoid posterior synechias. Phenylephrine (Neo-Synephrine), 10%, or 1% atropine is instilled by the surgeon at each dressing. With a patent iridectomy, this dilation is quite safe in almost all instances. The exception is the rare case of plateau iris in which dilation alone may result in a rise in pressure. Atropine has the advantage of tightening the pull of the zonules on the lens, resulting in a deeper anterior chamber. If there is much iritis, topical corticosteroids may be used. If the second eye has not been operated on and is receiving miotics, care must be taken that it is not given the mydriatic by mistake.

The patient is usually discharged from the hospital after 1 or 2 days. The medications can be stopped as soon as the slit lamp shows minimal iritis. Gonioscopy can be done at any time and should certainly be performed within two weeks so that the patient and the physician may know the probable prognosis. After three or four weeks, tonography may be performed to evaluate adequacy of the outflow channels and to determine whether or not miotics are likely to be needed. Tonometry is an important part of the long-term follow-up examination, since many cases after iridectomy require medications to control pressure.

Sector iridectomy

The actual incision into the anterior chamber needs to be a little larger than that for peripheral iridectomy in order to permit prolapse of the entire width of the iris. It is sometimes necessary to assist prolapse of the iris by hand-over-hand use of two forceps. In an iris bombé in which a sector iridectomy is desired, the incision may need to be as long as 3 mm to permit opening of forceps within the anterior chamber. When the iris is very friable, the best grasp on it can be made at the sphincter. A dull iris hook catching the pupillary margin may be the safest and surest way of pulling out the iris. Following are indications for a sector iridectomy.

1. *Inflammation.* In the presence of iritis or trauma a small peripheral iridectomy is likely to be closed by inflammatory products. Consequently the larger opening of a sector iridectomy is preferable. It also provides biopsy material for histologic or microbiologic investigations.

2. *Visual advantages.* If a pupillary membrane or nuclear cataract is present, material improvement of vision may result from a sector iridectomy. This is especially true if it proves necessary to use miotics postoperatively If trauma or keratitis has produced extensive scarring of the cornea, the sector iridectomy should be placed to take advantage of clear areas of cornea.

3. *Eyes with possible need of lens extraction.* If cataract extraction may be required in the future, a sector iridectomy with posterior synechialysis sets the stage.

4. *Aphakic pupillary block with pupillary membrane.* A peripheral iridectomy with discission by Vannas scissors through the central membrane and iris sphincter may solve both the pupillary block and the visual problem.

5. *Retinal detachment.* In cases with suspected detachment or when detachment is likely to occur, a large pupil permits adequate examination and treatment.

Basal iridectomy

Most surgical texts still stress the need for a basal iridectomy. In the past, relief of the obstruction in acute glaucoma was thought to come from exposing the trabecular meshwork in the area of the iridectomy. Therefore it was urged that the incision be placed near the scleral spur to cut or dialyze the root of the iris and to remove as large a piece of iris as possible.

Gonioscopy proves the fallacy of this reasoning. The iris tears loose at its thinnest spot near its insertion on the ciliary body, leaving a frill of iris behind. This often turns up, forming a small peripheral anterior synechia in the area of the iridectomy. The angle widens throughout its circumference because of the bypass of the pupillary block (Fig. 23-1). The incision needs to be near enough to the periphery to facilitate prolapse and to assure that posterior synechias to the lens cannot occlude it. A posteriorly placed incision invites disaster by injury to the ciliary body.

In a low percentage of patients ciliary processes are attached to posterior peripheral iris (Fig. 23-7). Foos finds a greater than 10% chance that a small portion of the posterior iris will contain ciliary processes. The excision of ciliary processes with an iridectomy may account for the occasional mild hemorrhage that occurs.

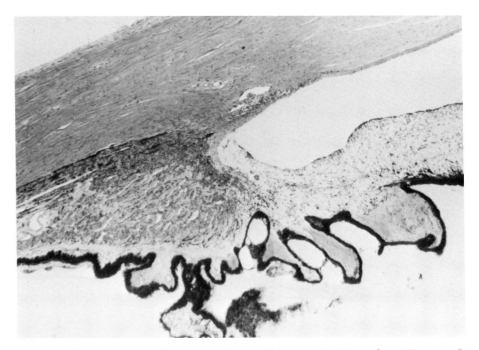

Fig. 23-7. Ciliary processes shown extending to the posterior iris surface. (Courtesy Dr. R. Y. Foos, Los Angeles.)

Transfixion

In iris bombé, it is sometimes safer to use transfixion of the iris rather than iridectomy to break the pupillary block. This is particularly true if the eye is congested and hemorrhage from dilated iris blood vessels is feared. Transfixion is accomplished by passing a Graefe knife across the anterior chamber from limbus to limbus, picking up the ballooned-up iris two to four times in the passage. Areas of excessive vascularity should be avoided. The knife must be kept in the normal plane of the iris to avoid damage to the lens.

If an anterior chamber is present in aphakic eyes, transfixion can be the procedure of choice. In addition to breaking the pupillary block by transfixion of the iris, discission of a pupillary membrane can be performed at the same time, and thus interruption of the pupillary block and visual improvement are accomplished in one procedure. If iris vitreous synechias extend to the base of the iris, discission of the hyaloid membrane may be required. If no anterior chamber is present transfixion is usually contraindicated.

Modification of iridectomy based on operating room gonioscopy

In the past, operating room gonioscopy has been of value in deciding whether to depend on an iridectomy or a filtering operation. The use of hyperosmotic agents and the Zeiss gonioscopic lens has permitted better evaluation of the extent of peripheral anterior synechias preoperatively. It has also been found that increased intraocular pressure after iridectomy can usually be controlled by medical therapy. Because of this, operating room gonioscopy is generally restricted to the occasional case in which the surgeon must know the degree of angle obstruction. It is also helpful if an iridectomy opening is not visible externally at the completion of surgery.

Lens extraction as an initial procedure

In phakic eyes both pupillary block and crowding of a shallow anterior chamber can be relieved by lens extraction. In occasional eyes with clear lenses the anterior chamber may be so shallow that primary lens extraction may be the safest antiglaucoma operation. This is particularly true if pressure cannot be restored to normal medically or if phakic malignant glaucoma has been precipitated by glaucoma surgery on the first eye. If the surgeon is undecided, a peripheral iridectomy can be performed, followed by operating room gonioscopy. If the angle has opened satisfactorily, the operation can be concluded. If not, the incision can be extended, sutures can be added as necessary, and lens extraction can be done.

Of course, if the angle-closure glaucoma is secondary to a swollen, cataractous lens, removal of the cataract is obligatory. If an eye with primary angle-closure glaucoma has significant lens changes, it is usually preferable to relieve the pupillary block by lens extraction rather than by peripheral iridectomy. The age and health of the patient as well as the type of cataract need to be considered. A nuclear cataract in an elderly patient is less likely to increase rapidly after iridectomy than is a posterior subcapsular opacity.

Laser iridotomy

Iridotomy by means of argon laser photocoagulation has recently been advocated by several authors. The procedure can be performed without anesthesia, although retrobulbar lidocaine is often used. Pilocarpine is administered to produce miosis, and the iris surface examined with the slit lamp about two thirds of the distance from the sphincter to the angle for an area where the stroma is somewhat thin. An area near the 10 or 2 o'clock position is selected, and four to six 50 to 100 μm coagulations, at 0.2-second exposure and about 300 mw power intensity, are placed in the region, surrounding an area about 1 mm in diameter. This tends to draw the iris taut and slightly elevated off the lens surface. The intensity is increased to 800 to 1000 mw, and the area bounded by the previous coagulation spots is treated to penetrate through the iris. This may require multiple applications. Penetration is marked by the sudden release of a small cloud of pigment. Postoperatively the patient is treated intensively with topical corticosteroids. Repeated treatments at weekly intervals may be required if a penetrating iridotomy is not produced.

The procedure has the obvious advantage of avoiding an operative procedure and can be performed as an outpatient technique. Disadvantages include the frequent necessity for multiple treatments, the great difficulty in producing iridotomies in eyes with brown irides, the possibility of lenticular opacities at the iridotomy site, and the creation of a retinal burn at the time of iris penetration by the laser beam. The beam should be directed obliquely to avoid the possibility of a retinal burn near the posterior pole. At the present time, argon laser iridotomy is not recommended as a replacement for iridectomy in uncomplicated cases.

Laser iridotomy is of great benefit in instances of incomplete iridectomy where only stromal tissue was removed, leaving the pigment epithelium intact. Small, 50 μm applications at 300 mw power intensity produce an immediate opening in the pigment epithelium and establish patency of the iridectomy.

CILIARY-BLOCK GLAUCOMA (MALIGNANT GLAUCOMA)
Phakic ciliary-block glaucoma

After glaucoma surgery, particularly filtering procedures in eyes with chronic angle-closure, the vitreous humor and lens may move forward, retaining the pupillary block. Within hours to days or years of the initial surgery, the anterior chamber is found to be flat and the tension high. Conventional procedures such as iridectomy or the various filtering operations fail to relieve the flat chamber and increased pressure. Such a condition in the past has usually resulted in loss of the eye. Prompt diagnosis and proper treatment salvage many of these eyes.

The surgeon should immediately start intravenous mannitol plus acetazolamide (Diamox). Local therapy should consist of a 4% solution of atropine and a 10% solution of phenylephrine (Neo-Synephrine), used at frequent intervals for 2 hours and then four times a day thereafter if the anterior chamber forms. If the anterior chamber does not form in 3 to 5 days or cannot be maintained in the future by reasonable therapy, vitreous aspiration becomes the operation of choice. The longer the delay and the more procedures tried before vitreous aspiration, the less likely is a cure, particularly in inflamed or high-pressure eyes.

Procedure

Vitreous aspiration is performed as follows. A scleral incision is made 4 mm behind the limbus in both inferior quadrants between the muscles to be sure that no choroidal bleeding is present. Diathermy is applied to the area around the temporal posterior sclerotomy. Before entering the vitreous, a paracentesis is performed. An 18-gauge blunt needle with depth-indicator marks is inserted 12 mm, and 1 to 1.5 ml of vitreous is removed by a 2 ml syringe. The anterior chamber is deepened with 0.5 ml of isotonic sodium chloride solution and then air through the paracentesis incision. The anterior chamber should be as deep as in a myopic eye. No sutures are necessary.

Postoperatively the eye is maintained on 4% atropine and 10% phenylephrine. This method of management according to Simmons cures over 90% of ciliary-block glaucomas. If vitreous aspiration does not cure the malignant process, lens extraction is indicated.

Aphakic ciliary-block glaucoma

After lens removal, it may be impossible to re-form the anterior chamber or the anterior chamber may collapse in a few days, and the pressure again elevates. This resembles aphakic pupillary block. Unfortunately, in ciliary-block glaucoma, iridectomy is not curative, since aqueous humor collects in or behind the vitreous body. The collection must be tapped by an incision into the vitreous body before the aqueous humor can again drain into the anterior chamber.

Method

The pressure is lowered preoperatively by hyperosmotic agents and acetazolamide. Because in most cases it is impossible clinically to differentiate aphakic pupillary block from ciliary-block glaucoma, an iridectomy should be performed first. If iridectomy is ineffective, the vitreous face should be incised. With a Ziegler knife-needle, discission of the anterior hyaloid membrane is performed just as for a secondary cataract. Usually the anterior chamber begins to form promptly. The anterior chamber should then be filled with balanced salt solution or air. Care must be taken, since air will follow vitreous channels behind the iris, complicating postoperative management. Such eyes may need no further treatment.

If aphakic ciliary-block glaucoma is unresponsive to discission of the vitreous face, further surgery is necessary. Either through the pupil or iridectomy, 0.5 ml of vitreous must be aspirated with a large needle. Posterior sclerotomy and vitreous aspiration or anterior vitrectomy may be indicated in some aphakic cases.

As a rule, these eyes also have damage to the trabecular meshwork, and peripheral anterior synechias. All forms of medical therapy should be used to keep the eye normotensive. Cyclodialysis, guarded thermal sclerostomy, or external trabeculectomy may be successful if additional surgery becomes necessary.

In a few of these eyes, after days or weeks, the re-formed anterior chamber again collapses and tension rises abruptly. A fresh vitreous condensation may be blocking aqueous flow, and another discission may be successful. However, in some eyes the aqueous humor appears to continue to flow behind the detached vitreous humor. An attempt can be made with a Wheeler knife to cut completely through the detached vitreous body, whose posterior upper surface usually lies just in front of the middle of the vitreous cavity. This is a dangerous type of surgery and may lead to retinal detachment. Nevertheless, when necessary, its use has retained vision in a number of eyes that would otherwise have been lost.

CHAPTER 24

Filtering procedures

When pressures cannot be held at a level low enough to protect the optic nerve from damage and pupillary block is no longer a factor, surgery to create new outflow channels is required. Included are a variety of operations that endeavor to maintain an opening for aqueous drainage from the anterior chamber into the subconjunctival space of eyes with no pupillary block. The opening must be of sufficient size to normalize intraocular pressure but not large enough to produce hypotony. The attempt of the surgeon to produce an adequate outflow channel frequently reduces outflow resistance to zero, resulting in excessive aqueous outflow and exhaustion of the ciliary body. Methods are needed to reduce aqueous outflow but to maintain the filtering area in the initial postoperative period. When successful, there is alteration of the subconjunctival collagenous tissue with fragmentation of fibrils, forming a thin, relatively acellular, lacy matrix (Fig. 24-1).

The aqueous humor appears to escape from the bleb by two main routes: first, by diffusion through the episcleral tissues and conjunctiva and, second, by absorption into the subconjunctival and episcleral blood vessels. The transconjunctival route can be demonstrated by the Seidel fluorescein test. Subconjunctival absorption is occasionally verified by visualization of an aqueous-filled capillary biomicroscopically. Trabeculectomies and some trabeculotomies appear to function mainly by filtration, as shown by fluorescein studies and pathologic specimens. Other routes of outflow may be through a cleft into the suprachoroidal space, through surgically opened scleral collector channels or the cut ends of Schlemm's canal. Thin-walled blebs that are covered mainly by conjunctiva are dangerous because of the risk of bacterial invasion followed by intraocular infection. The trephine bleb has been particularly susceptible to this complication. Patients should be told the symptoms of conjunctivitis and urged to report to an ophthalmologist for prompt therapy if infection begins.

Satisfactory pressure control can be expected in 60% to 85% of eyes, depending on the condition of the eye and the skill with which the surgery is done. In the young the percentage of success is around 30% to 35%. No one procedure has yet been proved better than another. The theoretic requirements for

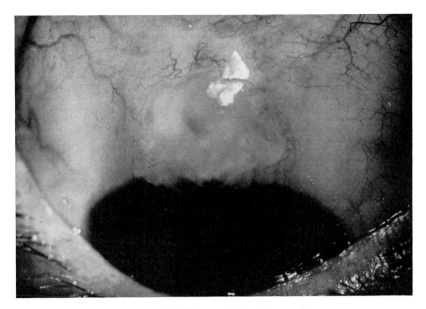

Fig. 24-1. Successful filtration bleb after a sclerectomy.

the development of new drainage channels of proper resistance make it surprising that the success rate is as good as it is. The main reason for avoiding filtering surgery, if at all possible, is the damage produced by that surgery to the inner eye, whether satisfactory pressure control is achieved or not. This includes complications of flat anterior chambers, anterior and posterior synechias, incarceration of ciliary processes, vitreous, iris, and lens in the filtration wound, acceleration of cataract formation, hypotony, infection, hemorrhage, malignant glaucoma, and bleb rupture.

CONJUNCTIVAL INCISION AND FLAP

Since all the filtering operations require a similar conjunctival incision and flap, its preparation and closure will be detailed now for all subsequent operations.

Conjunctival incision (Fig. 24-2)

It is best to have the operative site concealed by the upper lid but placed medial to the 12 o'clock meridian so that the opposite quadrant is available for subsequent surgery if needed. Because of the frequency of cataracts or their subsequent development in these eyes, the nasal quadrant is preferable. The cataract can then be removed at a later time by a temporal section without interfering with the filtering bleb.

A subconjunctival injection of as much as 0.5 ml should be used, which may contain an anesthetic agent. The tissue is thus ballooned out so that the superior rectus suture can be placed very high in the fornix. This simplifies the dissection

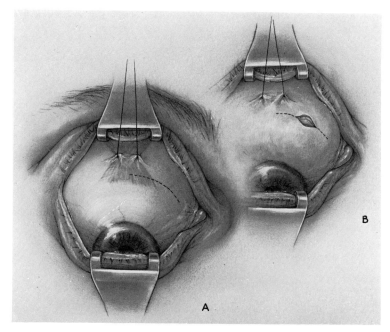

Fig. 24-2. Conjunctival incision for all operations to promote external drainage. **A,** Superior rectus suture placed as high as possible. **B,** Conjunctival incision.

and permits a high conjunctival section at least 8 mm from the limbus. The incision should be carried directly down through Tenon's membrane to the sclera at a point away from the superior rectus muscle to avoid bleeding from the muscle. The incision can be then enlarged sufficiently by blunt dissection to permit easy exposure of 4 mm of the limbus.

Excision of Tenon's capsule

Particularly in young persons and blacks, the subconjunctival connective tissue and Tenon's capsule form an extremely bulky layer. It has been suggested that removal of this connective tissue increases the probability of successful filtration. Proof of this statement remains open to question. If it is necessary to remove Tenon's capsule, an injection of fluid between Tenon's membrane and the conjunctiva will facilitate the difficult separation. After elevating the conjunctiva, a portion of Tenon's capsule can be dissected from the sclera and excised. Care should be taken not to buttonhole the conjunctiva.

Closure of the incision (Fig. 24-7)

There are several methods of closing conjunctival incisions. A round needle rather than a cutting edge is preferred to avoid enlarging puncture wounds in the conjunctiva. Suturing can be done in two layers or in one layer if care is taken to pick up both tissues each time a stitch is taken. A continuous suture is used, with the bites placed close together. In the center of the incision one bite may be taken into superficial scleral tissue. This prevents the flap from retracting downward toward the incision.

Conjunctival closure can be performed in the following way when early postoperative outflow is excessive, as occurs in, for example, thermal sclerostomies or trephination procedures. Before the suture is pulled up preparatory to tying the ends together in a purse-string fashion, a lacrimal needle on a syringe or anterior chamber irrigator may be slid between the lips of the incision down to the sclera. Balanced salt soluton is forced under the flap to test for leaks. The two ends of the continuous suture are then tied together tightly enough to create a line of demarcation for the bleb. This excludes the incision line from the aqueous humor under the bleb in the all-important early postoperative period. Sutures are removed in 5 to 10 days.

Conjunctival wounds are also closed with a continuous 7-0 silk suture pulled snug, but allowed to remain untied at both ends. This technique is applied when there is less concern with hypotony and a flat anterior chamber.

In spite of remarks suggesting tight wound closure by standard methods, some surgeons have suggested that conjunctival wound approximation with one to three interrupted silk sutures is adequate. This technique has the advantage of reduced inflammation because of less suture material used. No fistulas have been seen with the use of this method.

IRIDENCLEISIS

An ab externo incision is placed at the corneoscleral sulcus in wide-angled eyes. In eyes with narrow angles it is moved forward to place it between the sulcus and the conjunctival reflection. The incision is beveled forward slightly toward the anterior chamber. The entrance into the anterior chamber is only approximately 2 mm in length if the iris can be made to prolapse spontaneously. If not, it must be enlarged to at least 3 mm to provide room for a smooth iris forceps to be opened inside the eye. To avoid injury to the lens there should be no teeth on these forceps. The forceps have best control if the iris is grasped at or near the sphincter. If only one pillar is to be incarcerated, the surgeon pulls the iris out until the pupillary margin is visible and then runs the de Wecker scissors under the iris to its base to do a complete vertical iridotomy beside the forceps. The iris is then wedged firmly in the incision and dropped. With a double-pillar iris incarceration, the assistant should grasp the iris beside the surgeon's forceps. The radial iridotomy is similarly done between the two forceps, and both pillars are incarcerated in opposite edges of the incision. The disadvantage of the double-pillar incarceration is that it tends to give an updrawn pupil. However, two pillars may increase slightly the chance of success. Also, if further surgery becomes necessary and a cyclodialysis is done below at some later date, the pull of the updrawn pupil may help to hold open the cyclodialysis cleft.

If the iris is found to be of very poor texture, tearing easily, it is not likely to hold an incision open. In such a situation, the procedure should be converted to a sclerectomy either with or without iris incarceration.

There are two main advantages of iridencleisis. First, the anterior chamber is less likely to remain collapsed postoperatively than in sclerectomy or trephination. Second, it is simple. There are several disadvantages. First, the incarceration of iris tissue is contrary to normally accepted surgical principles, and sympathetic ophthalmia is probably more common with it than with other procedures. Second, there may be an induced irregular corneal astigmatism that can decrease vision by as much as one or two lines. Astigmatism is more common with the double-pillar iris incarceration. Third, it disfigures the pupil.

SCLERECTOMY

The conjunctival section is made as described for iridencleisis.

The tissue to be excised is always the limbal tissue, but the ab externo incision must be varied, depending on whether the sclerectomy is to be performed on the anterior or posterior lips of the incision.

Scissors sclerectomy. Some surgeons make two parallel ab externo incisions 0.5 mm apart, extending for 4 mm along the limbus. After one of these incisions has entered the anterior chamber, the entire corneoscleral strip is excised by scissors, and thus the sclerectomy is completed.

Posterior lip sclerectomy (Figs. 24-3 to 24-7). The ab externo incision is placed

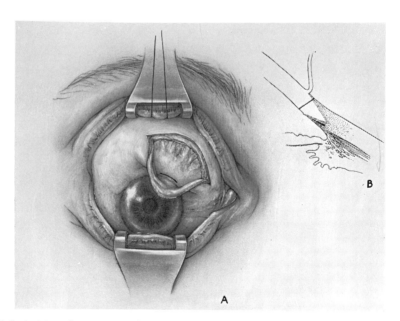

Fig. 24-3. Incision for posterior lip sclerectomy. **A,** Conjunctival and external limbal incision. **B,** Cross section of the limbal incision for a posterior lip sclerectomy. The incision for iridencleisis and thermal sclerostomy is placed 1 mm more posterior to the conjunctival reflection.

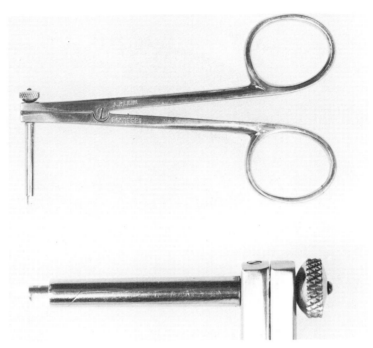

Fig. 24-4. Walser punch. Higher magnification (below) shows rotating 1 mm blade for convenient placement during sclerectomy.

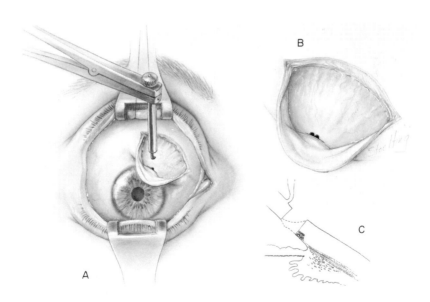

Fig. 24-5. Posterior lip sclerectomy with Walser punch. **A,** Single punch sclerectomy. **B,** Double punch sclerectomies. **C,** Cross section showing area excised. Dotted lines show incomplete excision of tissue that frequently occurs. Excised tissue may include trabeculum and Schlemm's canal.

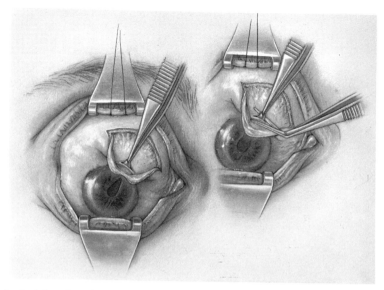

Fig. 24-6. Peripheral iridectomy after any of the operations for creating new outflow channels.

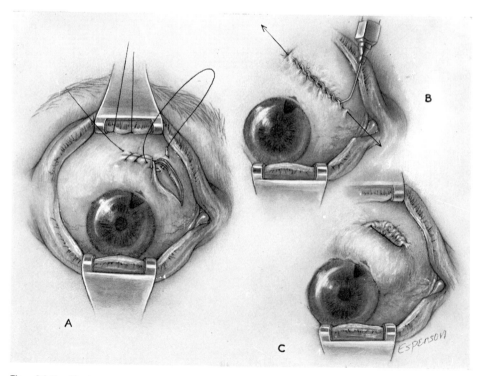

Fig. 24-7. Closing conjunctiva and Tenon's capsule. **A,** Running black silk suture with central bite picking up episcleral tissue to prevent retraction of the flap. **B,** Straightening suture and injecting isotonic sodium chloride solution under the flap. **C,** Snug tying of the suture, retaining the solution under the flap.

just behind the point of reflection of the conjunctiva in the anterior limbus. It is beveled forward somewhat more than for other procedures. The length of the incision must be at least 3 to 4 mm to permit a 1 mm punch to be slid easily under the back lip of the incision. The safest and easiest instrument available for this purpose is the Walser punch. With this punch, the size of the scleral bite is limited to 1 mm, and the cutting blade can be inserted into the anterior chamber through a small incision. One or two 1 mm bites side by side are adequate. One must inspect this opening carefully. Not infrequently the outer sclera is excised, but the punch slips off before the trabecular limbal tissues are excised, and a full-thickness opening is not made. As in the trephine operation, the specimen removed provides ideal opportunities for studying the pathology, histology, and electron microscopic appearance of freshly excised trabecular meshwork in glaucomatous eyes (Fig. 24-9). After sclerectomy, the iris usually prolapses into the opening. If it does not, it should be grasped gently by forceps, and in either case a peripheral iridectomy should be performed. Closure of the conjunctival incision is as described for iridencleisis.

Anterior lip sclerectomy. The ab externo incision must be placed back at the corneoscleral sulcus to permit room for the removal of the tissue between the incision and the conjunctival reflection. Otherwise the procedure is the same. Scissors can also be used, a 0.5 mm semicircle of tissue being excised. Buttonholing of the conjunctival flap while cutting out the scleral fragment is the principal danger of anterior lip sclerectomy.

THERMAL SCLEROSTOMY

The ab externo incision is placed as for iridencleisis. All bleeding is carefully controlled by cautery. As the 2 mm incision is deepened, its edges are seared to produce shrinkage, with care taken to have that shrinkage extend into the depths of the incision. Some operators advise actually entering the anterior chamber with the cautery, as in the Preziosi procedure. A peripheral iridectomy is performed on the prolapsed iris, much as in the simple iridectomy procedure.

The success rate of thermal sclerostomy appears to be about the same as that of sclerectomy with a punch. There is some uncertainty as to the amount of tissue destroyed. In some eyes the intraocular pressure is elevated for 1 or 2 days after the operation, and in these eyes the inner aspects of the incision may not be patent. Some of them develop filtration later. In other eyes drainage is excessive, with prolonged collapse of the anterior chamber and formation of synechias.

Guarded thermal sclerostomy (Fig. 24-8)

A guarded thermal sclerostomy provides a logical method of reducing the complications of filtering surgery. Aqueous production is reportedly reduced by surgical trauma to the eye; the added effect of an initially excessive outflow through the sclerostomy further decreases aqueous secretion by exhausting the ciliary body. More physiologic levels of aqueous production may be maintained if the size of the surgical filtering area is decreased initially with a double-armed guard suture. This approach is especially useful on shallow-chambered eyes where there is a greater susceptibility to flat chambers and malignant glaucoma. If the incidence of hypotony, flat anterior chambers, and choroidal detachment is reduced, the complications of cataract, synechias, and filtration failure are minimized.

The procedure is similar to that of the standard thermal sclerostomy. However, when the 3 mm long limbal incision is two thirds of the corneal depth, a horizontally placed 6-0 silk mattress suture is inserted across the groove. The free ends of the suture must be on the corneal side of the incision, 2 mm anterior to the conjunctival insertion. To complete the sclerostomy, the suture is withdrawn from the incision and may be used to support and separate the wound. The anterior chamber is entered with alternate applications of cautery and deepening of the incision with a No. 67 Beaver blade. Iridectomy is performed. The anterior chamber is deepened with balanced salt solution after the guard suture is pulled up. The suture is then secured with a single bowknot. There should be enough leakage through the sclerostomy to allow shallowing of the anterior chamber when moderate pressure is applied to the cornea. The suture is easily untied and adjusted as needed.

Postoperative visits are usually more frequent, and judgments must be made concerning the suture adjustment. Generally, if the pressure remains normal (6 to 16 mm Hg) and the anterior chamber deep and if the bleb appears ade-

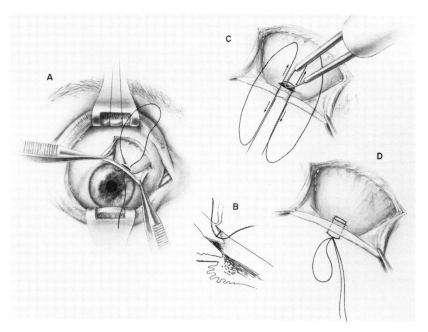

Fig. 24-8. Guarded thermal sclerostomy. **A,** Insertion of guard suture through limbal incision. **B,** Cross section showing suture in position. **C,** Suture loops retracted for additional cautery. **D,** Suture may be tied with a single bowknot, which can be adjusted as necessary during the early postoperative period.

quate, no adjustment is made, and the suture is loosened in 3 to 5 days. It is then removed 2 days later if conditions are satisfactory. If the chamber is flat and the eye hypotonous, the suture is tightened. Often the anterior chamber will deepen dramatically 1 to 2 hours after the tightening of the suture. When the chamber is deep, the pressure high, and the bleb small, the suture needs loosening even though this may be on the first postoperative day.

Thermal sclerostomy under a scleral flap

Since the development of trabeculectomy (p. 392), the use of a lamellar scleral flap has been applied to the techniques for other filtering procedures including thermal sclerostomy. After creation of a scleral flap carried forward into clear cornea, a sclerostomy is performed with cautery into the anterior chamber at about the level of Schwalbe's line. The opening in Descemet's membrane may be enlarged with the tip of a razor-blade knife. An iridectomy is performed, and the scleral flap sutured closed with one or two sutures. The conjunctival incision is closed in routine fashion. This technique combines the advantages of trabeculectomy with the ease of performance of thermal sclerostomy. The results appear equal to those of the other procedures.

TREPHINATION

It is difficult to criticize a well-performed trephine operation. It is clean, neat surgery, which has a high success rate. However, it is much more difficult for occa-

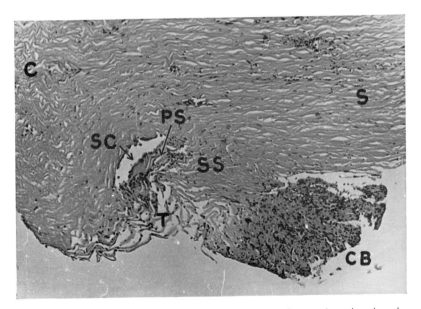

Fig. 24-9. Trephine button. *C*, Cornea; *SC*, Schlemm's canal; *PS*, altered trabecular meshwork of chronic glaucoma; *SS*, scleral spur; *S*, sclera; *CB*, ciliary body; *T*, trabecular meshwork.

sional operators to perform. Disastrous errors can occur at the time of surgery, such as misplacement of the trephine, buttonhole of the flap, injury to the lens or ciliary body, and incomplete removal of the corneoscleral button. The large opening produced by trephination invites hypotony, flat anterior chamber, and incarceration of intraocular tissue, particularly in the crowded segment of narrow-angle eyes (Fig. 24-9). Although similar complications can occur with other operations, they are less frequent and more easily avoided.

Postoperatively, gonioscopy usually reveals peripheral anterior synechias to the back lip of the trephine opening (Fig. 24-10, *A*). The size of the opening permits prolapse of intraocular tissues. These may include iris, one or more ciliary pro-

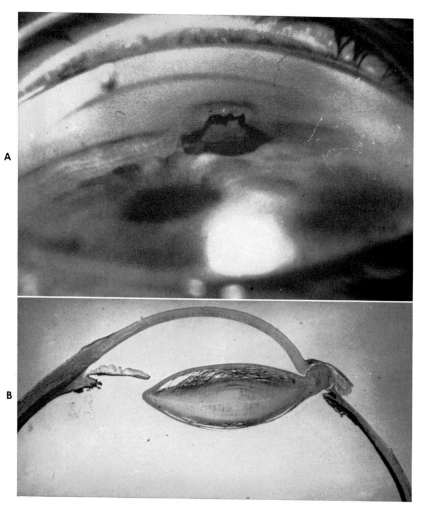

Fig. 24-10. A, Goniophotograph of a trephine opening with peripheral anterior synechias to trabecular meshwork and to the posterior lip of the trephine opening. Externally, a filtering bleb is present. **B,** Prolapse of lens into a trephine opening. (**B** courtesy Dr. P. Cibis, St. Louis.)

cesses, and occasionally lens or even vitreous (Fig. 24-10, *B*). If only part of the opening is occluded, the operation may still be a success. In the successful trephination the bleb is covered partly by split peripheral cornea and the thinnest area of the conjunctiva. This results in a thin-walled bleb. There is persistent danger of infection of the bleb, with resulting intraocular infection. The patient must be warned to report for emergency treatment of any conjunctivitis.

In an attempt to avoid the thin-walled bleb, most surgeons use the trephine only in wide-angled eyes and avoid dissection of the episcleral tissue into the cornea.

If for any reason trephination is to be done in a narrow-angle eye, it is necessary to split into clear corneal tissue under Bowman's membrane approximately 1 mm; otherwise, the back edge of the trephine may damage the ciliary body.

Procedure (Fig. 24-11)

After the conjunctival flap has been prepared, 1.5 mm trephine is held at right angles to the corneal surface and is then tipped ever so slightly, so that the corneal edge of the incision cuts into the anterior chamber first. The anterior edge of the trephine blade is held snugly against the reflected base of the conjunctival

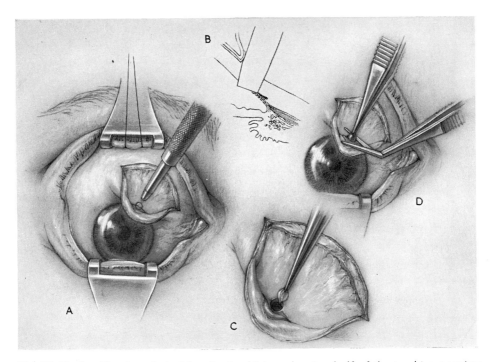

Fig. 24-11. Trephination. **A,** Incision for trephining, showing half of the trephine opening in split corneal tissue and half in limbal tissue. **B,** Cross section of trephination. **C,** Trephine button hinged posteriorly, ready to be excised, followed by iridectomy. **D,** Peripheral iridectomy.

flap. After the cut is started by twirling the blade with the fingers, it is periodically checked for position and direction and for depth of the trephine blade, care being taken to replace the blade exactly in the former cut.

When the blade enters the chamber, the pupil will elongate suddenly as the peripheral iris starts to prolapse. The trephine is lifted away immediately. If perfectly placed, the trephine cuts a neat corneoscleral button that hangs like a trapdoor by its last few inner fibers to the back of the trephine incision. The dark iris tissue is pushed out in a small bleb. If possible, the trephine button is removed by picking it up with forceps and completing the cut with small scissors. A peripheral iridectomy is then done, and the iris is reposited by gentle washing with an anterior chamber irrigator.

If the chamber has not been entered in sufficient area to complete the cut with scissors, it is occasionally possible to cut further with the trephine by tilting it away from the entrance point. If the iris is already beginning to prolapse, it is dangerous to use the trephine further. The tip of a keratome or Graefe knife, carefully controlled as to depth of incision, can sometimes extend most of the incision into the anterior chamber. It is often most difficult to excise the inner layers.

Many surgeons using the trephine procedure perform the operation under a lamellar scleral flap. This provides a safer technique and a much more easily performed operation. The closure of the flap is the same as for the other filtering operations.

TRABECULECTOMY (TRABECULOCANALECTOMY)
(Figs. 24-12 and 24-13 and Plate 6)

Trabeculectomy is one of the recent developments in glaucoma surgery; long-term results are thus not clearly determined. Successful control of pressure appears to be equal to that of older filtering procedures. Proponents of trabeculectomy say its major advantages lie in the fact that it leads to fewer complications. This is certainly true during surgery and the early postoperative period. The lower complication rate has encouraged many surgeons to use trabeculectomy as a primary procedure in open-angle glaucoma. Certainly it can be used as a secondary procedure if one favors the older filtering procedures. Trabeculectomy may be an advantage in aphakic glaucoma, in glaucoma with a shallow anterior chamber, as part of a combined procedure with cataract extraction when the patient desires possible contact lens wear, in glaucoma in the young and the black population, and, as stated above, when other procedures have failed.

Either general or local anesthesia can be used. Initially a large, limbus-based conjunctival flap is dissected in the superior nasal quadrant. Other quadrants are used when prior surgery or disease has damaged the primary site. A rectangular or triangular (Fig. 24-13) scleral flap is made with a No. 67 Beaver blade or razor blade knife, 6 mm long at the limbus to a point 3 to 6 mm in back of the limbus. The limbus-based scleral flap is about one-half the scleral thickness. With the flap elevated, a block of corneoscleral tissue approximately 1.5 × 4.0 mm is

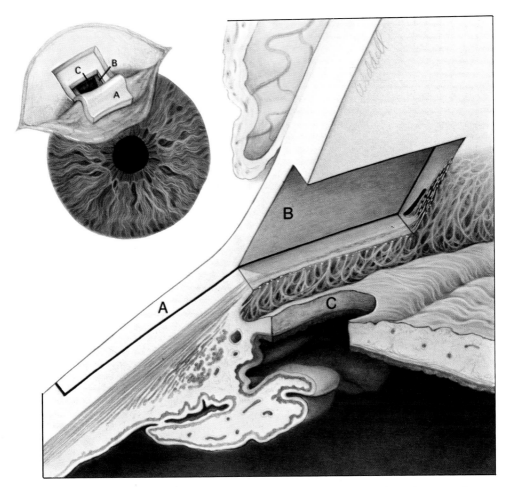

Plate 6. Trabeculectomy. Limbus-based conjunctival flap is dissected as shown to form a scleral flap, **A**, 6 mm wide near the limbus. The block excision (1.5 × 3 mm) at area **B**, anterior to scleral spur, will include trabeculum, Schlemm's canal, and peripheral cornea. **C**, Peripheral iridectomy is performed.

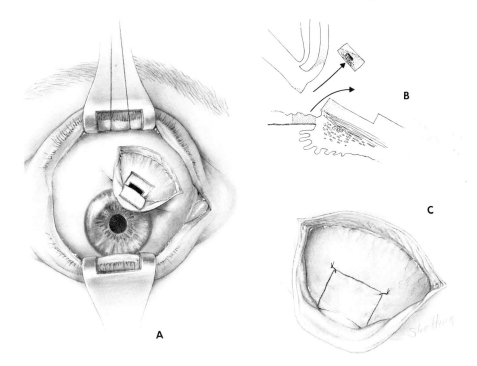

Fig. 24-12. Trabeculectomy. **A,** Anterior, and, **B,** cross-section views of scleral flap dissected forward with block removal of Schlemm's canal and trabecular tissue. Peripheral iridectomy illustrated. **C,** Scleral flap resutured.

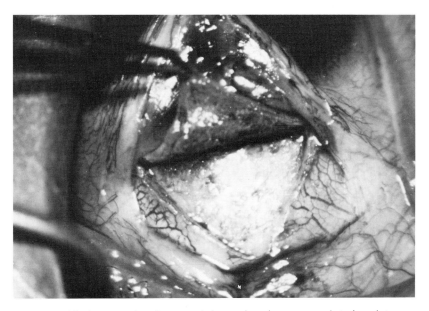

Fig. 24-13. Modified triangular flap used for trabeculectomy and trabeculotomy procedures.

planned for excision. This section usually includes Schlemm's canal and trabecular meshwork. Identification is made by the color change at the corneal-scleral junction. Schlemm's canal and the scleral spur just behind it are located at the beginning of the transition from white sclera to clear cornea. Here tissues appear a bluish gray. The area to be excised is first outlined with a superficial incision. The posterior incision for the block excision is made at the transitional zone. The anterior incision is made 1.5 mm anterior and the lateral incisions 3 to 4 mm apart at each side. The anterior chamber is then entered from the anterior incision. Vannas scissors, Colibri forceps and a No. 67 Beaver blade knife can be used to complete the lateral incisions until the tissue block is folded back to expose the anterior chamber angle. With the iris root and scleral spur thus visualized, the posterior excision is completed with angled Vannas scissors. As noted previously (p. 389), cautery rather than excision may be used with equal success to create the opening into the anterior chamber.

A cautery unit will be needed for bleeding areas, particularly in the inflamed eye. Peripheral iridectomy is cautiously performed, taking care to avoid the tendency to make a very peripheral incision where ciliary processes, ciliary body, or the major arterial circle of the iris could be incised.

The scleral flap is closed with interrupted 8-0 virgin silk sutures. Sufficient sutures are inserted to maintain a deep anterior chamber. One to five sutures may be necessary. The conjunctiva is sutured with interrupted 8-0 silk or 10-0 nylon.

Postoperatively, unless unusual complications of flat anterior chamber or hyphema are present, there is little reason to limit the patient's activity. Progressive ambulation can begin the first day, with dismissal on the second or third day. If subconjunctival steroids were not injected at surgery, topical steroids are instilled at 2- to 4-hour intervals. Usually neither miotics nor cycloplegics are needed in the initial postoperative stages. If inflammation or synechias form, dilation is indicated.

Visible blebs form in most patients, most of which are diffuse or located posteriorly. For this reason, trabeculectomy can be performed more safely in the inferior two thirds of the eye. Multicystic blebs are unusual, and the incidence of infection may be less than with other procedures. A contact lens may be worn more safely, but the potential risk of infection still remains.

SETON OPERATIONS

There has always been interest in devising a seton which could be counted on to maintain an opening between the anterior chamber and the subconjunctival space. Horsehair, silk, and metal sutures, tantalum mesh, tubes of gold, platinum, polyethylene, Gelfilm, and silicone have been used. All these procedures have initial successes, but most of them end in fibrosis and failure.

COMPLICATIONS

In addition to the general principles of postoperative care described in Chapter 21, filtering procedures have several complications in common.

Buttonholing the conjunctival flap

Accidental buttonholing of the conjunctival flap is a disconcerting complication of filtering surgery. Aqueous flowing through the conjunctival opening prevents healing, and the fistula can result in prolonged absence of the anterior chamber.

If a small buttonhole is noted at the time of surgery, it is usually possible to make the corneoscleral incision to one side of the opening or the other. It is often better to close the incision by pulling the whole conjunctival flap to one side and suturing it far away from the bleb area. However, if the buttonhole is large, it may be necessary to close it directly by sutures. Particularly in trephination and anterior lip sclerectomy, a buttonhole can be made at the limbus directly over the filtering incision. In this case it is possible to do a peritomy, denude the corneal epithelium below the incision, and sew the conjunctiva to the raw cornea. Occasionally it is necessary to use sliding flaps of conjunctiva to close larger openings.

Persistent flat chamber

Persistent flat chamber is a frequent occurrence after all varieties of filtering procedures, particularly those that produce large openings. Various methods may be used, such as limited activity or bed rest, mydriatic cycloplegics, miotics, carbonic anhydrase inhibitors, and hyperosmotic agents. Pressure dressings are simple to apply and should be tried before surgical intervention. If the chamber fails to re-form in about 10 days, efforts are made to re-form it with air, often combined with drainage of suprachoroidal fluid (Chapter 25). This should be done sooner if the eye is irritated and the bleb does not appear to contain much aqueous. Such an eye will develop extensive peripheral anterior synechias and posterior synechias. The hypotony causes shutdown of aqueous production, which jeopardizes bleb formation.

A horizontal mattress suture can be used to close a scleral fistula in order to re-form the anterior chamber and flatten choroidal detachments. The conjunctival flap over the scleral fistula is gently reopened to place a 6-0 silk suture in the same manner as the guard suture used with thermal sclerostomy. The suture is removed when more physiologic conditions prevail. Gentle massage may be required to reestablish outflow.

In a few cases a temporary soft contact lens is used to reduce aqueous outflow by flattening the bleb over the sclerostomy site. The anterior chamber will deepen, with a rise in pressure that reattaches the choroid. When aqueous secretion is increased and fibrosis of the conjunctival bleb area progresses, the pressure will remain in the normal range without the lens. This may require several days.

Cataract formation

Filtering operations, even when performed as carefully as possible, are followed by cataracts in about one third of the patients. Rapid changes can occur if the lens is damaged by instruments or incarceration into the incision or if the anterior chamber is collapsed for any period of time. When the changes are sufficient to impair vision, cataract extraction becomes necessary (Chapters 25 and 27).

Scarring down of the bleb (Fig. 24-14)

All filtering procedures are subject to the complication of scarring down of the bleb at any time. Tonography often demonstrates a progressive decrease in outflow facility before elevations of intraocular pressure are noted. The bleb appears more fibrous and smaller and contains less fluid. Pressure builds up to the low twenties. It is not uncommon to find a moundlike, thick-walled vascular bleb with well-defined borders in an eye with a high pressure. This represents exteriorization of the anterior chamber. Aqueous communicates through the fistula with the anterior chamber and "walled-off" bleb. Blebs of this character rarely function and require revision (Chapter 27). Massage of the bleb by the patient can sometimes keep aqueous filtering through the subconjunctival tissues and should be carried out postoperatively in most filtering operations.

If closure of the bleb seems imminent, vacuum should be applied to the bleb by means of a perilimbal suction cup set at –55 mm Hg for 5 minutes, once or twice a day. This may suck aqueous humor into the subconjunctival tissues or even into the cup. It may reestablish filtration. If no progress is made in a few days, a subconjunctival incision of the fibrous wall of the bleb by a Graefe knife may reinstitute successful filtration. Total revision of the bleb has proved useful in a number of cases (Chapter 27).

In some instances when filtration seems to have failed, medical therapy may still provide reasonable control. If tension remains elevated, reoperation may be necessary.

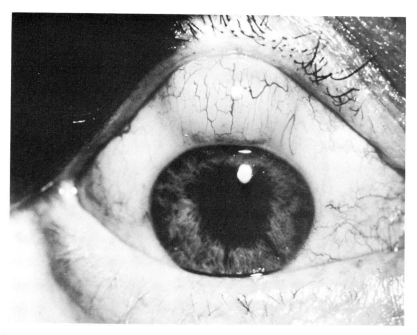

Fig. 24-14. Thick-walled, nonfunctioning vascular bleb from postoperative sclerectomy.

Late infection

Any bleb can become infected. Bacteria then have a direct path into the inside of the eye, and intraocular infection can result. The more thin-walled the bleb, the greater the risk of this complication. Patients should be warned to consult an ophthalmologist whenever they have conjunctivitis. Aspiration of the bleb may be necessary to identify the infecting organism.

Ruptured bleb

Particularly in large, thin-walled blebs, traumatic or spontaneous rupture can occur with or without collapse of the anterior chamber. The presence of the fistula can often be demonstrated by the Seidel fluorescein test. Local antibiotics should be used to prevent infection. A pressure dressing plus oral acetazolamide (Diamox) to decrease aqueous flow and time will sometimes result in closure of the opening.

A type of "tissue glue" (Fig. 24-15) has been used in some instances to correct a conjunctival fistula. The technique is simple and as an office procedure requires fluorescein for the Seidel test to locate the conjunctival hole, applicators to dry the conjunctiva, and tissue glue such as N-octyl-2-cyanoacrylate. The glue applied with a glass rod dries rapidly, forming a rough crystalline surface that adheres to the underlying tissues for 2 to 4 days until the bleb reepithelizes. Oint-

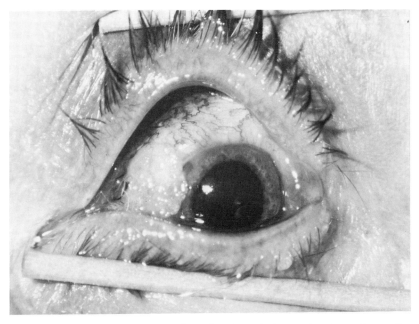

Fig. 24-15. Photograph shows area of application of tissue glue to seal superior nasal conjunctival fistula over limbus. Anterior chamber was flat 7 days. Forty-five minutes after application of glue, anterior chamber deepened. The bleb has continued to function well.

ment should be instilled frequently to reduce irritation by the glue. If the fistula seals, the anterior chamber will often deepen within 1 hour of application. The fistula may recur either because the reepithelized bleb is too thin and ruptures or because the glue forms a cork in the hole, which reopens when the glue is removed. Until recently, the tissue glue has been available on an investigational basis. A similar preparation is sold as a household adhesive under the commercial name of Super Glue. The sterility, effectiveness, and applicability of this preparation for ruptured filtering blebs is unknown.

Other complications

Other complications such as hyphema, iritis, persistent hypotony, and malignant glaucoma are discussed in Chapters 25 and 27.

POSTOPERATIVE MANAGEMENT

There is no need for the strict postoperative regimen used in treatment of postcataract extraction. The patient may be up and in a chair and have lavatory privileges immediately and is usually dismissed in 2 or 3 days. Sutures are removed in 5 to 10 days.

Postoperative iritis is treated by 1% atropine solution instilled daily and corticosteroid drops or ointment containing an antibiotic if the iritis is severe. Massage of the bleb is done daily if the anterior chamber has re-formed and with increasing vigor and frequency if there is a tendency for the bleb to flatten. Systemic steroids are occasionally used postoperatively.

25

Other surgical procedures

CYCLODIALYSIS

The popularity of cyclodialysis as a primary procedure has declined in recent years, and it is now used mainly in aphakic glaucoma and occasionally as a re-operation after failure of some other type of glaucoma operation.

Cyclodialysis is effective in lowering the intraocular pressure when a patent opening is produced between the anterior chamber and the suprachoroidal space (Plate 6, *G,* and Reel III-6). The aqueous humor drains into this suprachoroidal cleft and spreads widely between the choroid and the sclera. This often results in some shallowing of the anterior chamber. The decrease in pressure seems to be caused at first by a profound depression in aqueous production, as shown by fluorometry. At later times some of these eyes demonstrate improved outflow facility and normalized aqueous flow. It is remarkable how abrupt a rise in pressure may occur if the cleft is suddenly occluded. The mechanism of pressure reduction by cyclodialysis is still not thoroughly understood.

Incision (Fig. 25-1)

It should be remembered that the ciliary arteries perforate the sclera 4 to 8 mm from the limbus in the regions of the extraocular muscle insertions. To avoid bleeding, the scleral incision for the cyclodialysis is placed in front of the muscle insertions, 3 mm from the limbus. The dialysis can then be performed in the relatively avascular quadrants between the muscles. If the anterior chamber contains vitreous, posterior sclerotomy with vitreous aspiration and re-formation of the anterior chamber are necessary before cyclodialysis.

When possible, the cyclodialysis is done above so that any bleeding drains away from the cleft. Blood in the cleft often leads to fibrosis and closure. The conjunctival incision is made 5 to 6 mm in length, 5 mm from the limbus and concentric with it. The conjunctiva is undermined toward the cornea. At a distance of 3 mm from the limbus the scleral incision is begun, slanting slightly toward the anterior chamber to facilitate introduction of the spatula. When the incision is halfway through the sclera, a McLean type of suture of 6-0 silk is placed and

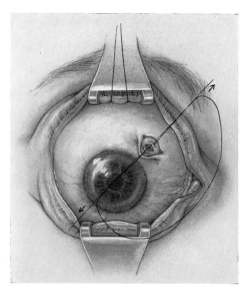

Fig. 25-1. Cyclodialysis. Conjunctival and scleral incision.

pulled out to hold the lips of the incision apart. The suture is placed deeper than the similar cataract suture; its purpose is to lift the deeper sclera away from the ciliary body and to facilitate passage of the spatula. It is later used in wound closure.

The inner scleral incision need be little more than 1.5 mm in length to admit the Elschnig spatula, which is 1 mm in width and very thin. Other spatulas are too thick and wide. The incision is slowly deepened as the assistant opens and lifts the incision by pulling on the loops of the suture. When close to the suprachoroidal space, only the tip of the knife is used. The surgeon can usually feel the grating or ticking sensation of the knife tip passing over scleral fibers. When this ceases, the suprachoroidal space has been reached, although often the opening is not large enough to admit the spatula. The few remaining fibrils of sclera must be severed. If effort is needed to pass the spatula through the incision, it is not yet completely in the suprachoroidal space.

Dialysis (Fig. 25-2)

Once the tip of the spatula is slid into the incision, it must be held closely against the inner sclera to avoid perforating the ciliary body. Before entering the anterior chamber, one may dialyze the suprachoroidal space and pause 1 to 2 minutes for bleeding to subside. To further reduce hemorrhage, epinephrine 1:20,000 can be injected into the dialyzed suprachoroidal space. This maneuver is necessary if the eye is inflamed. When the location of the spatula tip is questioned, the tip should be advanced toward the chamber until it appears in the chamber angle. The blade is then pulled slightly back and turned parallel with the limbus and slid along the suprachoroidal space until it is entirely hidden. The blade has a longer radius of curvature than the eye, and if the tip is held firmly up against the sclera, it will

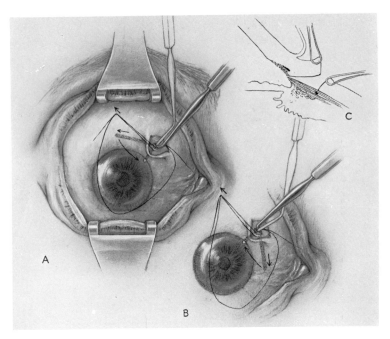

Fig. 25-2. Cyclodialysis. **A,** Inverse cyclodialysis, showing insertion of Elschnig spatula, rotation past the scleral spur to produce the dialysis, and withdrawal of spatula to avoid damage to Descemet's membrane. **B,** Inverse cyclodialysis of the opposite side. **C,** Cross section to show placement of suture, incision, and area of cyclodialysis.

periodically butt into the inner sclera and will not move until the tip is slightly depressed. The course of the spatula should be followed by moving the tip back and forth slightly as it is moved into the eye, care being taken to avoid hitting the scleral spur.

Now, by rotating the handle, the side of the spatula is slid against the attachment of the ciliary body to the scleral spur. Unusual pressure should not be applied. Usually the spatula slides easily into the anterior chamber. To avoid injury to Descemet's membrane, the spatula should not be held up against the inner cornea. There should be no fuzzy covering of peripheral anterior synechias, trabecular meshwork, or superficial iris on the spatula blade. It should look clear and bright through the cornea.

If the spatula does not cut through easily into the anterior chamber, several maneuvers are helpful. Keeping the spatula tip close to the spur, withdraw the blade at least halfway so that the tip of the spatula can be used to work its way into the chamber. If it still does not appear, the assistant should take a muscle hook and with massagelike pressure squeeze the limbal tissues between the hook and the spatula. Even with dense peripheral anterior synechias this maneuver will eventually work the tip of the spatula into the chamber. The cyclodialysis can usually be completed by withdrawing the tip of the spatula and performing the dialysis in segments.

Rather than rotating the spatula into the anterior chamber, some surgeons prefer to use a multiple-thrust method by repeatedly advancing the tip of the spatula into the chamber angle. Adjacent thrusts with the tip open a cleft, usually smaller than with the method just described, but with reduced risk of hemorrhage.

Completion of cyclodialysis (Fig. 25-3)

A Randolph spatula on a syringe or a Goldstein anterior chamber irrigator, with a gold lacrimal needle bent to match the curve of the Elschnig spatula, may be used to inject a balanced salt solution into the anterior chamber. This should be done promptly, especially if any bleeding from the dialysis has occurred. Flushing is continued until all bleeding has stopped. Building up the intraocular pressure by single-tying the suture around the needle as solution is being forced into the eye will help stop venous ooze. Refilling the whole anterior chamber with air can be dangerous because of the risk of air blockade of the pupil.

The two ends of the double-arm McLean suture should be passed through the upper and lower edges of the conjunctival incision. Tying the suture closes both the scleral and conjunctival openings. The eye is patched.

Cyclodialysis with iridectomy

In aphakic glaucoma with pupillary block, combined cyclodialysis and iridectomy are often indicated. Separate, properly placed incisions for each procedure

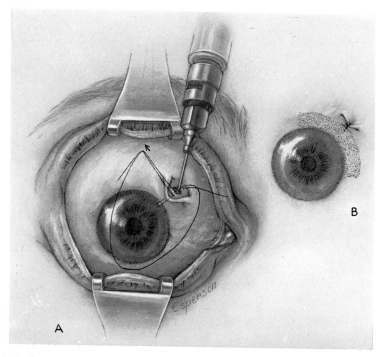

Fig. 25-3. Cyclodialysis. **A,** Injection of isotonic sodium chloride solution to flush out blood and re-form the anterior chamber. **B,** Suture tied. Stippling shows the area of the cyclodialysis.

are preferable. A single incision is either too posterior for safe iridectomy or too anterior for cyclodialysis. The cyclodialysis incision and dialysing sweep to the spur can be completed without entering the anterior chamber. This permits bleeding to subside while iridectomy is being performed. The iridectomy incision is closed by tying the McLean suture, and the anterior chamber is refilled. The cyclodialysis is then completed as described.

Postoperative care (Fig. 25-4)

The presence of blood in the cleft favors fibroblastic ingrowth and closure. The patient's head should be kept turned away from the dialysis area so that blood can drain out of the cleft in the immediate postoperative period. The pupil should be miotic for the first few days to hold open the cleft but should be moved daily with phenylephrine (Neo-Synephrine), as is done with an iridectomy, to avoid posterior synechias. If there is much iritis, corticosteroids topically are indicated. In the absence of bleeding, the patient may be discharged from the hospital on the third or fourth day, although delayed bleeding can occur up to one week postoperatively.

The suture is removed at the end of one week. At that time gonioscopy can be done. If there is no suprachoroidal cleft, one may predict recurrence of increased intraocular pressure in four to six weeks. If there is a cleft, the chance of initial success is excellent, although connective tissue ingrowth can close it at any time in the future. There are some apparent clefts that fail to normalize intraocular pressure as a consequence of retroplaced attachment of the ciliary body behind the scleral spur. Miotics may be required on a permanent basis to keep the cleft open.

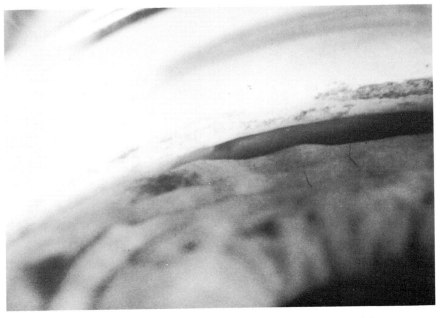

Fig. 25-4. Goniophotograph of functioning cyclodialysis cleft.

Complications

Complications associated with cyclodialysis are hemorrhage, iritis, hypotony, late closure of cleft, and cataract formation.

Hemorrhage

Severe bleeding is unusual if the incision and dialysis are in front of the anterior ciliary arteries, 3 mm from the limbus. Although it is safe to go farther back in the areas between the recti muscles, little is gained, since the only real attachment of ciliary body to sclera is at the spur. With the attachment severed, the cleft should form without any passage of spatulas through the suprachoroidal space. If bleeding is severe during the operation, a small paracentesis made opposite the cleft can be used to flush out the blood. The addition of epinephrine 1:20,000 helps control bleeding. A No. 27 needle on a Luer syringe is used to inject solution through the paracentesis into the anterior chamber. At the same time the surgeon keeps the spatula turned on edge so that the solution will carry the blood out through the scleral incision.

Delayed hemorrhage is difficult to handle and is usually permitted to absorb spontaneously. If pressure goes above 40 mm Hg, bloodstaining of the cornea becomes a danger. Pressure reduction by acetazolamide (Diamox), hyperosmotic agents, and miotics is helpful. Evacuation of the hemorrhage by a small ab externo incision may become necessary. If a large, rubbery, black clot is present, a larger incision is needed to remove it. A suitable number of corneoscleral sutures should be preplaced for closure.

Iritis

Postoperative iritis is always present. Mydriatics and corticosteroids may be necessary. Considerable care must be employed to avoid posterior synechias; the pupil should be kept miotic most of the time in the first few days to help keep the cleft pulled open.

Hypotony

There is more danger of prolonged hypotony after cyclodialysis than with any other procedure, particularly in patients less than 45 years of age. This seems to be due to the fact that the aqueous humor in the open suprachoroidal cleft causes an overly extensive choroidal separation, with suppression of aqueous production. The extent of this separation is not related to the size of the dialysis, for a small cleft may cause as profound hypotony as does a large one. Vision is reduced by edema of the optic nerve and the macula. The sudden postoperative drop in vision from 20/20 to 20/200 is disconcerting to both patient and surgeon. Often as tension builds up above 10 mm Hg (Schiøtz), vision will be restored. Restoration to 20/40 was seen in one eye that had had hypotony for ten years, but such success is unusual. External diathermy or cyclocryotherapy can be used to partially close an overfunctioning cyclodialysis. A lamellar scleral flap may be turned and penetrating diathermy applied in the bed of the flap to induce cleft closure. After diathermy, external plumbage with a silicone strip sutured to the sclera over the cleft has been recommended.

Late closure of cyclodialysis cleft

Closure of a dialysis cleft can be caused by ingrowth of connective tissue and reattachment of the ciliary body, sometimes at a point behind the spur. The closure can be abrupt, leading to a sudden, acute rise of pressure with symptoms much like those of an acute angle-closure glaucoma. Sometimes miotics will reopen the cleft, with prompt normalization of pressure. Such an eye should be kept on miotics, as should eyes with very narrow clefts.

Cataract formation

Cataracts seem to be produced or hastened by cyclodialysis more than by other glaucoma operations, barring direct injury to the lens. This is thought to be due to the reduced aqueous production and perhaps to some change in aqueous composition. When necessary, lens extraction is done well away from the cleft or with a shelving incision whose inner edge is well anterior to the cleft.

TRABECULOTOMY (EXTERNAL) (Plate 7; Figs. 25-5 and 25-6)

Published results of external trabeculotomy in infantile and juvenile glaucoma are excellent, with a reported success rate of about 90%. Long-term results, how-

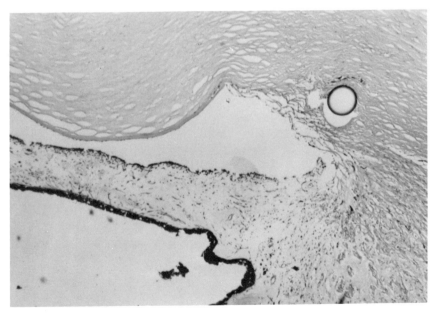

Fig. 25-5. Pathologic specimen showing the suture correctly placed in Schlemm's canal.

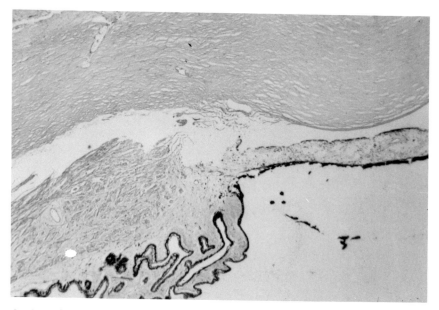

Fig. 25-6. Pathologic specimen demonstrating one of the complications of trabeculotomy. The probe missed Schlemm's canal and had actually entered the suprachoroidal space.

ever, have not been clearly established. Although some surgeons claim excellent results, others indicate discouragement by lack of success. The difficult operation depends on introduction of a probe into Schlemm's canal. The inner wall of the canal and trabeculum are ruptured by rotation of the probe into the anterior chamber. Successful probing of Schlemm's canal can be accomplished (Fig. 25-5), but pathologic specimens often refute claims of success (Fig. 25-6).

The operating microscope is essential, particularly for locating and probing Schlemm's canal. The easiest and most precise approach to external trabeculotomy is from beneath a scleral flap where landmarks and canal are discernible. This approach has an added advantage because it allows the surgeon the option of a trabeculectomy if the trabeculotomy attempt fails. The conjunctival and

---

Plate 7. Trabeculotomy. **A,** Sclera is exposed by formation of a limbus-based conjunctival flap. A thick scleral flap can then be dissected forward so that it is hinged at the cornea. **B,** Meticulous dissection of remaining sclera over Schlemm's canal is performed under high magnification through a radial incision at the transitional white-to-blue-white color change between the sclera and cornea. **C,** Entrance to the canal is verified by inserting a 5-0 nylon suture and threading it a short distance. Probing is made easier if the canal is further exposed at the entry site with the Vannas scissors. **D,** Probe is gently passed along the canal with little resistance for 6 to 10 mm. **E,** Gonioscopically the probe is barely visible through the trabecular meshwork. **F,** By rotating the probe internally, trabeculum is ruptured, and the probe appears in the anterior chamber with minimal bleeding.

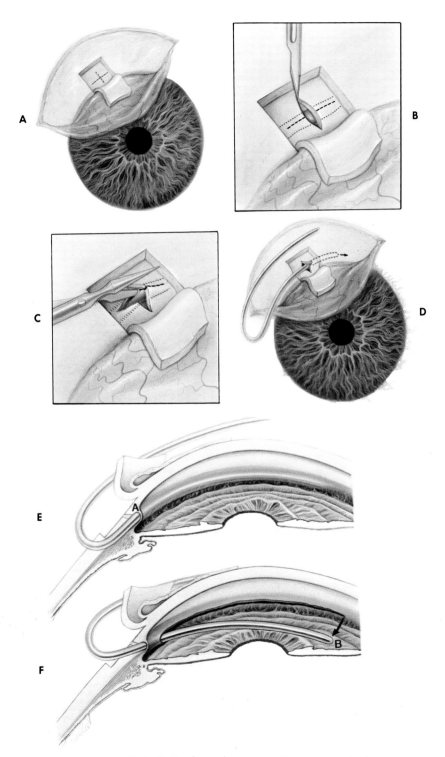

Plate 7. For legend see opposite page.

scleral flap incisions are as described in the procedure for trabeculectomy. A radial incision, approximately 2 mm in length, should be made at the blue-grey transitional line, using a 16× or 25× magnification on the operating microscope. Slow and meticulous dissection is performed by spreading tissues as this incision is deepened. The trabecular tissue that separates the canal from the anterior chamber is thin and tenuous, making it easy at this point to pass the knife or probe prematurely into the anterior chamber. The eye then softens, and an adequate trabeculotomy is almost impossible.

The canal, when approached in the appropriate manner, appears as a slightly pigmented depression or a translucent, grayish white trough with, on occasion, blood slowly seeping from the open ends. A 5-0 nylon suture, beveled with scissors, should pass through this opened area smoothly (Fig. 25-7). A Harms or McPherson trabeculotome with gentle manipulation is allowed to follow the course of the canal previously tested with the suture. The probe is inserted 5 to 8 mm and then rotated into the anterior chamber. The same probing technique is attempted in the opposite direction, although this tends to be more difficult unless the eye is again made firm by air instillation into the anterior chamber. A small amount of blood usually appears in the probed area of the anterior chamber. After successful probing, the scleral flap is replaced with interrupted 8-0 or 10-0 sutures.

Postoperatively topical steroids are used. Pilocarpine is also recommended by some authors. Patients are ambulated on the first postoperative day and are usually

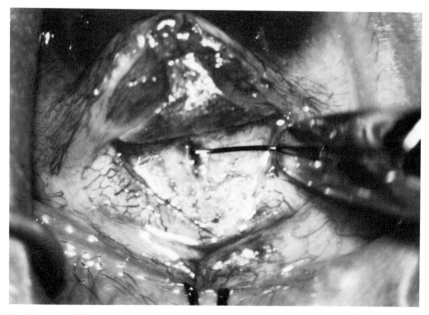

Fig. 25-7. Here a 5-0 nylon suture, beveled with scissors, is used to test the approach to the canal. If Schlemm's canal has been correctly located, the suture should pass through this opened area smoothly.

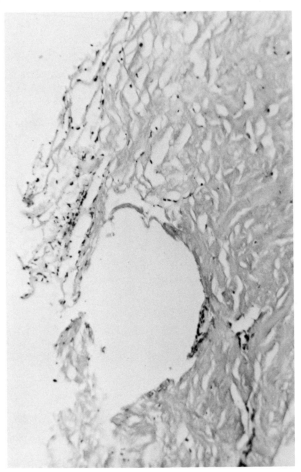

Fig. 25-8. Pathologic specimen shows block section of Schlemm's canal and trabeculum after Harms trabeculotomy. Schlemm's canal is dilated from the probe, and trabeculum is ruptured. Often pathologic specimens show the probe mistakenly threaded in corneal or scleral tissue.

dismissed from the hospital 1 to 2 days after surgery. Gonioscopy can be performed postoperatively to verify the trabeculotomy incision.

External trabeculotomy, rather than goniotomy, is indicated in infantile glaucoma when angle structures cannot be visualized through a cloudy cornea. It may also be a surgical choice in young patients with open-angle or secondary glaucoma. Fair to poor results have been reported by some authors in adults with open-angle glaucoma.

LASER TRABECULOTOMY

Multiple laser applications have been used to produce openings in the trabecular meshwork in an effort to improve outflow facility and lower intraocular pressure. The procedure is still in its research stages. Lowering of intraocular pressure

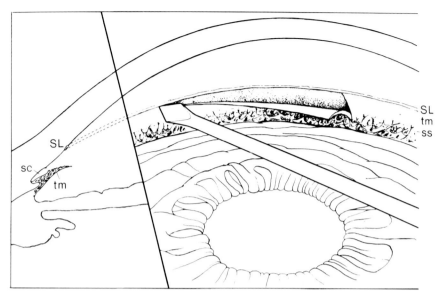

Fig. 25-9. Trabeculodialysis. Using the spade-shaped goniotomy knife, the trabeculum is incised at Schwalbe's line and disinserted from the scleral sulcus. Vertical relaxing incisions at the extremes of the incision allow the trabecular flap to fall away from the scleral wall. *sc*, Schlemm's canal; *SL*, Schwalbe's line; *tm*, trabecular meshwork; *ss*, scleral spur.

is at best temporary, usually lasting two to three months. Furthermore, tissue damage and inflammation with subsequent scarring may have the opposite of the desired effect and produce pressure elevation in some instances. Although the technique may eventually prove useful, it cannot be recommended in its present state.

TRABECULODIALYSIS (Fig. 25-9)

Glaucoma secondary to inflammation, pigmentation, and exfoliation responds occasionally to trabeculodialysis. The procedure initially advocated by Haas resembles the goniotomy procedure in infants. A moderately deep incision is made with the Swan knife at the anterior portion of the trabeculum while viewed through a Barkan lens. Incised trabeculum falls away from the angle wall as a sheet, and the iris root moves posteriorly.

Complications include hemorrhage and reactivation of inflammation. Like goniotomy, the procedure is relatively atraumatic, and failure does not jeopardize the success of other more extensive procedures. Success and complication rates have yet to be determined in a large series of eyes.

SINUSOTOMY

Krasnov in Moscow reported a surgical procedure for the "intrascleral" form of open-angle glaucoma, in which obstruction to aqueous outflow is believed to be in scleral tissue peripheral to Schlemm's canal rather than in trabeculum. If the uncontrolled glaucoma is due to intrascleral retention, Schlemm's canal is externalized by surgically unroofing or opening tissue to allow free aqueous flow to subconjunctival tissues. This procedure has been discarded by most surgeons, including its proponent.

CYCLOCRYOTHERAPY (Fig. 25-10)

Cryo-applications to sclera overlying the ciliary body may lower intraocular pressure by producing damage to the ciliary epithelium, thereby reducing aqueous secretion. A retrobulbar anesthetic is used. In neovascular glaucoma, eight to twelve equally spaced applications are made about 4 mm from the limbus, between the rectus muscles. For open-angle glaucoma, only the inferior half of the eye is usually treated. The retina probe (rather than the smaller cataract probe) is used; the tip is held against the conjunctiva, and the temperature lowered to –70° to –80° C for a period of 30 to 60 seconds. The probe is allowed to warm until the ice-ball thaws and is then removed. Experimental studies indicate that greater tissue damage is produced by a freeze-thaw-refreeze technique. Because of this, a second application of 15 to 20 seconds is often placed over the original area of treatment. The procedure is immediately followed by a transient, marked elevation in intraocular pressure and moderate to severe pain requiring strong analgesics. This is particularly true in the treatment of neovascular glaucoma. Hospitalization is usually not necessary for cyclocryotherapy, especially when used in uninflamed eyes.

Good pressure control has been maintained in some patients for up to three years postoperatively. However, there are patients unresponsive to repeated applications. Intraocular hemorrhage has been reported with too rigorous treatment. Iritis is common as a postoperative finding, but phthisis is rare. The use of cold applications has eliminated the problems of scleral necrosis associated with diathermy procedures and largely eliminated the latter operations.

There are several situations in which cyclocryotherapy is useful, among which are neovascular glaucoma, absolute glaucoma, traumatic transient glaucoma, and open-angle glaucoma where intraocular surgery is contraindicated. Relief of pain is usually possible even when intraocular pressure is not normalized.

CYCLODIATHERMY

Indications for cyclodiathermy are similar to those for cryotherapy. The ciliary body is damaged with a high-frequency current to diminish aqueous secretion.

A 2 mm conjunctival incision is made 4 mm from the limbus with conjunctival scissors. A spatula is then passed over the ciliary body area, separating conjunctiva and sclera as far as possible. If the spatula catches on Tenon's capsule, scissors may be required to produce a tract along which the insulated 0.5 mm electrode of Pischel or Kronfeld can be passed. The electrode is slid in sideways as far as possible and then is turned so that the point engages the sclera. A single or double

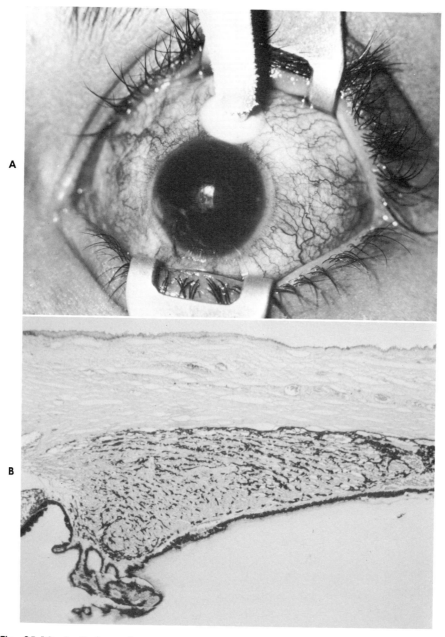

Fig. 25-10. A, Cyclocryotherapy application. **B,** Photomicrograph 5 days after cyclocryo-therapy to ciliary body of monkey, showing dilated vessels, edema, and extravasated blood.

line of diathermy punctures of the sclera are placed 4 to 6 mm from the limbus, using 50 ma of current for 3 seconds, much as is done in retinal detachment surgery. The electrode is then reintroduced in the opposite direction, and another row of diathermy punctures is placed. This permits more than half the sclera to be treated with a conjunctival incision so tiny that usually no suture is needed. The opposite half can be treated at a later time. The coagulation should not be brought closer than 2 mm from the limbus.

Iritis, bullous keratopathy, phthisis bulbi, and sympathetic ophthalmia are among the serious complications that have been reported, but they are fortunately rare.

RETROBULBAR ALCOHOL INJECTION

In the past, retrobulbar alcohol injection was used quite frequently. It is now used less often, mainly because other procedures have proved more effective. Nevertheless, it still has a place in late glaucoma for management of the blind, painful eye. A standard retrobulbar block is given, and the needle left in place a few minutes until the anesthetic is effective. Through the same needle, 0.5 to 1.0 ml of absolute alcohol is injected. Postoperatively, ptosis and conjunctival chemosis or injection may develop but are usually of only short duration.

GLAUCOMA AND CATARACTS

Senile lens changes tend to occur among members of the same age group as does primary glaucoma. As a result, coexistence of these diseases in the same patient is common. As previously stated, progressive visual field loss caused by lens changes must not be mistaken for increasing glaucoma damage. Neither should the physician overlook open-angle glaucoma in his preoccupation with an obvious cataract.

Glaucoma surgery leads to a higher incidence of cataracts than occurs in unoperated eyes. Cataracts rapidly develop if the lens is injured during surgery—for example, by toothed forceps, incarceration of the lens in a filtration wound, and prolonged absence of the anterior chamber. Lens changes months or years after a glaucoma operation may have no connection with the original surgery. Alteration in the rate of aqueous production and in the quality of aqueous humor can be factors. This is particularly true after cyclodialysis. It is unlikely that iridectomy adds serious risk of cataract formation.

Management of cataracts in eyes with glaucoma
Narrow-angle glaucoma

If a cataract is present in an eye with angle closure, lens extraction is often the procedure of choice, even with the patient having 20/50 vision. One alternative is a full iridectomy, which aids vision and also permits the use of miotics. The cataract extraction deepens the anterior chamber, widens the angle, and lessens the risk of malignant glaucoma. If angle closure is merely threatened or if combined-mechanism glaucoma exists, lens extraction may be indicated when the cataract reduces vision to the 20/70 level or less.

Open-angle glaucoma

The visual acuity of an eye with a cataract, especially a nuclear opacity, is made much worse by the use of miotics. It may be possible to postpone cataract extraction in a glaucomatous eye by using miotics infrequently or only at bedtime. Pressure control can usually be achieved by the additional use of epinephrine and acetazolamide (Diamox). Better pupillary dilation is obtained with phenylephrine (Neo-Synephrine) than with epinephrine, but the pressure reduction is usually less. To minimize postoperative reaction when cataract extraction becomes necessary, it is wise to stop strong miotics and use pilocarpine for three weeks before surgery. At surgery, posterior synechias should be swept free with a spatula.

Uncontrolled open-angle glaucoma with cataract

Uncontrolled open-angle glaucoma in a patient with immature cataracts presents a difficult management problem. If a filtering operation is performed on an eye with immature lens opacities, rapid progression of the opacities can be expected. The surgeon may be pleased with the reduction in pressure, but the patient is usually less than enthusiastic about the reduction in visual acuity. Furthermore, when lens extraction becomes necessary, the functional integrity of a filtering bleb is lost in about 50% of patients. For these reasons, when lens opacities are significant, it is usually wise to remove the lens first and deal with the glaucoma later in the aphakic eye. To facilitate lens removal, a full iridectomy and rarely an inferior sphincterotomy may be needed. This also provides a large pupil that will not interfere with vision even if miotics are needed postoperatively. An alternative method to create a large pupil is the performance of four or five sphincterotomies evenly placed around the pupil. This provides a large pupillary opening, which will not become miotic if antiglaucoma therapy is later required. Blunt corneal scissors are used to avoid rupture of the lens capsule.

In a series of 100 eyes with coexisting cataract and glaucoma, the pressure was harder to control postoperatively than preoperatively in only 10%. In many eyes, it was easier to control. Another totally independent study provided strikingly similar results. Thus 89% of 100 glaucomatous eyes were as well or better controlled one year after cataract surgery, whereas only 11% were less well controlled. In eyes considered to be under poor glaucoma control before cataract extraction, 58% could be more adequately controlled one year afterward. Cyclodialysis or thermal sclerostomy is generally reserved for those few cases that cannot be controlled medically after cataract extraction.

Combined procedure

Combining cataract extraction with filtering surgery may eliminate the need for a second operation to control glaucoma at a later date. The combined procedure has been recommended by some surgeons in patients needing cataract extraction with proved, medically uncontrolled glaucoma and in uncontrolled open-angle glaucoma patients with minor lens opacities likely to progress after filtering surgery. It should be emphasized that additional risk is inherent in this surgery. A postoperative flat anterior chamber quite common to filtering procedures is especially hazardous after cataract extraction. The large limbal cataract wound further weakened by cautery has a greater chance of rupturing. One must also consider that cataract extraction alone may make the glaucoma easier to control postoperatively. Nevertheless, surprisingly few serious complications of the combined procedure have been reported. If the surgeon finds such a procedure necessary, the cataract surgery must be modified.

Trabeculectomy with cataract extraction. Postoperative flat anterior chambers and hypotony are significantly less frequent with trabeculectomy than with other filtering procedures. A reasonably safe approach, then, would be to use the trabeculectomy with cataract extraction when a combined procedure is indicated.

For this, a large, limbus-based conjunctival flap is needed. The split-thickness, triangular scleral flap can be dissected to the limbus and peripheral cornea as described in the initial stages of the standard trabeculectomy (Chapter 24). A limbal groove is made at each side of the scleral flap for preplaced sutures. Trabeculectomy tissue is excised in the usual way, and the cataract incision is completed. The usual peripheral iridectomy and lens extraction are performed. The scleral and corneal wounds are closed with 8-0 silk or 10-0 nylon interrupted sutures. After instillation of balanced salt solution to deepen the anterior chamber, the wound and anterior chamber depth should be checked carefully for excessive wound leak.

If the trabeculectomy is performed with cautery, it is possible to delay the filtering part of the operation until the cataract operation has been completed. If the extraction has gone well, the trabeculectomy is then performed. If any complications have occurred, the scleral flap can be sutured closed without any fistulizing procedure performed.

Cataract extraction with limbal cauterization. The second technique for combined procedure is as follows. A large, limbus-based conjuctival flap is used. The filtering fistula is prepared with light applications of thermal cautery to 2 to 3 mm of the superior nasal scleral lip of the cataract incision. Sutures are placed at each side of the cauterized area and can be inserted as a guard suture recommended with thermal sclerostomy. A peripheral rather than a full iridectomy near the limbal wound is more likely to check vitreous. If a full iridectomy is needed for the cataract extraction, it should be performed elsewhere. The procedure can be modified by touching the cautery to two small areas between sutures along the cataract incision instead of cauterizing one large area. Buried 8-0 silk sutures help to prevent dehiscence of the large, slow-healing cataract wound and increase the probability of filtration.

The conjunctiva is sutured with running or interrupted 7-0 silk sutures. Close postoperative supervision is required, and gentle eye massage may be performed by the surgeon to maintain a fistula.

• • •

Although the statistical success with combined procedures appears satisfying, a separate analysis showed that 55% of 100 glaucoma patients were better controlled after cataract extraction alone. This is not significantly different from the results of combined procedures.

Cataract extraction after glaucoma surgery

The technique (Chapter 27) has many modifications dependent on a variety of factors such as the level of intraocular pressure control, the quality of a bleb if present, the degree of synechia formation, and the routine used by the surgeon.

EXPULSIVE HEMORRHAGE

Subchoroidal expulsive hemorrhage has been known to follow almost any intraocular surgery but is most common after cataract extraction. During surgery or in a few hours or days postoperatively the patient has severe ocular pain and shocklike symptoms. The eye becomes firm; the increased intraocular pressure breaks open the wound; vitreous, retina, choroid, and blood are extruded, and the eye is usually lost. This rare but devastating complication is more common in eyes with advanced glaucoma, especially if the patient is hypertensive and arteriosclerotic. Prophylaxis is best accomplished by presurgical normalization of both blood pressure and intraocular pressure.

Only by prompt and bold surgery can such eyes be saved. A T-shaped or L-shaped posterior sclerotomy over the pars plana of the ciliary body will exteriorize the bleeding. Diathermy to the scleral edges will help hold open the incision and will facilitate the escape of blood, even if bleeding should continue for several days. If blood is not obtained with the first temporal sclerotomy, a nasal incision should be made. If an ophthalmoscope is promptly available, an accurate incision can be made into the dark mound that marks the bleeding site. However, speed is usually more important than accuracy.

With the eye softened by the sclerotomy, vitreous can be excised, and the wound can be closed by additional sutures. Re-forming the anterior chamber with physiologic salt solution will increase the intraocular pressure and express the remaining unclotted blood through the sclerotomy incision.

CHAPTER 26

Surgery for congenital glaucoma

GONIOTOMY

The only truly satisfactory operation for congenital glaucoma is goniotomy. An improvement in the decreased facility of outflow is obtained by successful surgery, probably by restoring outflow through Schlemm's canal. The increased facility can be maintained for long periods or even indefinitely. However, recurrences of increased pressure in some of the children originally operated on by Barkan thirty years ago make the lifetime prognosis for these eyes still in doubt. Just as is true with all other glaucomas medically or surgically treated or spontaneously arrested, all individuals with congenital glaucoma should have periodic checkups. The operation itself is as safe as an iridectomy when done under gonioscopic visualization by a trained surgeon and does not materially damage the eye for other types of surgery.

Method

Preoperative measures

The preoperative care and examination under anesthesia have been discussed in Chapter 17 and are summarized here.

Medication. If the diagnosis is in doubt, no miotics or acetazolamide (Diamox) is given. If the pressure is obviously elevated, a miotic such as 2% pilocarpine should be given every 6 hours plus three times in the 30 minutes immediately preceding surgery. Acetazolamide can be given every 6 hours in a dosage of 5 to 10 mg/kg body weight intramuscularly, or it can be included in the child's feedings.

Anesthesia. General anesthesia is necessary to standardize the pressure taking unless ketamine is used.

Examination under anesthesia (Fig. 26-1). The horizontal diameter of the cornea from limbus to limbus should be measured by calipers and recorded. Tonometry should be performed, preferably with the hand-held applanation tonometer or with the Schiøtz tonometer. Tonographic results are considered unreliable by most observers, and tonography is used only infrequently. Gonioscopy is done, preceded, if necessary for visualization of the angle, by removal of the corneal

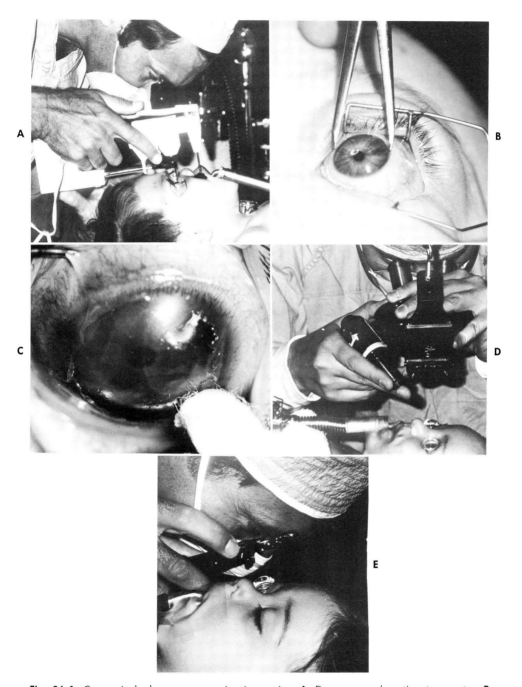

Fig. 26-1. Congenital glaucoma examination series. **A**, Draeger applanation tonometer. **B**, Corneal measurement. **C**, Epithelium removal. **D**, Gonioscopy. **E**, Ophthalmoscopy with smooth-domed lens.

epithelium down to Bowman's membrane. In borderline degrees of corneal edema, it is tempting to avoid this unpleasant procedure. However, safety of goniotomy depends on good visibility, and epithelial haze can be expected to increase after the diagnostic and surgical contact lenses have been used. If a great deal of edema is present, a sheet of epithelium comes off easily. Otherwise, considerable pressure on the curet or the side of the No. 15 Bard-Parker blade may be needed to start peeling off the epithelial layer. Scrubbing the cornea with an applicator soaked in 70% ethyl alcohol loosens the epithelium and makes its removal much easier; however, it increases postoperative discomfort.

With severe corneal edema, only the junction point of the iris to the trabecular meshwork may be visible, but this is enough to orient the position of the goniotomy incision. Usually it is possible to tell the height of the iris and to see any abnormal vascularization, and often a perfectly clear view of the angle is obtained. If there is extreme haziness, trabeculotomy ab externo is indicated.

The diagnostic Koeppe lens for operating room gonioscopy should be smooth-domed and should not have a dimple on its surface. This permits a surprisingly clear view of the optic disc if the cornea has moderate clarity and the pupil is at all dilated. Dilation of the pupil should not be done deliberately if surgery is contemplated. Ophthalmoscopy with a dilated pupil can await a future examination. If the pupil is not miotic, 2% pilocarpine solution should be used to fill the diagnostic Koeppe lens. The pupil may then be small by the time of surgery.

Surgical technique

Attention to details is of utmost importance in goniotomy.

Fixation of the eye. The eyelashes are trimmed. Two Elschnig forceps with locks are firmly applied to the superior and inferior rectus muscles. It is easier to pick up these tendons when the lid and fornix are held out of the way with a muscle hook while the eye is turned with forceps. No speculum is used, for it would be in the way of the forceps throughout the procedure. Sutures under the tendons will not slip off but otherwise are inferior to forceps. If exposure is difficult, a cathotomy is most helpful.

Surgical contact lens (Fig. 26-2). The patient's head is turned 45° away from the surgeon so that he can be operating "downhill," thus avoiding bubbles under the Barkan surgical contact lens. The surgeon's left forefinger holds the contact lens against the eye. The Elschnig forceps under that left hand must be rotated out of the way. A drop of isotonic sodium chloride solution is placed under the contact lens. The lens is rotated away from the near limbus so that there will be ample room to make the corneal incision. Other gonioscopic lenses such as the Swan and Worst lenses may be used instead of the Barkan surgical contact lens.

Light and magnification (Fig. 26-3). A Zeiss zoom-lens operating microscope gives excellent magnification and lighting for this surgery, and the exact depth of the incision can be controlled by its use. The 10× to 16× magnifications seem most satisfactory. When the microscope is set to observe the trabecular meshwork, it is

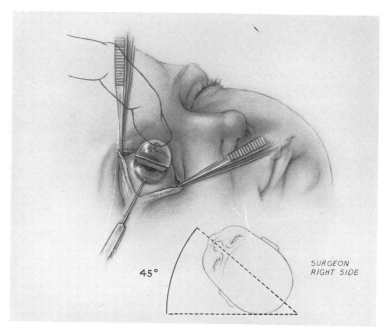

Fig. 26-2. Goniotomy, showing position of child's head turned away from surgeon at 45° away from the vertical. The eye is fixated by two locking Elschnig forceps in the superior and inferior rectus muscles.

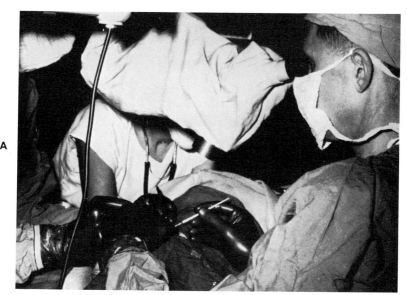

Continued.

Fig. 26-3. A, Goniotomy with the use of the Zeiss lens operating microscope. **B,** Goniotomy using Welch-Allyn lamp and loupe. **C,** Position of surgical contract lens and knife. (**A** and **C** from Shaffer, R. N.: Amer. J. Ophthal. **47:**90, 1959.)

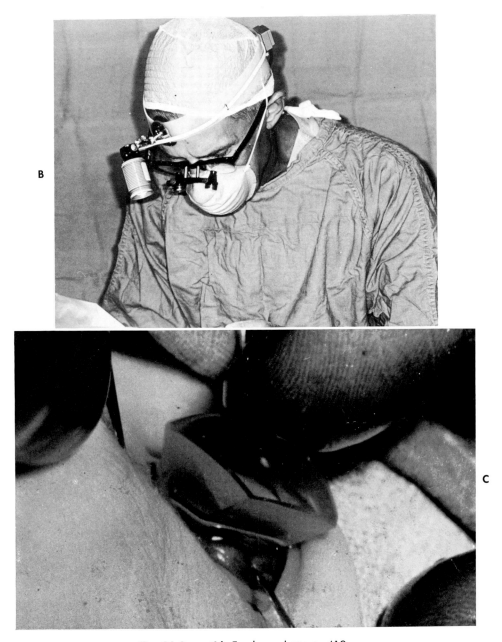

Fig. 26-3, cont'd. For legend see p. 419.

not in good position to control the puncture incision and passage of the knife blade across the anterior chamber. This should be done under very low magnification and with the help and guidance of the assistant. Once the blade is beyond the pupil, the microscopic view is excellent although mobility is limited.

When the patient's cornea is irregularly hazy, the usual 2.5× loupe is preferable. Illumination is obtained by a Welch-Allyn head lamp focused to a 2 to 3 cm wide beam at working distance. In this way the surgeon is free to move the light and visual axis in any direction to achieve maximal visual clarity. He should stand for this surgery, to permit complete mobility. In this way the goniotomy is more easily done, and there is less danger of accidental injury to the lens.

Positioning of the eye. The assistant must hold the eye so that the plane of the iris is absolutely parallel with the direction in which the knife thrust is to be made. The eye should be lifted upward from the orbit to permit maximum exposure. It should then be rotated so that the incision can be made as far away from the horizontal axis as possible. This permits a second goniotomy to be done from the temporal side if the first one fails.

Puncture (Figs. 26-2 and 26-3, C). The contact lens is held against the cornea

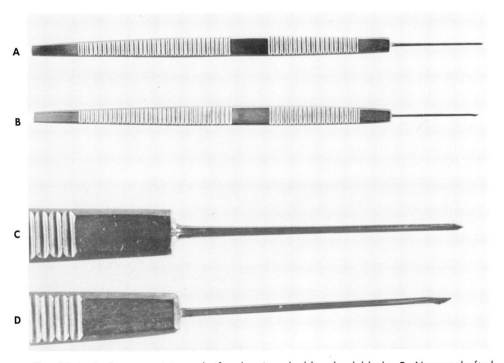

Fig. 26-4. A, Swan goniotomy knife, showing double-edged blade. **B,** Narrow-shafted, modified Barkan goniotomy knife. **C** and **D,** Enlarged views of **A** and **B.** (From Shaffer, R. N., and Weiss, D. I.: Congenital and pediatric glaucomas, St. Louis, 1970, The C. V. Mosby Co.)

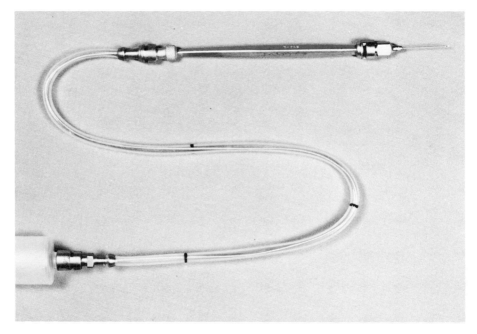

Fig. 26-5. Needle-knife for goniotomy.

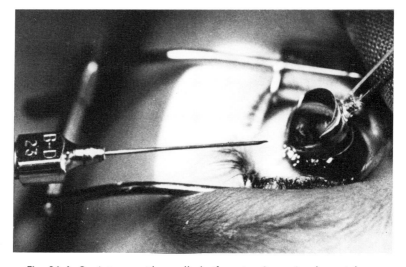

Fig. 26-6. Goniotomy with needle-knife, using Swan-Jacob goniolens.

but several millimeters away from the lateral limbus. The goniotomy knife is placed against the cornea 1 to 2 mm inside the limbus. The assistant needs to hold the eye against this point to provide support, for it is necessary to enter the cornea obliquely to avoid aqueous escape during and after the procedure. A Swan goniotomy knife with thin, straight shaft helps further to prevent aqueous leak when the instrument is withdrawn. The knife is constructed with a double edge so that the trabeculotomy can be made in opposite directions without rotating the blade (Fig. 26-4). The blade must be carried evenly across the anterior chamber to the far side of the pupil with a slight alternating rotative motion. This part of the procedure can be done more leisurely with a goniotomy needle-knife connected to a syringe containing balanced salt solution (Figs. 26-5 and 26-6). With the bevel down, the anterior chamber may be deepened at will by fluid injection. This is useful not only when crossing the chamber but also for placing the iris–trabecular meshwork attachment under stretch for easier and more bloodless surgery. There is now plenty of time to position the blade exactly against the trabecular meshwork, under magnification.

Goniotomy (Figs. 26-7 and 26-8 and Plate 8). The knife tip should engage the trabecular meshwork just below Schwalbe's line and should barely enter the meshwork. At least the back four fifths of the blade must remain visible to avoid a scleral incision, which would result in scarring or accidental goniopuncture. It is

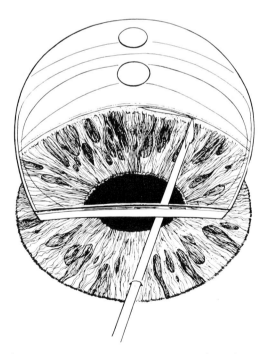

Fig. 26-7. Drawing showing goniotomy incision as seen through a surgical contact lens. (From Shaffer, R. N.: Amer. J. Ophthal. **47**:90, 1959.)

often necessary to rotate the knife handle around its axis to get the blade far enough into the angle without producing a marked dimple in the cornea at the point of entry. Such a dimple allows a bubble to enter under the contact lens unless the lens is rotated away from the entry puncture site. With the knife tip engaged, the contact lens can be moved about to give optimum visibility. Then, with the use of the puncture site as the fulcrum, a 60° trabeculotomy is done as indicated in Fig. 26-7. The knife blade is then repositioned, and the incision is carried 60° in the other direction. If more than 60° in one direction is attempted, aqueous humor

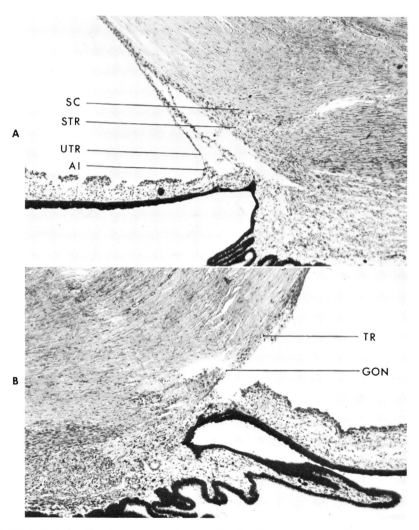

Fig. 26-8. A, Infantile glaucoma angle. **B,** Infantile glaucoma angle, showing the opposite side of the same eye after goniotomy. *SC,* Schlemm's canal; *STR,* trabecular meshwork; *AI,* hypoplastic iris; *UTR,* Barkan's membrane; *GON,* incision. (Courtesy Dr. L. Christensen, Portland, Ore.)

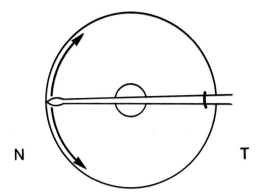

N T

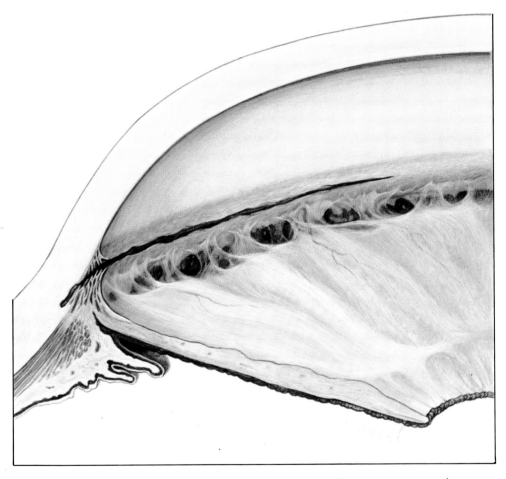

Plate 8. Goniotomy. Through a temporal corneal incision, *T*, a goniotomy can be performed nasally, *N*. The illustrated gonioscopic cross section shows the exact location of the incision in the abnormal trabecular meshwork.

is likely to leak from the entry site, and it is also difficult to maintain accurate visual control of the knife tip. An incision that goes back into the anterior ciliary body will produce severe and possibly disastrous bleeding. One that goes anterior to Schwalbe's line is useless therapeutically. One that goes into the sclera tends to fail because of fibrous proliferation. These are the reasons why visual control is so essential.

As can be seen in Fig. 26-9, two thirds of the circumference may be goniotomized from the temporal side in two procedures. If the pressure and outflow facility are still not normalized, the technically more difficult temporal goniotomy, with the knife passed over the bridge of the nose, can be done as the third operation.

Removal of knife. The knife should be removed smoothly and quickly with its handle kept parallel to the iris to avoid the lens. The needle-knife may be removed more leisurely, maintaining a deep anterior chamber and intraocular pressure by fluid injection. The side of the blade should be pressed toward the corneal incision to avoid enlarging it.

Turning of patient's head. The patient's head should now be turned 180° toward the surgeon. This places the goniotomy incision up and the puncture site down. If the eye is soft and the anterior chamber is collapsed, a slow flow of venous blood may now run down from the goniotomy incision and out the puncture wound.

Irrigating and maintaining the anterior chamber (Fig. 26-10). After withdrawal of the goniotomy knife the corneal wound tends to leak aqueous. To maintain the anterior chamber, the Barkan lens can be slipped over the puncture site. "Self-sealing" characteristics of the cornea will reduce and eventually prevent aqueous from escaping through the corneal wound. If ocular pressure and normal corneal depth can be maintained, bleeding will be minimized. If necessary, physiologic saline solution is instilled with a flat needle to irrigate blood from the anterior chamber and to deepen the chamber at the close of the procedure. A normal pressure reduces or prevents hemorrhage from the goniotomy incision. When the anterior chamber does not hold saline, air may be necessary but should not fill more than one half the anterior chamber. An aluminum shield is taped only over the operated eye.

Postsurgical technique

Position of head. When possible, the patient's head is kept turned toward the side of the puncture wound for the first 8 hours. This keeps the goniotomy incision upward so that blood can run away from it. Usually this position can be accomplished by a pillow propped behind the baby's back or by a wristlet fastened to the bed, holding the baby's body toward that side. Within 3 days any blood present has usually disappeared from the anterior chamber. The child is dismissed in 2 to 3 days if the eye looks satisfactory.

Reexamination. The child is reexamined four to six weeks after the goniotomy, with all equipment prepared to proceed with another goniotomy if the

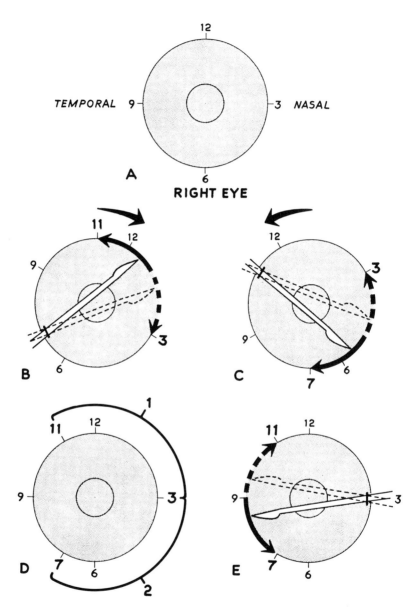

Fig. 26-9. Diagram showing method of doing two goniotomies from the temporal side. The third goniotomy is done over the patient's nose from the nasal side. **A,** Right eye. **B,** Eye rotated clockwise for first goniotomy. **C,** Eye rotated counterclockwise for second goniotomy if needed. **D,** Nasal area that has been goniotomized in **B** and **C,** with the knife entering from the temporal side. **E,** If a third goniotomy is needed, it must be performed temporally with the knife crossing the nose to puncture the cornea nasally. (From Shaffer, R. N.: Amer. J. Ophthal. **47:**90, 1959.)

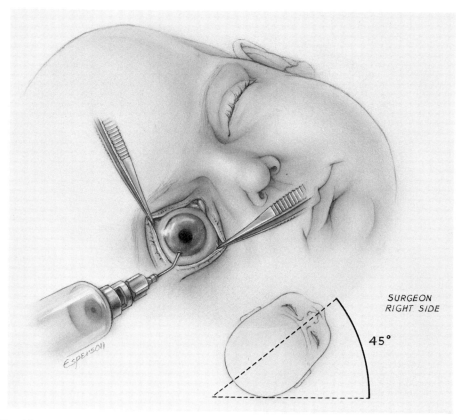

SURGEON
RIGHT SIDE

45°

Fig. 26-10. Irrigation of anterior chamber with head turned away from goniotomy incision.

pressure is elevated or if the cornea and disc show deterioration. Symptoms must also be considered in evaluating the need for reoperation. If pressure is controlled, the child is rechecked in two months; then at three- to four-month intervals for one year, twice in the next year, and yearly thereafter.

Practice goniotomy (Figs. 26-11 to 26-13)

The two essentials in performing skillful and safe goniotomies are thorough knowledge of the gonioscopic appearance of the infant angle and adequate practice in the technique of goniotomy under gonioscopic control. A good gonioscopist can quickly acquire a knowledge of the infant angle by gonioscoping babies who are under anesthesia for some other purpose. The surgical skill can be obtained by practicing on animal eyes fastened by toweling and thumbtacks to a wooden block. The various stages in performing goniotomy on a cat's eye are illustrated in Figs. 26-11 to 26-13.

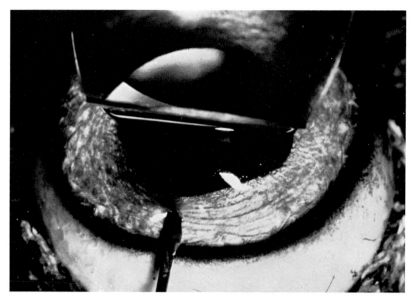

Fig. 26-11. Position of puncture in goniotomy. This photograph was taken from the surgeon's position. Although the knife blade appears at the bottom, the eye is turned away from the surgeon, as shown in Fig. 26-2. The knife is directed downward at a 45° angle from the vertical. (From Shaffer, R. N.: Amer. J. Ophthal. **47**:90, 1959.)

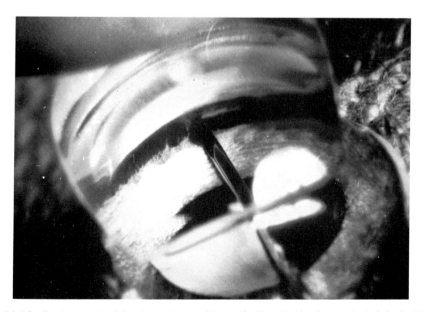

Fig. 26-12. Goniotomy incision in cat's eye (From Shaffer, R. N.: Amer. J. Ophthal. **47**:90, 1959.)

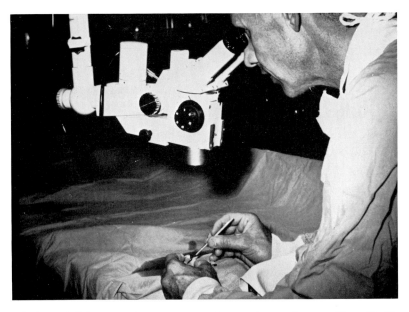

Fig. 26-13. Use of Zeiss operating microscope in practice goniotomy. (From Shaffer, R. N.: Amer. J. Ophthal. **47**:90, 1959.)

Evaluation of goniotomy

In early infantile glaucoma, goniotomy is usually successful. Three goniotomies should be done in different areas of the eye before resorting to more mutilating procedures. In eyes with glaucoma present at birth, multiple goniotomies will cure 25% to 50% of the patients. In those eyes in which glaucoma appears between the second and twelfth months, nearly 90% can be arrested by multiple goniotomies, with half of them needing only one operation. In trained hands the risks of goniotomies are negligible. Most of the complications are from injury to lens or ciliary body by improperly performed incisions. Hemorrhage can occur, and of course infection is always a possibility. An external trabeculotomy or trabeculectomy is indicated when three internal goniotomies have failed. There have been relatively few successes with goniotomy when the corneal diameter exceeds 15 mm. Nevertheless, it is still worth trying.

GONIOPUNCTURE

Goniopuncture may be used either alone or in conjunction with goniotomy. Its purpose is to produce filtration by a tiny puncture through the trabecular meshwork into the subconjunctival space. Preoperative treatment and examination are the same as for goniotomy.

The eye is prepared and fixated as for goniotomy. The actual goniopuncture can be made in any area of the eye but is usually placed at 6 o'clock. The conjunctiva is ballooned up by an injection of isotonic sodium chloride solution at this point to avoid injury when the knife comes into the subconjunctival space. The initial incision is made in the upper temporal cornea just inside the limbus. The knife blade is passed across the anterior chamber to engage the meshwork at the 6 o'clock position. It is passed through the limbal tissues and can be seen under the conjunctiva. The blade is then drawn back into the anterior chamber and withdrawn. There will be additional ballooning of the conjunctiva by aqueous humor, and the anterior chamber will rapidly collapse.

After infancy, goniopuncture is done with a larger knife than the normal goniotomy knife. After the age of 25 to 30 years, goniopuncture seems to be ineffective. The operation is done by Scheie without a contact lens. However, it seems desirable for the occasional operator to take advantage of visual gonioscopic control as described for goniotomy.

In our practice, goniotomy has been used alone rather than combined with goniopuncture. The addition of the goniopuncture has the disadvantage of collapsing the anterior chamber, which may produce peripheral anterior synechias to the goniotomy incision. Consequently, goniopuncture is reserved as a secondary procedure for those eyes in which repeated goniotomy has failed. It is also useful to reduce intraocular pressure and clear the cornea for later goniotomy.

CHAPTER **27**

Reoperation

The subject of reoperation in glaucoma is always distasteful, carrying as it does the stigma of failure. The disappointment of the patient and the surgeon must not be allowed to interfere with a realistic appraisal of the new situation. If medical therapy is unable to maintain pressure at a level that the optic nerve can tolerate, a surgical procedure is again indicated. If the primary operation has failed because of technical difficulties, it may be repeated. If failure is the result of new problems such as peripheral anterior synechias or the finding of poorly functioning outflow channels after an iridectomy, the reoperation must be planned to circumvent these problems.

In operations to provide new outflow channels, the surgical opening is far larger than is needed for aqueous outflow. Also, as a consequence of the surgical insult and secretory exhaustion, there is suppression of aqueous production for a variable period of time. The postoperative hypotony persists until aqueous production is at least partially restored and the healing of the surgical incision has produced sufficient resistance to aqueous outflow. The pressure is determined by the outflow facility through the filtering area and the rate of aqueous secretion. If a reasonable balance is not established, intraocular pressure may rise above normal. This often means that the new outflow channels have been closed by scar tissue. Sometimes, with massage and miotics or suctioning a bleb, a small drainage channel can be maintained, and pressure falls to normal in a few days. More often a rise in pressure means that the filtering bleb will disappear as fibrous tissue seals the opening.

A marked overgrowth of connective tissue can form a lump that may mistakenly be called a bleb. Occasionally connective tissue walls off a bleb, forming a thick-walled blister communicating with the anterior chamber. It is sometimes possible to regain drainage by performing a subconjunctival discission or excision of the side wall of this blister.

When pressure becomes elevated after a cyclodialysis, it is almost certain evidence that the suprachoroidal cleft has closed (Chapter 25).

POSTERIOR SCLEROTOMY

Posterior sclerotomy lowers the pressure of the vitreous chamber by removal of vitreous humor or subvitreal fluid and thus provides more room in the anterior segment. Full local anesthesia or general anesthesia is needed. The opening should be made in the pars plana of the ciliary body just anterior to the ora serrata and should be placed between the recti muscles to avoid the ciliary arteries. The inferior temporal quadrant is the most convenient location. The use of hyperosmotic agents has made posterior sclerotomy unnecessary in most instances.

The oldest and simplest technique is to hold a Graefe knife with its blade 6 mm from, and perpendicular to, the limbus and then thrust it through conjunctiva, sclera, and pars plana into the center of the eye. It is then turned at right angles to stretch the incision. Ordinarily the solid anterior condensation of vitreous humor does not escape. The knife must be far enough into the eye to reach the semiliquid vitreous humor.

A safer sclerotomy can be achieved by a scratch incision 6 mm from the limbus in a quadrant between the muscle insertions This is gradually deepened to the suprachoroidal space. The incision is rimmed by diathermy, and the vitreous aspirated through a No. 18 to 22 needle mounted on a 2 ml Luer syringe. The small conjunctival incision can then be closed by one suture.

CORRECTION OF HYPOTONY

After all intraocular operations, the sudden drop in tension leads to choroidal edema or choroidal separation. This may be a flat disinsertion that is clinically undetectable, or it may appear as one or more gray balloons in the peripheral fundus as seen ophthalmoscopically. Hypotony is usually accompanied by marked decrease in aqueous production.

In glaucoma surgery, a flat anterior chamber often accompanies the choroidal separation. In filtering operations, the large limbal opening permits rapid loss of aqueous, and the decreased aqueous production delays restoration of the anterior chamber. An inadvertent cyclodialysis can occur while external filtration surgery is being attempted. If fluorescein injected into the anterior chamber appears in fluid drained from an incision over the ciliary body, cyclodialysis is present. Gonioscopy frequently reveals the cyclodialysis cleft. This is a space-occupying lesion of the posterior eye, and a shallow anterior chamber can result. Especially with cyclodialysis the accompanying hypotony can be so profound as to cause edema of the macula and optic disc, with severe loss of central vision.

It should be remembered that choroidal separation is commonly the result of a flat anterior chamber and not the initiating cause. The true cause of the flat chamber is either the limbal or suprachoroidal surgical opening. The persistence of the collapse is aided by the large limbal opening and suppression of aqueous production and occasionally by an actual conjunctival fistula.

The decision to re-form an anterior chamber must be made within one or two weeks. The timing depends on the appearance of the eye. If there is little inflammation and a good bleb is present, delay is permissible; if the eye is inflamed, vision is poor, and failure of the bleb is likely, prompt intervention is indicated.

AIR INJECTION INTO ANTERIOR CHAMBER

As a general rule, the use of air in the anterior chamber should be avoided. Air deepens only the central portion of the chamber, which can leave the periphery flat and the angle closed. Injected balanced salt solution deepens both peripheral and central chamber.

Air injection into the anterior chamber is one effective method of reducing a wound leak. With a sharp, sterile No. 30 needle on a Luer syringe filled with air, paracentesis can be performed, carefully working the needle into the potential space between cornea and iris. With such soft eyes, it is often easier to make a preliminary opening for the needle with a Ziegler knife. Some fluorescein dried on the knife beforehand will stain the path of the paracentesis, making the opening easier to find. It is also helpful to have the edges of the needle rounded off to keep the sharpened tip from starting a new corneal tract. Good light and magnification such as are obtained with the Zeiss operating microscope are essential. With the tip of the needle in the chamber, air is injected. This builds up the intraocular pressure. The surface tension of the air restricts its running out through any fistulous opening that may be present. In the few days needed to absorb the air, the opening may be reduced in size, and aqueous production may be increased to a point that the chamber remains formed.

In the absence of an anterior chamber, the Seidel fluorescein test is often negative. To determine the position of a postcataract wound leak or a conjunctival fistula after an external drainage operation, the paracentesis incision is most useful. Sterile, fluorescein-stained physiologic saline solution is injected into the anterior chamber under moderate pressure. Its appearance externally identifies the site of the leak, which must be closed. In an external drainage operation the prognosis for spontaneous re-formation of the anterior chamber is good if the solution runs out under the conjunctiva but does not appear externally.

DRAINAGE OF SUBCHOROIDAL FLUID WITH FLUID RESTORATION OF THE ANTERIOR CHAMBER (Fig. 27-1)

A most effective method of correcting hypotomy is by drainage of the choroidal fluid through a posterior sclerotomy and restoration of the anterior chamber by balanced salt solution. A corneal paracentesis is first prepared for future injection, the incision being marked by fluorescein. In the lower temporal quadrant 6 mm from the limbus, a scleral trapdoor is cut down to the choroid and is hinged by its last few fibers at the back. When the knife cuts through, there is generally an outpouring of straw-colored fluid, which continues to flow as the intraocular pressure is built up by injection of balanced salt solution into the anterior chamber. Usually no closure of the incision is made. In a very soft eye, two mattress sutures 3 mm apart and opposed to each other will hold out the sclera while the incision is

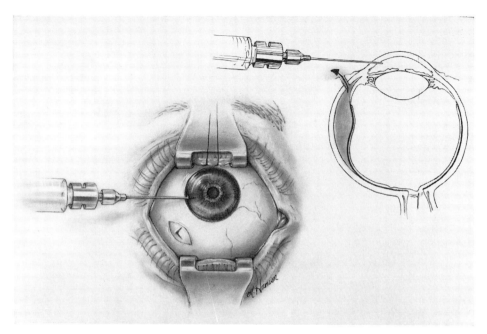

Fig. 27-1. Posterior sclerotomy and injection into the anterior chamber.

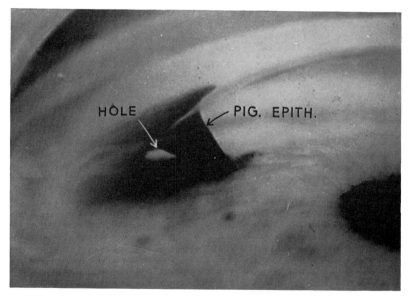

Fig. 27-2. Goniophotograph showing a hole in the pigmented epithelium produced by a discission needle. Case history: A 48-year-old woman had an iridectomy of the left eye done for acute angle-closure glaucoma with complete cure. A prophylactic peripheral iridectomy was performed on the right eye. Repeated subacute attacks occurred in this eye. Examination showed slitlike to closed angles and a peripheral iridectomy through which the intact pigmented epithelium of the iris bulged up and was attached to the cornea. The angle opened in most areas following the discission of the pigmented epithelium.

done between them. Air injection is sometimes required to deepen the anterior chamber when a large wound leak is present. If the procedure fails, it may be repeated in another quadrant. By closing only the corneoscleral fistula, a choroidal detachment will sometimes disappear within hours if the pressure rises and the anterior chamber deepens. A sclerotomy may be unnecessary.

REOPERATION AFTER SURGERY TO BREAK PUPILLARY BLOCK

When glaucoma surgery becomes necessary after an iridectomy has been done, one must be certain that no element of pupillary block remains. This is determined gonioscopically by seeing that the iridectomy opening is not occluded by the posterior iris pigment layer (Fig. 27-2), by fibrous tissue, or by adhesions to lens, vitreous humor, or cornea. With these factors eliminated, the choice of surgery then depends on whatever secondary factors are responsible for the pressure elevation.

Occasionally only the iris stroma is excised during an iridectomy, leaving the pigment epithelium intact and resulting in failure to break pupillary block. A discission of the pigment epithelium may be necessary to complete the iridectomy. The argon laser provides an effective alternative. The pigment epithelium absorbs the laser energy and almost disintegrates. The procedure is much easier to perform than laser iridectomy.

Plateau iris

If tension elevation occurs with pupillary dilation despite a patent iridectomy and the angles can be seen to be as narrow as before, the plateau iris syndrome is probably present (Chapter 12). Miotics are usually sufficiently effective to hold the iris away from the trabecular meshwork.

Peripheral anterior synechias
Cyclodialysis

In the absence of pupillary block, if peripheral anterior synechias represent the only block to outflow, medical treatment is indicated if at all possible. If it is not successful, cyclodialysis can be effective. Care must be used to avoid tearing the iris loose as the spatula comes into the chamber (Chapter 25). The advantage of cyclodialysis is that it frees the angle and may give some access of aqueous humor to Schlemm's canal even if a suprachoroidal cleft is not formed. It also opens the angle so that a subsequent external filtering procedure can be done more effectively in the area freed of peripheral anterior synechias.

Filtering surgery

If intraocular pressure cannot be controlled medically after an iridectomy, some form of filtering procedure is required. If the eye has a shallow chamber, an iridencleisis has some advantages. If the iridectomy has been done under a conjunctival flap, the surgery should be performed in a quadrant away from the iridectomy to avoid the area of conjunctival scarring. If no flap was used, the iridectomy site is most convenient. Usually it is easiest to do a sphincterotomy through the existing iridectomy and incarcerate one pillar of iris. Most surgeons now prefer thermal sclerostomy or trabeculectomy. If a tertiary procedure is required, cyclodialysis can be done opposite the filtering procedure.

REOPERATION AFTER FILTERING SURGERY

It is discouraging to find patients in the early postoperative period with gradually increasing pressures. For many reasons additional manipulation of the operative area is usually avoided. Before the patient is subjected to another filtering procedure with further tissue destruction, it is advisable to make every effort to reestablish the function of the failing bleb.

Suction cup (Fig. 27-3)

In early stages of bleb failure a perilimbal suction cup can be applied. The cup is positioned so that the cuff surrounds the bleb; with the pressure reduced to −55 mm Hg, the length of application should be 5 minutes, and the procedure must be done under careful observation. During the procedure the anterior chamber may noticeably shallow while aqueous appears in the plastic cup as the intra-

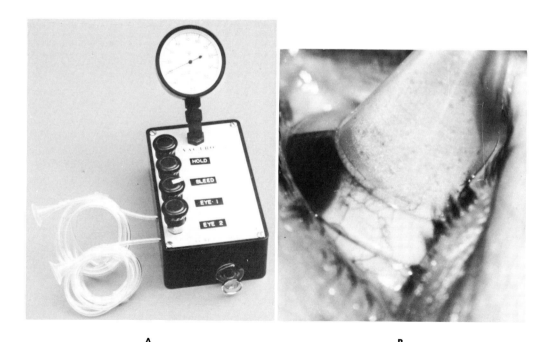

A   B

Fig. 27-3. Suction of failing bleb. A, Equipment. B, Method of application of perilimbal suction cup in patient with elevated pressures and cystic bleb.

ocular pressure decreases. It may be necessary to perform frequent applications to permanently establish filtration. Although not always successful, the procedure is easy to perform and occasionally salvages a failing filtering operation.

Bleb revision

The procedure of bleb revision frequently alters the course of a failing filtering bleb. Failure begins often at the periphery of the bleb where fibrosis limits diffusion and absorption of aqueous. The corneal fistula will usually close after the bleb has scarred down on the sclera. Patency of the translimbal opening is established when pressure applied to the cornea visibly increases the bleb volume and when fluorescein injection into the bleb leaks into the anterior chamber. If exteriorization of the anterior chamber exists and pressure is elevated, revision should be attempted. This salvages the successful corneoscleral fistula and preserves room for any additional filtering operations if they become necessary.

The revision is performed as follows. A retrobulbar anesthetic is used, and balanced salt solution or local anesthetic is injected under the conjunctiva beside the bleb to show its limits and facilitate dissection. The previous conjunctival incision is reopened and the conjunctiva elevated to the resistant bleb wall. If thinning of the bleb is desired, Tenon's membrane may be dissected from the sclera and removed. When the bleb wall is entered, aqueous will escape and the anterior chamber will shallow. The entire bleb wall should be incised, and any remaining fibrous ridge excised with scissors. Cautery is applied to the corneoscleral incision if the fistula appears inadequate. The conjunctiva is closed by the usual suturing technique of filtering operations.

Failing trabeculectomies can be revised by loosening the scleral flap along the original incision. The tissue can be cauterized or corrections can be made to improve the chances for filtration.

During the postoperative phase there is an opportunity to alter the regimen from that used previously. Topical or systemic steroids may be administered, and more attention given to eye massage.

Repeated filtering procedures

If there has been no technical reason for failure of the first operation, a rational choice of reoperation becomes very difficult. It may be wise to shift to another type of filtering operation in the hope of a more favorable response by the eye. If peripheral anterior synechias are present, a cyclodialysis may free the angle, making subsequent filtering surgery easier even if no suprachoroidal cleft is formed. If an iridencleisis has been done, again cyclodialysis is advisable, performed opposite the iridencleisis incision. Reoperation by any of the external filtering procedures probably has at least a 50% chance of being successful. Such operations should always be placed where there is unscarred conjunctiva and under the upper or lower lid if possible. Trabeculectomy or external trabeculotomy must be considered if other procedures have failed.

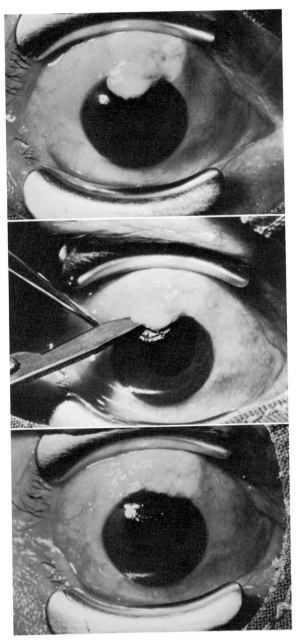

Fig. 27-4. Method of removal of migrating corneal bleb. Using sharp dissection the bleb is elevated from the cornea and excised at the limbus with scissors.

Management of corneal bleb (Fig. 27-4)

Occasionally, after a successful operation for external drainage, the conjunctival bleb will dissect down into the cornea. Here it forms a translucent white blister, which slowly extends toward the central cornea. Pathologically, this blister is largely acellular and filled with amorphous material. It can be removed by dissecting it off the cornea like a pterygium. When the limbus is reached, the tissue can be excised without collapsing the filtering bleb.

REOPERATION AFTER CYCLODIALYSIS
Aphakic glaucoma

If aphakic glaucoma was the reason for the cyclodialysis, the procedure can be repeated one or two times before resorting to external filtering procedures. Care should be taken to avoid scarring down conjunctiva. Any form of external filtering procedure has a chance of success in aphakic eyes but often fails because of vitreous incarceration. At the present time trabeculectomy or guarded thermal sclerostomy seems to be the safest operation because the external opening is not large and only a small peripheral iridectomy is needed. Often the iris will not prolapse spontaneously and must be picked up with forceps or a sharp iris buttonhook to perform the iridectomy. Cyclocryotherapy or cyclodiathermy is a poor last choice.

External diathermy to close cyclodialysis cleft

It is sometimes possible to limit the extent of a cyclodialysis cleft by producing fibrous tissue by a technique similar to cyclodiathermy except that the coagulation points run backward from the limbus along both edges of the cleft. Usually there will be only a small decrease in the extent of the cleft, and repeat diathermy is needed. Before each procedure the cleft must be accurately localized by gonioscopy. The retrobulbar anesthetic will occasionally paralyze one of the oblique muscles more than another, and the resulting torsion turns the cleft to a position that would be quite unsuspected by the surgeon if he did not use gonioscopy during the operation. Complete closure may result in an abrupt tension rise and may even require an external filtering operation for control.

REOPERATION AFTER GONIOTOMY

Ordinarily three goniotomies should be tried before one resorts to other procedures unless the eye seems unfavorable for goniotomy because of its size or angle appearance. If it is thought that Schlemm's canal is not available for drainage, goniopuncture is the safest external filtering operation that one can use. Reported success with trabeculectomies and external trabeculotomies provides the surgeon with a potentially useful procedure for infants who have failed to respond to goniotomies. If it fails, thermal sclerostomy or other external filtering procedures can be used. Thin sclera, however, makes the procedure difficult and dangerous. Blood vessels looping forward in the angle can hemorrhage when inadvertently cut during trabeculectomy. Cyclodialysis has a very low success rate in the congenital glaucomas. Cyclodiathermy and cyclocryotherapy are used as a last resort.

CATARACT OPERATION AFTER GLAUCOMA SURGERY

A routine cataract extraction technique can be used after an iridectomy and after failure of a filtering procedure or cyclodialysis. The scarring of subconjunctival tissues and accompanying bleeding increase the difficulty. The groove for McLean sutures should be placed away from a previous limbal scar to avoid premature entrance into the anterior chamber. A spatula should be passed between the iris and the lens to divide posterior synechias before lens removal is undertaken.

After successful iridectomy

No change in surgical technique is required for cataract extraction. After the limbal incision, a spatula should be passed between the iris and the lens to be sure that no posterior synechias are present to interfere with the lens delivery. If a full iridectomy is desired, the peripheral iridectomy can be enlarged by doing a sphincterotomy.

After successful surgery to open new outflow channels

The integrity of a functioning antiglaucoma operation is threatened by lens extraction, whatever method is used. It seems logical to protect the function of the bleb by placing incisions away from the site of the glaucoma operation. Although many techniques have been advocated, no one procedure is superior to others. If a bleb or cyclodialysis cleft is in the upper nasal quadrant, a temporal cataract incision is easily performed (Fig. 27-5). If the glaucoma surgery was at the 12 o'clock position, a corneal incision can be made (Fig. 27-6), or the lens may be removed by a limbal incision of the lower cornea (Fig. 27-7). In the latter instance an inferior sphincterotomy will facilitate extraction. A limbus-based conjunctival flap through the original incision and bleb area (Fig. 27-8) can be used with equal success, especially if the bleb is large and succulent. In all these cases posterior synechias must be dialysed.

The preservation of a functioning filtering procedure depends on a free flow of aqueous in the postoperative period. For this reason air should not be used to reform the anterior chamber, since it tends to form a tamponade against the inner glaucoma incision.

No one approach has been clearly proved superior. The choice of procedure depends on the skill and adaptability of the surgeon at performing techniques that are not customary, the appearance of the bleb, the level of pressure control, and other factors that require judgment. No matter how skillfully such surgery is done, about 50% of successful filtration areas may diminish postoperatively.

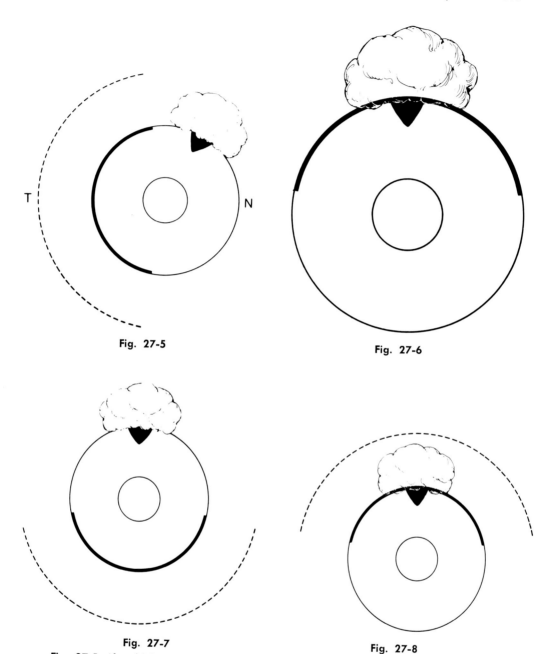

Fig. 27-5.

Fig. 27-6.

Fig. 27-7.

Fig. 27-8.

Fig. 27-5. If a bleb or cyclodialysis cleft is in the upper nasal quadrant, a temporal cataract incision is easily performed.

Fig. 27-6. If the glaucoma surgery was performed at the 12 o'clock position, a corneal incision can be made as shown.

Fig. 27-7. Here cataract extraction is performed through a limbal incision of the lower cornea.

Fig. 27-8. Here a limbus-based conjunctival flap through the original incision and bleb area is used.

After successful cyclodialysis

The cataract incision and extraction can be performed as usual if the cyclodialysis cleft is below. If it is above, the incision should be beveled sufficiently that the inner incision line is well in front of Schwalbe's line. By this method most suprachoroidal clefts can be maintained.

REOPERATION ON THE BLIND, PAINFUL EYE

The only rational operation on the blind, painful eye is enucleation. If it is absolutely certain that no tumor is present in the eye, a retrobulbar injection of 1 ml of absolute alcohol, either with brief general anesthetic or after previous retrobulbar lidocaine (Xylocaine) block, is permissible. Even with the retrobulbar anesthetic, pain is severe for 2 or 3 minutes.

Cyclocryotherapy has proved useful in some cases. Cyclodiathermy will sometimes stop pain. However, sympathetic ophthalmia has been reported after its use. Patients with blindness and pain are often reluctant to have enucleation and welcome a simple procedure such as cyclocryotherapy relatively free of complications.

X-ray treatment will sometimes stop the pain of absolute glaucoma. Up to 1000 R are given in divided doses. Relief, if it occurs, is delayed two to four weeks. Relief may occur spontaneously without x-ray treatment.

It deserves reemphasis: the only operation sure to relieve pain completely and

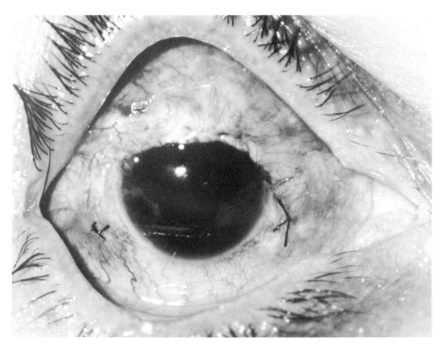

Fig. 27-9. Method of repair of conjunctival fistula by suturing flap to deepithelized cornea with 10-0 virgin silk.

permanently is enucleation. There is little excuse for risking sympathetic oph-thalmia in a seeing eye by doing intraocular procedures on its fellow blind eye. Furthermore, there is considerable danger of overlooking an intraocular tumor in such an eye.

LATE FISTULA FORMATION

As noted in Chapter 25, a thin-walled bleb can perforate either spontaneously or after minor trauma. Infection should be avoided by the use of antibiotic agents. If the fistula does not close by pressure dressings, tissue glue, or administration of oral acetazolamide (Diamox), surgical intervention is required.

When surgery is indicated, a sliding flap of conjunctiva is mobilized by parallel vertical incisions into the upper cul-de-sac and pulled over the bleb area (Fig. 27-9). The thin epithelium may be treated with alcohol or 35% tincture of iodine to promote adhesion of the flap. If it is actually necrotic, the bleb tissue is excised. A lamellar removal of superficial corneal tissue at the limbus is performed. The flap is fastened to this area and to adjacent conjunctiva with interrupted 9-0 silk mattress sutures. The flap must not be under stretch, or it will retract.

One procedure that has proved effective requires the insertion of a tongue of Tenon's capsule beneath the bleb. The tongue pedicle incised superior to the bleb is everted down into the elevated bleb and sutured to the corneal margin. Tenon's tissue will plug the external fistula, hopefully retaining the filtering area.

There is considerable risk of destroying the function of the filtering area by such a plastic procedure. Adjacent limbal areas should be spared for future surgery, if it is needed. For this same reason no treatment of hypotonous eyes is advisable if the epithelium is intact over a thin-walled bleb when the anterior chamber is formed and vision is not materially reduced.

References–Section VII

Allen, L., and Burian, H. M.: Trabeculotomy ab externo, Amer. J. Ophthal. **53:**19, 1962.

Allen, L., and others: A new concept of the development of the anterior chamber angle, Arch. Ophthal. **53:**783, 1955.

Barkan, O.: Present status of goniotomy, Amer. J. Ophthal. **36:**445, 1953.

Barkan, O.: Surgery of congenital glaucoma, Amer. J. Ophthal. **36:**1523, 1953.

Barkan, O., and others: Symposium: The infantile form of congenital glaucoma, Trans. Amer. Acad. Ophthal. Otolaryng. **59:**322, 1955.

Bietti, G. B.: Surgical intervention on ciliary body, J.A.M.A. **142:**889, 1950.

Bigger, J. F., and Becker, B.: Cataracts and open-angle glaucoma. The effect of uncomplicated cataract extraction on glaucoma control, Trans. Amer. Acad. Ophthal. Otolaryng. **75:**260, 1971.

Cairns, J. E.: Trabeculectomy, Amer. J. Ophthal. **66:**673, 1968.

Cairns, J. E.: Trabeculectomy, Trans. Amer. Acad. Ophthal. Otolaryng. **76:**384, 1972.

Chandler, A.: Peripheral iridectomy, Arch. Ophthal. **72:**804, 1964.

Dannheim, R.: Trabeculotomy, Trans. Amer. Acad. Ophthal. Otolaryng. **76:**375, 1972.

de Roeth, A., Jr.: Cryosurgery for glaucoma. In Cryosurgery, Int. Ophthal. Clin. **7**(2): 351, 1967.

Fitzgerald, J. R., and McCarthy, J. L.: Surgery of the filtering bleb, Arch. Ophthal. **68:** 453, 1962.

Harms, H.: Glaukom-Operationen am Schlemm'sschen Kanal. Sitzungsbericht der 114. Versammlung des Vereins Rhein-Uiestz Augenärzte, 1966.

Harms, H., and Dannheim, R.: Epicritical consideration of 300 cases of trabeculotomy ab externo, Oxford Ophthalmological Congress, July, 1969.

Iliff, C. E.: Flap perforation in glaucoma surgery sealed by a tissue patch, Arch. Ophthal. **71:**215, 1964.

Krasnov, M. M.: Externalization of Schlemm's canal (sinusotomy) in glaucoma, Brit. J. Ophthal. **52:**157, 1968.

Krasnov, M. M.: Microsurgery of glaucoma, Amer. J. Ophthal. **67:**857, 1969.

Kupfer, C.: Gonioscopy in infants and children. In Apt, L., editor: Diagnostic procedures in pediatric ophthalmology, London, 1963, J. A. Churchill, Ltd.

Mann, I.: The development of the human eye, ed. 2, New York, 1950, Grune & Stratton, Inc.

Maumenee, A. E.: The pathogenesis of congenital glaucoma, Amer. J. Ophthal. **47:**827, 1959.

Maumenee, A. E., and Stark, W. J.: Management of persistent hypotony after planned or inadvertent cyclodialysis, Amer. J. Ophthal. **71:**320, 1971.

McLean, J. M., and Lincoff, H. A.: Cryosurgery of the ciliary body, Trans. Amer. Ophthal. Soc. **62:**384, 1964.

Portney, G. L., and Purcell, T. W.: Surgical repair of cyclodialysis induced hypotony, Ophthalmic Surg. **5:**30, 1974.

Ridgway, A. E.: Trabeculectomy, Brit. J. Ophthal. **58:**680, 1974.

Scheie, H. G.: The management of infantile glaucoma, Arch. Ophthal. **62:**35, 1959.

Scheie, H. G.: Goniopuncture: an evaluation after eleven years, Arch. Ophthal. **65:**38, 1961.

Shaffer, R. N., and Weiss, D. I.: Concerning

cyclodialysis and hyptony, Arch. Ophthal. **68**:25, 1962.

Simmons, R. J.: Malignant glaucoma, Brit. J. Ophthal. **56**:263, 1972.

Sira, I. B., and Ticho, U.: Excision of Tenon's capsule in fistulizing operations on Africans, Amer. J. Ophthal. **68**:336, 1969.

Smith, R.: A new technique for opening of the canal of Schlemm, Brit. J. Ophthal. **44**:370, 1960.

Smith, R. J. H.: Recent advances in the surgical treatment of glaucoma, Brit. J. Ophthal. **58**:478, 1974.

Spaeth, G. L., Joseph, N. H., and Fernandes, E.: Trabeculectomy: a reevaluation after three years and a comparison with Scheie's procedure, Trans. Amer. Acad. Ophthal. Otolaryng. **70**:349, 1975.

Stocher, F. W.: Combined cataract extraction and sclerae cauterization, Arch. Ophthal. **72**:503, 1964.

Strachan, I. M.: A method of trabeculotomy with some preliminary results, Brit. J. Ophthal. **51**:539, 1967.

Sugar, H. S.: The glaucomas, New York, 1957, Hoeber Medical Division, Harper & Row, Publishers.

Sugar, H. S.: Complications, repair and reoperation of antiglaucoma filtering blebs, Amer. J. Ophthal. **63**:825, 1967.

Swan, K. C.: Reopening of nonfunctioning filters—simplified surgical techniques, Trans. Amer. Acad. Ophthal. Otolaryng. **79**:342, 1975.

Walser, E.: Über eine Kombinationsoperation "Iridektomie-Sklerektomie" beim Primärglaukom, Klin. Mbl. Augenheilk. **145**:720, 1964.

Worst, J. G. F.: The cause and treatment of congenital glaucoma, Trans. Amer. Acad. Ophthal. Otolaryng. **68**:766, 1964.

Iridectomy in advanced angle-closure glaucoma (Figs. 29-13 and 29-14)

Excellent response to echothiophate iodide (Phospholine iodide) in a patient no longer responsive to pilocarpine (Fig. 29-15)

Decreased ocular rigidity after echothiophate iodide (Fig. 29-16)

Responsiveness to pilocarpine after resistance to echothiophate iodide (Fig. 29-17)

Typical response to carbonic anhydrase inhibitors (Fig. 29-18)

Cardiac irregularity with topical epinephrine (Fig. 29-19)

Repeated tonograms over a period of six years (Fig. 29-20)

Successful filtering operation (Fig. 29-21)

Examples of artifacts in the tonographic tracing (Figs. 29-22 to 29-26)

CHAPTER 30 **GONIOSCOPIC EXAMPLES**

Grade 3 to 4, open angle; iris processes; blood in Schlemm's canal (Fig. 30-1, Reel I-1)

Slitlike narrow angle; closure imminent (Fig. 30-2, Reel I-2)

Grade 3, peripheral anterior synechias (Fig. 30-3, Reel I-3)

Closed angle preceding iridectomy (Fig. 30-4, Reel I-4)

Opened angle following iridectomy (Fig. 30-5, Reel I-5)

Iridocyclitis; Grade 3; small peripheral anterior synechias (PAS) (Fig. 30-6, Reel I-6)

Iridocyclitis; partial angle closure by peripheral anterior synechias (PAS) (Fig. 30-7, Reel I-7)

Acute granulomatous iridocyclitis (Fig. 30-8, Reel II-1)

Rubeosis iridis; anterior synechias (Fig. 30-9, Reel II-2)

Essential iris atrophy; anterior synechias (Fig. 30-10, Reel II-3)

Exfoliation syndrome (Fig. 30-11, Reel II-4)

Krukenberg's spindle; pigmentary glaucoma (Fig. 30-12, Reel II-5)

Pigmentary glaucoma (Fig. 30-13, Reel II-6)

Infantile glaucoma (Fig. 30-14, Reel II-7)

Aniridia (Fig. 30-15, Reel III-1)

Axenfeld's syndrome (Fig. 30-16, Reel III-2)

Melanoma of iris (Fig. 30-17, Reel III-3)

Pigment cyst of iris (Fig. 30-18, Reel III-4)

Foreign body (Fig. 30-19, Reel III-5)

Cyclodialysis (Fig. 30-20, Reel III-6)

Detached Descemet's membrane (Fig. 30-21, Reel III-7)

Tables for tonography and tonometry

SIMPLIFIED TONOGRAPHY TABLE

Table 28-1 is a great convenience in the interpretation of tonograms. It gives at a glance the intraocular pressure, P_0, and the outflow facility, C. In the derivation of this table the assumption is made that the eye is of average ocular rigidity (0.0215), that it has a normal radius of curvature of the cornea (7.8 mm anterior surface), and that the application of the tonometer produces a rise in episcleral venous pressure of 1.25 mm Hg.

Table 28-1. Simplified tonography table for eyes of average ocular rigidity

Initial reading		ΔR (change in scale reading)									
P_0	R	0	0.50	1.00	1.50	2.00	2.50	3.00	3.50	4.00	4.50	5.00
					5.5-gram weight							
21	4.00	0	0.04	0.08	0.13	0.18	0.24	0.30	0.37	0.45	0.54	0.63
20	4.25	0	0.04	0.08	0.13	0.18	0.24	0.30	0.36	0.43	0.52	0.60
19	4.50	0	0.04	0.08	0.12	0.17	0.23	0.29	0.35	0.42	0.50	0.58
18	4.75	0	0.04	0.08	0.12	0.17	0.23	0.28	0.34	0.41	0.48	0.56
17	5.00	0	0.04	0.08	0.12	0.17	0.22	0.27	0.33	0.40	0.47	0.54
17	5.25	0	0.04	0.08	0.12	0.17	0.22	0.27	0.33	0.39	0.46	0.53
16	5.50	0	0.04	0.08	0.12	0.16	0.21	0.26	0.32	0.38	0.45	0.52
15	5.75	0	0.04	0.08	0.12	0.16	0.21	0.26	0.32	0.38	0.44	0.50
15	6.00	0	0.03	0.07	0.11	0.15	0.20	0.25	0.31	0.37	0.43	0.49
14	6.25	0	0.03	0.07	0.11	0.15	0.20	0.25	0.31	0.37	0.43	0.49
13	6.50	0	0.03	0.07	0.11	0.15	0.20	0.25	0.30	0.36	0.42	0.48
13	6.75	0	0.03	0.07	0.11	0.15	0.20	0.24	0.30	0.36	0.41	0.47
12	7.00	0	0.03	0.07	0.11	0.15	0.20	0.24	0.29	0.35	0.40	0.46
11	7.50	0	0.03	0.07	0.11	0.15	0.19	0.24	0.29	0.34	0.39	0.45
10	8.00	0	0.03	0.07	0.11	0.15	0.19	0.24	0.29	0.34	0.39	0.45
9	8.50	0	0.03	0.07	0.11	0.15	0.19	0.23	0.28	0.33	0.39	0.44
9	9.00	0	0.03	0.07	0.11	0.15	0.19	0.23	0.28	0.33	0.38	0.44

Continued.

Table 28-1. Simplified tonography table for eyes of average ocular rigidity—cont'd

Initial reading		ΔR (change in scale reading)										
P_o	R	0	0.50	1.00	1.50	2.00	2.50	3.00	3.50	4.00	4.50	5.00
						7.5-gram weight						
30	4.00	0	0.03	0.06	0.10	0.15	0.20	0.25	0.32	0.39	0.46	0.55
29	4.25	0	0.03	0.06	0.10	0.15	0.19	0.25	0.30	0.37	0.44	0.52
28	4.50	0	0.03	0.06	0.10	0.14	0.18	0.24	0.29	0.35	0.42	0.50
27	4.75	0	0.03	0.06	0.10	0.14	0.18	0.23	0.28	0.34	0.40	0.47
26	5.00	0	0.03	0.06	0.10	0.13	0.17	0.22	0.27	0.33	0.39	0.45
25	5.25	0	0.03	0.06	0.10	0.13	0.17	0.22	0.27	0.32	0.38	0.43
24	5.50	0	0.03	0.06	0.09	0.13	0.16	0.21	0.26	0.31	0.37	0.42
23	5.75	0	0.03	0.06	0.09	0.13	0.16	0.21	0.26	0.31	0.36	0.41
22	6.00	0	0.03	0.06	0.09	0.12	0.16	0.20	0.25	0.30	0.35	0.40
21	6.25	0	0.03	0.06	0.09	0.12	0.16	0.20	0.25	0.29	0.34	0.39
20	6.50	0	0.03	0.05	0.09	0.12	0.15	0.19	0.24	0.28	0.33	0.38
19	6.75	0	0.03	0.05	0.09	0.12	0.15	0.19	0.24	0.28	0.33	0.38
18	7.00	0	0.03	0.05	0.08	0.12	0.15	0.19	0.23	0.27	0.32	0.37
17	7.50	0	0.03	0.05	0.08	0.12	0.15	0.19	0.23	0.27	0.31	0.36
16	8.00	0	0.03	0.05	0.08	0.11	0.15	0.18	0.22	0.26	0.30	0.35
14	8.50	0	0.03	0.05	0.08	0.11	0.15	0.18	0.22	0.26	0.30	0.35
13	9.00	0	0.03	0.05	0.08	0.11	0.15	0.18	0.22	0.25	0.29	0.34
12	9.50	0	0.03	0.05	0.08	0.11	0.15	0.18	0.22	0.25	0.29	0.34
						10.0-gram weight						
43	4.00	0	0.02	0.05	0.08	0.12	0.17	0.22	0.28	0.35	0.43	0.52
42	4.25	0	0.02	0.05	0.08	0.12	0.17	0.21	0.26	0.33	0.40	0.48
40	4.50	0	0.02	0.05	0.07	0.11	0.16	0.20	0.25	0.31	0.38	0.44
38	4.75	0	0.02	0.05	0.07	0.11	0.16	0.20	0.24	0.29	0.36	0.42
37	5.00	0	0.02	0.05	0.07	0.10	0.15	0.19	0.23	0.28	0.34	0.40
36	5.25	0	0.02	0.05	0.07	0.10	0.15	0.19	0.23	0.27	0.32	0.38
34	5.50	0	0.02	0.05	0.07	0.10	0.14	0.18	0.22	0.26	0.31	0.36
33	5.75	0	0.02	0.05	0.07	0.10	0.14	0.18	0.22	0.25	0.30	0.34
32	6.00	0	0.02	0.04	0.07	0.10	0.13	0.17	0.21	0.24	0.29	0.33
31	6.25	0	0.02	0.04	0.07	0.10	0.13	0.17	0.21	0.24	0.28	0.32
29	6.50	0	0.02	0.04	0.07	0.10	0.13	0.16	0.20	0.23	0.27	0.31
28	6.75	0	0.02	0.04	0.07	0.10	0.13	0.16	0.20	0.23	0.27	0.31
27	7.00	0	0.02	0.04	0.07	0.09	0.12	0.15	0.19	0.22	0.26	0.30
26	7.25	0	0.02	0.04	0.07	0.09	0.12	0.15	0.19	0.22	0.26	0.30
25	7.50	0	0.02	0.04	0.07	0.09	0.12	0.15	0.18	0.21	0.25	0.29
24	7.75	0	0.02	0.04	0.07	0.09	0.12	0.15	0.18	0.21	0.25	0.29
23	8.00	0	0.02	0.04	0.06	0.09	0.12	0.14	0.18	0.21	0.24	0.28
21	8.50	0	0.02	0.04	0.06	0.09	0.11	0.14	0.18	0.20	0.23	0.27
20	9.00	0	0.02	0.04	0.06	0.09	0.11	0.14	0.17	0.20	0.23	0.26
18	9.50	0	0.02	0.04	0.06	0.09	0.11	0.14	0.17	0.20	0.23	0.26
16	10.00	0	0.02	0.04	0.06	0.09	0.11	0.14	0.17	0.19	0.22	0.26
14	11.00	0	0.02	0.04	0.06	0.09	0.11	0.14	0.17	0.19	0.22	0.25

Values for intraocular pressure, P_0, for various scale readings, R, with the 5.5-, 7.5-, and 10-gram weights are presented in the left-hand column. The coefficient of outflow facility, C, is determined on the basis of the initial scale reading, R_1, and the number of scale units, ΔR, the tonometer has changed in 4 minutes. Thus, if the tonogram with the 5.5-gram weight began at a scale reading of 5.0 and reached a scale reading of 8.5 in 4 minutes ($\Delta R = 3.5$), the intraocular pressure is read as 17 mm Hg and the facility of outflow is 0.33.

Because of space limitations the table provides values only to the 0.5 scale unit. Therefore suitable interpolations may be necessary. In the example just given, if the final scale reading had been 8.25 ($\Delta R = 3.25$), the outflow facility would be estimated by interpolation as 0.30.

INTRAOCULAR PRESSURE TABLES (1955)

Table 28-2 presents the estimated pressure in the undisturbed eye, P_0, for various scale readings and plunger loads. The values assume normal ocular rigidity. If ocular rigidity is abnormal, the true pressure value can be obtained from Tables 28-8 and 28-9 by using two different plunger loads. It is more accurately estimated by applanation and Schiøtz readings, plotting the results on the Friedenwald nomogram (Figs. 28-1 and 28-2).

Table 28-2. Calibration scale for Schiøtz tonometers, P_0 (mm Hg), revised 1955

Scale reading	Plunger load			
	5.5 grams	7.5 grams	10 grams	15 grams
3.0	24.4	35.8	50.6	81.8
3.5	22.4	33.0	46.9	76.2
4.0	20.6	30.4	43.4	71.0
4.5	18.9	28.0	40.2	66.2
5.0	17.3	25.8	37.2	61.8
5.5	15.9	23.8	34.4	57.6
6.0	14.6	21.9	31.8	53.6
6.5	13.4	20.1	29.4	49.9
7.0	12.2	18.5	27.2	46.5
7.5	11.2	17.0	25.1	43.2
8.0	10.2	15.6	23.1	40.2
8.5	9.4	14.3	21.3	38.1
9.0	8.5	13.1	19.6	34.6
9.5	7.8	12.0	18.0	32.0
10.0	7.1	10.9	16.5	29.6

Table 28-3. Intraocular pressure during tonometry, P_t (mm Hg)

Scale reading	Plunger load			
	5.5 grams	7.5 grams	10 grams	15 grams
3.0	37.1	50.5	67.4	101.1
3.5	35.4	48.3	64.4	96.6
4.0	33.9	46.2	61.7	92.5
4.5	32.5	44.4	59.1	88.7
5.0	31.3	42.6	56.8	85.2
5.5	30.1	41.0	54.7	82.0
6.0	29.0	39.5	52.7	79.0
6.5	28.0	38.1	50.8	76.3
7.0	27.0	36.8	49.1	73.7
7.5	26.1	35.6	47.5	71.3
8.0	25.3	34.5	46.0	69.0
8.5	24.5	33.4	44.6	66.9
9.0	23.8	32.4	43.3	64.9
9.5	23.1	31.5	42.0	63.0
10.0	22.5	30.6	40.8	61.2
10.5	21.8	29.8	39.7	59.6
11.0	21.3	29.0	38.6	58.0
11.5	20.7	28.2	37.6	56.5
12.0	20.2	27.5	36.7	55.0
12.5	19.7	26.8	35.8	53.7
13.0	19.2	26.2	34.9	52.4
13.5	18.8	25.6	34.1	51.1
14.0	18.3	25.0	33.3	50.0
14.5	17.9	24.4	32.6	48.8
15.0	17.5	23.9	31.9	47.8

Table 28-3 presents in similar fashion the intraocular pressure with the tonometer in place, P_t. These are the P_0 and P_t values that are used in the denominator of the Grant formula for outflow facility.

VOLUME TABLES

The volume tables permit the estimation of the volume of fluid expressed from the eye during tonography, that is, the numerator ΔV of Grant's formula for outflow facility:

$$C = \frac{\Delta V}{4[P_{t_{av}} - (P_0 + 1.25)]}$$

From Table 28-4, ΔV values can be obtained by subtraction. This table assumes an average value for ocular rigidity (0.0215) and a radius of curvature of the anterior surface of the cornea of 7.8 mm.

Table 28-4. Change in ocular volume (ΔV in μl) for various plunger weights when tonometer reading falls from 0 to R

$$\Delta V = \frac{1}{0.0215} \log \frac{P_{t_0}}{P_{t_R}} + V_{c_R} - V_{c_0}*$$

Scale reading R	Plunger load			
	5.5 grams	7.5 grams	10 grams	15 grams
0.0	0.0	0.0	0.0	0.0
3.0	10.7	10.1	9.7	9.0
3.5	12.4	11.8	11.2	10.4
4.0	14.1	13.5	12.8	11.8
4.5	15.9	15.1	14.3	13.2
5.0	17.6	16.8	15.9	14.6
5.5	19.4	18.4	17.5	16.1
6.0	21.1	20.1	19.0	17.4
6.5	22.9	21.8	20.6	18.9
7.0	24.6	23.5	22.2	20.4
7.5	26.4	25.2	23.9	21.9
8.0	28.2	26.9	25.5	23.3
8.5	30.0	28.7	27.2	24.8
9.0	31.9	30.5	28.9	26.4
9.5	33.7	32.3	30.6	27.9
10.0	35.6	34.1	32.3	29.5
10.5	37.5	36.0	34.1	31.1
11.0	39.4	37.8	35.9	32.7
11.5	41.4	39.7	37.7	34.4
12.0	43.3	41.7	39.6	36.0
12.5	45.3	43.7	41.5	37.7
13.0	47.4	45.7	43.4	39.5
13.5	49.4	47.7	45.5	41.3
14.0	51.5	49.7	47.4	43.1
14.5	53.6	51.8	49.4	44.9
15.0	55.7	53.9	51.4	46.8

*Subscripts 0 and R refer to tonometer scale readings zero and R.

Table 28-5. Volume of corneal indentation, V_c (μl)

Scale reading	Plunger load			
	5.5 grams	*7.5 grams*	*10 grams*	*15 grams*
3.0	8.5	7.0	5.8	4.3
3.5	9.3	7.7	6.4	4.8
4.0	10.1	8.5	7.1	5.3
4.5	11.0	9.3	7.8	5.9
5.0	11.9	10.1	8.6	6.5
5.5	12.9	11.0	9.4	7.2
6.0	13.9	11.9	10.2	7.8
6.5	14.9	12.9	11.1	8.6
7.0	16.0	13.9	12.0	9.3
7.5	17.1	14.9	12.9	10.1
8.0	18.3	16.0	13.9	10.9
8.5	19.5	17.2	15.0	11.8
9.0	20.7	18.3	16.0	12.7
9.5	22.0	19.5	17.2	13.7
10.0	23.3	20.8	18.3	14.7
10.5	24.6	22.1	19.5	15.7
11.0	26.0	23.4	20.8	16.8
11.5	27.4	24.8	22.1	17.9
12.0	28.8	26.2	23.4	19.1
12.5	30.3	27.7	24.8	20.3
13.0	31.9	29.2	26.2	21.5
13.5	33.4	30.7	27.7	22.8
14.0	35.0	32.3	29.3	24.2
14.5	36.7	34.0	30.8	25.5
15.0	38.3	35.6	32.4	27.0

The change in volume, ΔV, is the sum of the decrease in ocular distention, ΔV_s, and the increase in corneal indentation, ΔV_c, during the 4 minutes of tonography. Table 28-5 provides estimates of the volume of corneal indentation, V_c, at various scale readings. From this table ΔV_c between any two scale readings can be obtained by subtraction.

If the radius of curvature of the anterior surface of the cornea differs from 7.8 mm, there is a small change in ΔV_c (Table 28-6).

If V_c = volume of corneal indentation for radius 7.8 mm

and V_{cr} = volume of corneal indentation corrected for radius, r,

then $V_{cr} = V_c + V_r$.

During tonography

$$\Delta V_{cr} = (V_{c_2} + V_{r_2}) - (V_{c_1} + V_{r_1}) = \Delta V_c + \Delta V_r,$$

where ΔV_c = change in volume of corneal indentation during tonography (radius 7.8) (see Table 28-5 for ΔV_C),

           $\Delta V_r = V_{r_2} - V_{r_1}$ = correction for radius, r,

and ΔV_{cr} = change in volume of corneal indentation during tonography corrected for radius, r.

Table 28-6. Change, V_r,* in volume of corneal indentation by tonometer with radius, r,† of curvature of cornea

Scale reading	V_r						
	6.5	*7.0*	*7.5*	*8.0*	*8.5*	*9.0*	*9.5*
			5.5-gram weight				
3	+ 3.1	+1.7	+0.6	-0.5	-1.2	-1.9	- 2.5
4	+ 3.7	+2.0	+0.7	-0.5	-1.4	-2.3	- 3.0
5	+ 4.4	+2.5	+0.9	-0.6	-1.7	-2.7	- 3.5
6	+ 5.2	+3.0	+1.0	-0.7	-2.0	-3.1	- 4.1
7	+ 6.1	+3.5	+1.1	-0.8	-2.3	-3.6	- 4.8
8	+ 7.2	+4.0	+1.3	-0.9	-2.6	-4.1	- 5.4
9	+ 8.4	+4.6	+1.4	-1.0	-2.9	-4.7	6.2
10	+ 9.7	+5.3	+1.6	-1.1	-3.3	-5.5	- 7.1
11	+11.1	+6.0	+1.7	-1.3	-3.9	-6.2	- 8.0
12	+12.5	+6.7	+1.9	-1.4	-4.4	-7.0	- 9.1
13	+14.2	+7.7	+2.3	-1.6	-5.0	-7.8	-10.3
14	+15.9	+8.7	+2.7	-1.7	-5.6	-8.5	-11.5
15	+18.1	+9.7	+3.0	-1.8	-6.2	-9.4	-12.8
			10-gram weight				
3	+1.4	+0.8	+0.3	-0.2	-0.5	-0.8	-1.2
4	+1.7	+0.9	+0.3	-0.3	-0.6	-1.0	-1.4
5	+2.0	+1.1	+0.4	-0.3	-0.7	-1.2	-1.6
6	+2.3	+1.3	+0.4	-0.3	-0.9	-1.4	-1.9
7	+2.6	+1.5	+0.5	-0.4	-1.0	-1.6	-2.2
8	+3.0	+1.7	+0.5	-0.4	-1.2	-1.9	-2.5
9	+3.5	+1.9	+0.6	-0.5	-1.4	-2.2	-2.8
10	+4.0	+2.2	+0.7	-0.6	-1.6	-2.5	-3.2
11	+4.5	+2.5	+0.8	-0.6	-1.7	-2.8	-3.6
12	+5.0	+2.8	+0.9	-0.7	-2.0	-3.1	-4.0
13	+5.6	+3.1	+1.1	-0.8	-2.2	-3.5	-4.4
14	+6.4	+3.4	+1.2	-0.9	-2.5	-3.9	-4.8
15	+7.2	+3.7	+1.4	-1.0	-2.7	-4.2	-5.3

*V_r = change in volume of corneal indentation for radius, r.
†r = radius of curvature of anterior corneal surface (mm).

Since $\Delta V = \Delta V_c + \Delta V_s$ (see Table 28-4 for ΔV),
to correct ΔV for radius, r,
   $\Delta V_{corr} = \Delta V + \Delta V_r$.

For example, in a tonogram with a 5.5-gram weight starting at scale reading 4.5 and reaching 6.5 at 4 minutes:
   for radius of corneal curvature 7.8 mm: $\Delta V = 7.0 \ \mu l$ (Table 28-4)

$$C = \frac{\Delta V}{4[P_{tav} - (P_0 + 1.25)]} = \frac{7.0}{4(30.25 - 20.25)} = 0.18;$$

   for radius of corneal curvature 7.0 mm; $\Delta V = 7.0 + 1.0 = 8.0$ (Table 28-6)

$$C = \frac{8.0}{4 \times 10} = 0.20.$$

Table 28-7 presents the values for the decrease in ocular distention during tonography, ΔV_{sav}. The values in this table are based on the assumption of a normal ocular rigidity (0.0215). ΔV_{sav} is obtained by subtraction of the values corresponding to the scale readings at the beginning and at the 4-minute value in the tonogram. If the rigidity of the individual eye, E, differs from the mean value, a corrected value for the decrease in ocular distention can be obtained as follows:

$$\Delta V_{scorr} = \Delta V_{sav} \times \frac{0.0215}{E}$$

The value for E may be obtained from Tables 28-8 and 28-9 or from the slope of the line resulting from plotting the applanation and Schiøtz tonometry values on the nomogram (Figs. 28-1 and 28-2). Then

$$C = \frac{\Delta V_c + \Delta V_{scorr}}{4[P_{tav} - (P_{0corr} + 1.25)]}$$

Table 28-7. Change in volume of ocular distention, ΔV_{sav} in μl,* for all plunger weights when the tonometer reading falls from 0 to R

$$\Delta V_{sav} = \frac{1}{0.0215} \log \frac{P_{t0}\dagger}{P_{tR}}$$

Scale reading R	ΔV_{sav} (E = 0.0215)	Scale reading R	ΔV_{sav} (E = 0.0215)
0.0	0.0	9.0	15.5
3.0	6.6	9.5	16.1
3.5	7.5	10.0	16.7
4.0	8.4	10.5	17.3
4.5	9.2	11.0	17.9
5.0	10.0	11.5	18.4
5.5	10.8	12.0	18.9
6.0	11.6	12.5	19.4
6.5	12.3	13.0	19.9
7.0	13.0	13.5	20.4
7.5	13.7	14.0	20.9
8.0	14.3	14.5	21.3
8.5	14.9	15.0	21.7

*To correct ΔV_{sav} for ocular rigidity, E, of individual eye:

$$\Delta V_{scorr} = \Delta V_{sav} \times \frac{0.0215}{E}$$

†Subscripts 0 and R refer to tonometer scale readings zero and R.

Table 28-8. Pressure and rigidity table for paired readings with 5.5- and 10.0-gram weights

Reading with 5.5-gram weight	Reading with 10.0-gram weight																		
	6.0	6.5	7.0	7.5	8.0	8.5	9.0	9.5	10.0	10.5	11.0	11.5	12.0	12.5	13.0	13.5	14.0	14.5	15.0
3.0	.0904	.0536	.0353	.0244	.0173	.0124	.0088	.0063	.0049	.0027	.0015								
	6	13	19	23	26	29	31	33	34	35	36								
3.5		.0877	.0526	.0350	.0244	.0176	.0127	.0094	.0068	.0048	.0033	.0021	.0011						
		7	12	17	21	24	27	29	31	32	33	34	35						
4.0			.0870	.0523	.0349	.0245	.0177	.0132	.0098	.0073	.0053	.0038	.0026	.0016					
			5	10	15	19	22	25	27	29	30	31	32	33					
4.5					.0517	.0346	.0244	.0180	.0135	.0102	.0076	.0057	.0042	.0030	.0020	.0012			
					9	14	18	21	23	25	27	28	29	30	31	32			
5.0						.0511	.0342	.0246	.0182	.0137	.0104	.0080	.0061	.0046	.0034	.0024	.0016		
						8	12	16	19	21	24	25	26	28	29	29	30		
5.5							.0498	.0341	.0245	.0182	.0138	.0106	.0082	.0063	.0049	.0037	.0027	.0019	.0013
							7	11	15	18	20	22	24	25	26	27	28	28	29
6.0								.0493	.0336	.0242	.0181	.0139	.0107	.0084	.0066	.0051	.0039	.0030	.0022
								6	10	13	16	19	21	22	24	25	26	26	27
6.5									.0486	.0332	.0240	.0181	.0139	.0109	.0085	.0067	.0053	.0042	.0032
									5	9	12	15	17	19	21	22	23	24	25
7.0										.0475	.0325	.0237	.0179	.0139	.0109	.0086	.0069	.0055	.0044
										5	8	11	14	16	18	20	21	22	23
7.5												.0320	.0233	.0178	.0138	.0109	.0086	.0070	.0056
												7	10	13	15	17	19	20	21
8.0													.0313	.0230	.0176	.0137	.0109	.0087	.0071
													7	10	12	14	16	18	19
8.5														.0307	.0226	.0173	.0136	.0108	.0088
														6	9	11	13	15	17
9.0															.0300	.0222	.0171	.0135	.0108
															6	8	11	13	14

Table 28-9. Pressure and rigidity table for paired readings with 7.5- and 15.0-gram weights

Each cell shows the value with its associated count (smaller number) as "value / count".

Reading with 7.5-gram weight	\ Reading with 15.0-gram weight → 6.5	7.0	7.5	8.0	8.5	9.0	9.5	10.0	10.5	11.0	11.5	12.0	12.5	13.0	13.5	14.0	14.5	15.0
3.0	.1145 / 8	.0705 / 16	.0480 / 23	.0343 / 29	.0252 / 34	.0189 / 37	.0143 / 40	.0108 / 43	.0082 / 44	.0061 / 46	.0044 / 47	.0031 / 48	.0020 / 49	.0011 / 50				
3.5		.1146 / 6	.0707 / 14	.0481 / 21	.0345 / 26	.0256 / 31	.0194 / 34	.0148 / 37	.0114 / 39	.0087 / 41	.0067 / 43	.0050 / 44	.0037 / 45	.0026 / 46	.0016 / 49			
4.0			.1146 / 6	.0710 / 12	.0481 / 18	.0347 / 24	.0259 / 28	.0197 / 32	.0152 / 34	.0118 / 37	.0092 / 39	.0071 / 40	.0055 / 42	.0041 / 43	.0031 / 44	.0021 / 44	.0014 / 45	
4.5					.0705 / 10	.0482 / 16	.0347 / 21	.0260 / 25	.0199 / 29	.0155 / 32	.0122 / 34	.0096 / 36	.0075 / 38	.0059 / 39	.0046 / 40	.0035 / 41	.0026 / 42	.0018 / 43
5.0						.0705 / 8	.0480 / 16	.0347 / 19	.0261 / 23	.0201 / 27	.0157 / 30	.0124 / 32	.0099 / 34	.0079 / 35	.0063 / 37	.0049 / 38	.0038 / 39	.0029 / 40
5.5							.0701 / 7	.0475 / 12	.0345 / 17	.0260 / 21	.0201 / 24	.0159 / 27	.0126 / 30	.0101 / 32	.0082 / 33	.0065 / 35	.0052 / 36	.0042 / 37
6.0								.0694 / 6	.0472 / 11	.0343 / 15	.0259 / 19	.0202 / 23	.0160 / 26	.0127 / 28	.0102 / 30	.0083 / 32	.0068 / 33	.0055 / 34
6.5										.0479 / 11	.0346 / 15	.0262 / 19	.0204 / 21	.0161 / 24	.0130 / 26	.0105 / 28	.0086 / 30	.0070 / 25
7.0											.0462 / 8	.0337 / 13	.0257 / 16	.0200 / 19	.0160 / 22	.0129 / 24	.0105 / 26	.0086 / 25
7.5												.0458 / 7	.0334 / 11	.0254 / 15	.0199 / 18	.0159 / 21	.0129 / 23	.0109 / 21
8.0													.0453 / 6	.0330 / 10	.0252 / 14	.0198 / 17	.0159 / 19	.0126 / 21
8.5														.0446 / 6	.0326 / 9	.0249 / 13	.0196 / 15	.0158 / 18
9.0															.0440 / 5	.0322 / 8	.0248 / 12	.0194 / 14

For example, we may use the values assumed in Table 6-2 and in Fig. 28-2. In a tonogram with a 5.5-gram weight that begins at scale reading 4.5 and reaches scale reading 6.5 at 4 minutes:

(1) If the ocular rigidity is *normal* (0.0215), then

ΔV_c = 3.9 μl (Table 28-5)

ΔV_s = 3.1 μl (Table 28-7)

P_{tav} = 30.25 mm Hg (Table 28-3)

P_0 = 19.0 mm Hg (Table 28-4)

$$C = \frac{3.9 + 3.1}{4[30.25 - (19.0 + 1.25)]}$$

C = 0.17

(2) If the ocular rigidity is *low* (e.g., 0.0135), then

$$\Delta V_{scorr} = 3.1 \times \frac{0.0215}{0.0135} = 4.9 \; \mu l$$

The values for ΔV_c and P_{tav} are not altered from those in the normal eye.

P_{0corr} = 23.0 mm Hg (Fig. 28-2)

$$C = \frac{3.9 + 4.9}{4[30.25 - (23.0 + 1.25)]}$$

C = 0.37

(3) If ocular rigidity is *elevated* (e.g., 0.0315), then

$$\Delta V_{scorr} = 3.1 \times \frac{0.0215}{0.0315} = 2.1 \; \mu l$$

The values for ΔV_c and P_{tav} are not altered from those in the normal eye.

P_{0corr} = 15.0 mm Hg (Fig. 28-2)

$$C = \frac{3.9 + 2.1}{4[30.25 - (15.0 + 1.25)]}$$

C = 0.11

FRIEDENWALD NOMOGRAM

The Friedenwald nomogram may be used for estimation of the true intraocular pressure, for the determination of ocular rigidity, and for the graphic estimation of outflow facility.

In Fig. 28-1 the data are presented for an eye with normal ocular rigidity. The pretonography applanation value was 19.5 mm Hg. Note that this is plotted at a volume of 0.5 μl. The tonogram with the 5.5-gram weight began at Schiøtz scale reading 4.5 and reached 6.5 at 4 minutes. By drawing a line through the applanation value and the Schiøtz scale reading, one determines the true P_0 as 19 mm Hg (the intercept on the pressure axis). The ocular rigidity coefficient, E, is the slope of this line. It may be estimated from the protractor provided. This is done by drawing a line (such as the broken line in Fig. 28-1) parallel to the

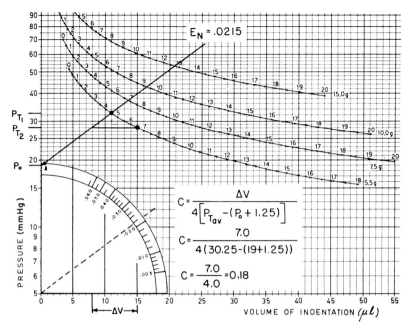

Fig. 28-1. Example of the use of the Friedenwald nomogram for estimating ocular rigidity and for calculating the tonographic outflow facility, C.

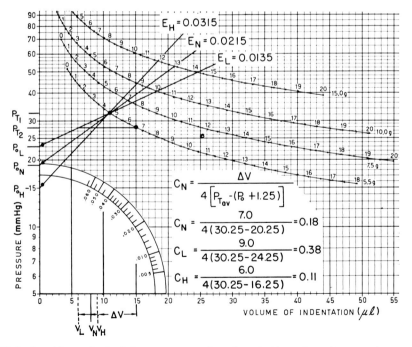

Fig. 28-2. Graphic method of determination of outflow facility, C, and intraocular pressure, P_0, for eyes with normal, N, high, H, and low, L, ocular rigidity.

line in question and through the origin of the nomogram as indicated. This is read from the intersection with the protractor scale as 0.0215.

The calculations for the tonogram are indicated in Fig. 28-1. ΔV is obtained from the difference between the volume values corresponding to the scale reading at 4 minutes and the volume at the intercept of the pressure line for this scale reading with the ocular rigidity line. The P_t values are read directly from the pressure axis and averaged. The values calculated for P_0 (19) and C (0.18) can be obtained much more readily from Table 28-1. However, this graphic method of measurement is of enormous advantage in those eyes that deviate from normal ocular rigidity (Fig. 28-2). The values obtained by the graphic method should be compared with those derived in Table 28-7 (Table 6-2).

CHAPTER **29**

Examples of tonograms

This chapter consists of informal accounts of patients selected from the tonography files presented briefly, with particular reference to the use of tonography in the diagnosis and management of their glaucoma problems.

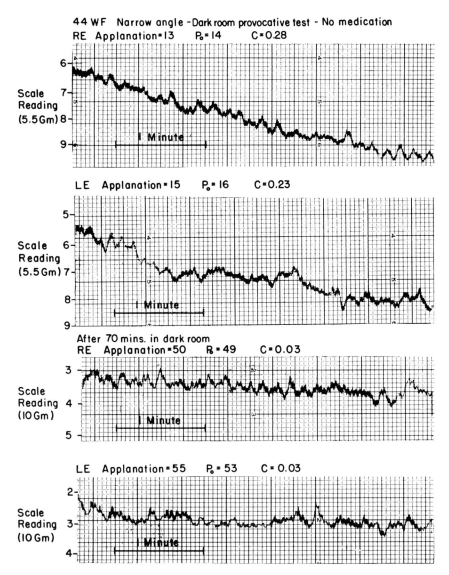

44 WF   Narrow angle - Dark room provocative test - No medication
RE Applanation=13   P₀=14   C=0.28

Scale Reading (5.5 Gm)

I Minute

LE   Applanation=15   P₀=16   C=0.23

Scale Reading (5.5 Gm)

I Minute

After 70 mins. in dark room
RE   Applanation=50   P₀=49   C=0.03

Scale Reading (10 Gm)

I Minute

LE   Applanation=55   P₀=53   C=0.03

Scale Reading (10 Gm)

I Minute

Fig. 29-1. Dark room provocative test. This 44-year-old white female was found on routine examination to have Grade 1 angles. She had no history of pain, inflammation, or halo vision, nor did she present evidence of field loss or cupping. Her pressures at initial examination were found to be well within normal limits. She was referred for a dark room provocative test. The initial tracings revealed normal pressures and outflow facilities in both eyes, as indicated in the upper two tracings. After 70 minutes in the dark room her pressures rose into the fifties with flat tracings (lower tracings). Gonioscopy at this time revealed completely occluded angles. She responded dramatically to the administration of pilocarpine, and bilateral peripheral iridectomies were performed.

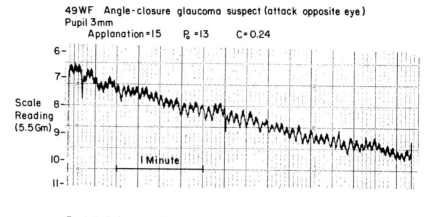

49WF Angle-closure glaucoma suspect (attack opposite eye)
Pupil 3mm
Applanation = 15 P_o = 13   C = 0.24

Scale
Reading
(5.5 Gm)

I Minute

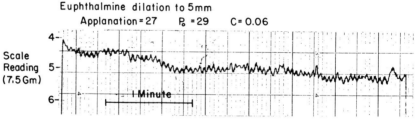

Euphthalmine dilation to 5mm
Applanation = 27 P_o = 29   C = 0.06

Scale
Reading
(7.5 Gm)

I Minute

Fig. 29-2. Positive eucatropine (Euphthalmine) dilation test. This 49-year-old white female had had an attack of angle-closure glaucoma in one eye, which had been cured by iridectomy. She was referred to the tonography laboratory for a eucatropine (Euphthalmine) dilation test on the unoperated eye. After dilation of the pupil from 3 to 5 mm with eucatropine, the pressure rose significantly and the outflow facility was decreased as illustrated. Gonioscopy at this time demonstrated an occluded angle. The administration of pilocarpine lowered the pressure promptly to 15 mm Hg, and the outflow facility measured 0.33. Subsequently, she had a peripheral iridectomy. Two years postoperatively, the pressure was 15 mm Hg, and the outflow facility 0.27 without therapy.

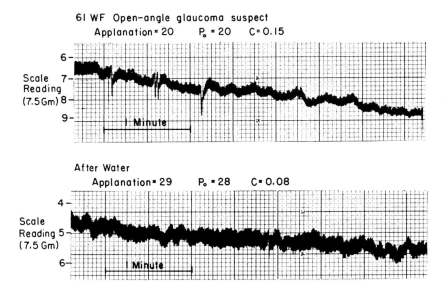

Fig. 29-3. Positive water provocative test. The patient, a 61-year-old white female, was referred because of repeated applanation readings above 20 mm Hg. She had normal optic nerve heads and no field loss. The tonogram before water drinking reproduced the referral pressure of 20 mm Hg, both by applanation and Schiøtz tonometry. The outflow facility was borderline at 0.15. After the patient drank a liter of water, intraocular pressure rose significantly to an applanation reading of 29 mm Hg. The outflow facility was decreased to 0.08. The abnormal tracing after water drinking suggested a diagnosis of glaucoma.

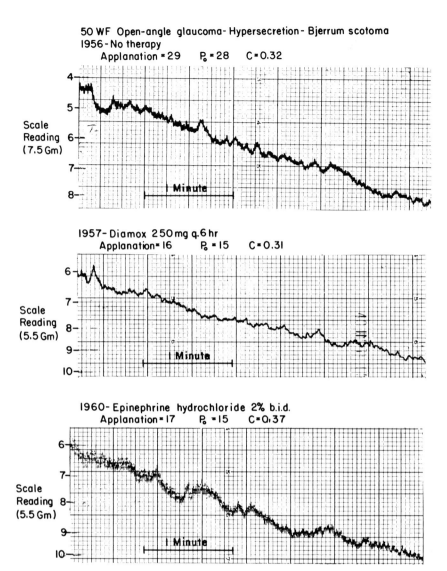

Fig. 29-4. Hypersecretion glaucoma controlled with acetazolamide (Diamox) or epinephrine. This 50-year-old white female was found to have elevated pressures, cupping, and Bjerrum's scotoma in 1956. The first tracing illustrates her status at that time, demonstrating pressures in the high twenties, with normal outflow facility. A diagnosis of hypersecretion glaucoma was made, and the patient was placed on acetazolamide, 250 mg every 6 hours. She remained under excellent pressure control. An example of her status at that time is illustrated in the second tracing obtained in 1957, with pressures in the midteens and an outflow facility of 0.31. In 1959 she had an attack of renal colic, and therefore acetazolamide was discontinued. She was placed on topical 2% epinephrine hydrochloride twice a day and has been maintained under excellent control for a period of over two years. The lower tracing was obtained in 1960 and demonstrates control with epinephrine.

Because of the systemic side effects of carbonic anhydrase inhibitors, it is probably wiser to control patients with hypersecretion glaucoma on topical epinephrine if this proves possible. Acetazolamide may then be reserved for those patients who fail to respond to epinephrine. The use of both agents together often produces a greater effect than either one alone.

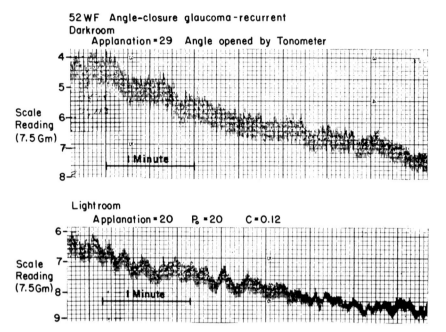

Fig. 29-5. Opening of a closed angle by the application of the tonometer. This 52-year-old white female had known angle-closure glaucoma with recurrent attacks. She was referred for evaluation of outflow facility. The initial applanation tonometry and tonogram were done in a darkened room. An applanation reading of 29 mm Hg was obtained. The tonogram started at 4.5/7.5. However, as noted from the tracing, there was a sudden increase in slope after the first 30 seconds. It was suspected that this was due to the pressure of the tonometer deepening the periphery of the anterior chamber and opening the angle. Tonography was therefore repeated 2 hours later in a well-lighted room and demonstrated a pressure of 20 mm Hg with an outflow facility of 0.12. The initial tracing could be confused with hypersecretion glaucoma, since the ocular rigidity appeared normal. This emphasizes the importance of gonioscopy if one is to interpret tonograms intelligently.

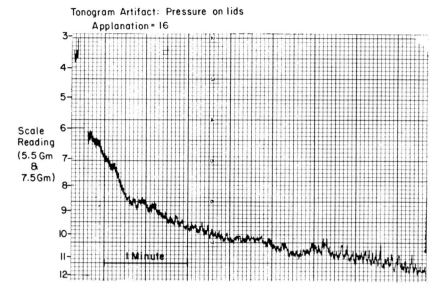

Fig. 29-6. **Tonographic artifact that can be misinterpreted as hypersecretion glaucoma.** The patient, a 45-year-old white female, was referred because of a Schiøtz reading of 3.0/5.5. On the initial tonograms, although the applanation reading was 16 mm Hg, the Schiøtz scale reading was 3.5/5.5. This necessitated changing to a 7.5-gram weight. The tracing with a 7.5-gram weight showed an initial sharp drop as illustrated. The technician commented on the difficulty of separating this patient's lids and suspected that the initial Schiøtz readings were false because of pressure on the eye by the techician's fingers. A subsequent tonogram showed a pressure of 16 mm Hg and an outflow facility of 0.25, and the patient had a negative water provocative test. This type of tracing emphasizes the importance of recognizing the artifact and also of avoiding any pressure on the patient's globe in separating the lids. In some individuals this proves most difficult.

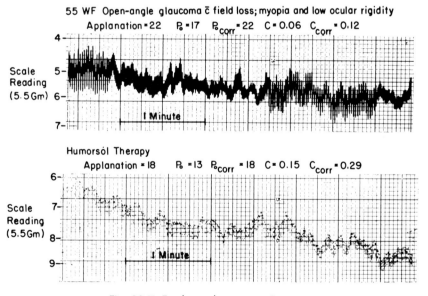

Fig. 29-7. For legend see opposite page.

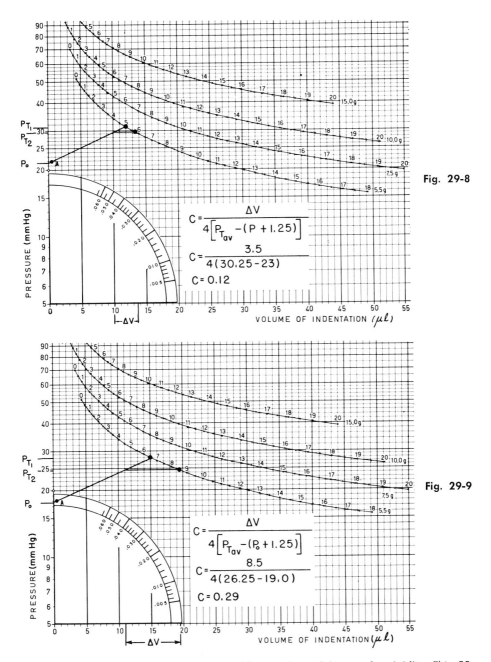

Fig. 29-8

Fig. 29-9

$$C = \frac{\Delta V}{4\left[P_{T_{av}} - (P + 1.25)\right]}$$

$$C = \frac{3.5}{4(30.25 - 23)}$$

$$C = 0.12$$

$$C = \frac{\Delta V}{4\left[P_{T_{av}} - (P_o + 1.25)\right]}$$

$$C = \frac{8.5}{4(26.25 - 19.0)}$$

$$C = 0.29$$

Figs. 29-7 to 29-9. Glaucoma in an eye with myopia and low ocular rigidity. This 55-year-old white female had been myopic all her life (5.00 to 6.00 D). Her intraocular pressure had been measured a number of times by Schiøtz tonometry. It had always been found to be within normal limits. It was not until she had extensive field loss that a diagnosis of glaucoma was suspected. A comparison of applanation and Schiøtz measurements revealed the low ocular rigidity. Her tonographic tracings were flat, and even when corrected for the low rigidity, outflow facilities were reduced markedly. On demecarium bromide (Humorsol) therapy she demonstrated an excellent response. The decreased ocular rigidity persisted, however. Her condition has remained under excellent control for a period of over two years without further field loss. Note the cardiac irregularities in the initial tracing. The corrections of these tracings for the low ocular rigidity are demonstrated in Figs. 29-8 and 29-9.

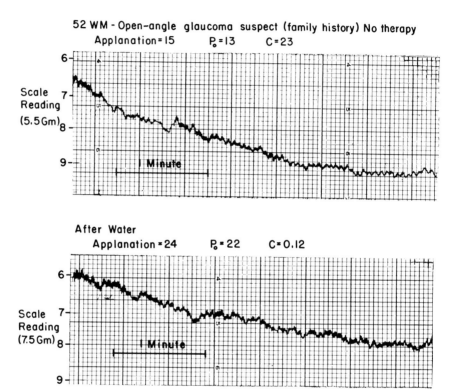

Fig. 29-10. Development of glaucoma in a patient with a family history of open-angle glaucoma. This 52-year-old man was referred because of a family history of open-angle glaucoma. All findings were within normal limits on initial examination. Tonography demonstrated a normal tonogram. However, after water drinking, the pressure rose to 24 mm Hg by applanation, and the outflow facility was 0.12. He was maintained on no therapy. One year later he demonstrated spontaneous pressure rises to the middle to high twenties and a flat tonographic tracing before water. He was placed on 2% pilocarpine every 6 hours. The last tracing demonstrates his status after three months of such therapy and illustrates an excellent response to pilocarpine.

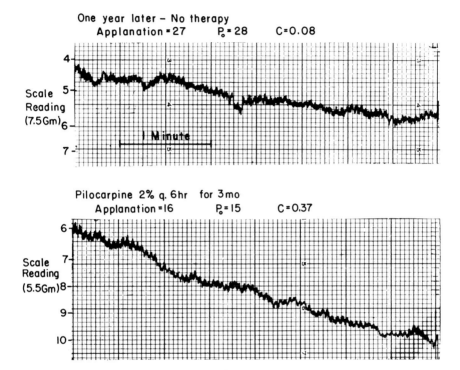

Fig. 29-10, cont'd. For legend see opposite page.

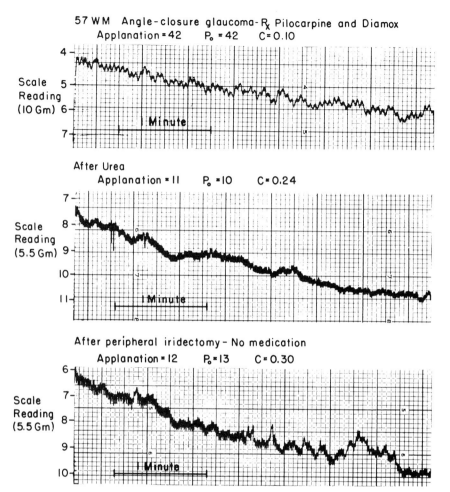

Fig. 29-11. Intravenous urea in angle-closure glaucoma. This 57-year-old white man was admitted to the hospital in an acute attack of angle-closure glaucoma. He had been in the attack for 48 hours and had been treated vigorously for over 12 hours with pilocarpine and intravenous and oral acetazolamide. His intraocular pressure failed to fall below 40 mm Hg. His outflow facility remained depressed. It was planned to perform an iridencleisis. After administration of urea his intraocular pressure fell promptly to readings that were too low to measure. Gonioscopy at this time revealed a slitlike opening in two areas of the angle. Surgery was therefore delayed, and he was maintained on miotics and acetazolamide. The next day the second tonographic tracing illustrated was obtained. The excellent outflow facility suggested that peripheral iridectomy be done. This procedure was performed 3 days later. Since the operation, he has been controlled for a period of over one year on no medication. The last tonogram demonstrates his excellent control one year after surgery.

This case demonstrates successful opening of an angle after the lowering of intraocular pressure by urea, permitting peripheral iridectomy rather than a filtering procedure to be done.

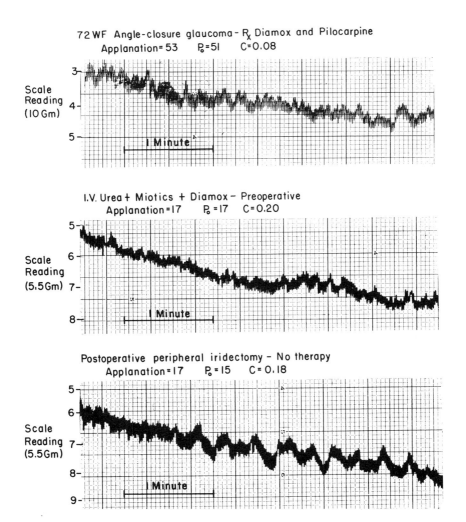

72 WF Angle-closure glaucoma - R$_x$ Diamox and Pilocarpine
Applanation= 53   P$_o$=51   C=0.08

Scale
Reading
(10 Gm)

3 —
4 —
5 —

I Minute

I.V. Urea + Miotics + Diamox — Preoperative
Applanation = 17   P$_o$ = 17   C=0.20

Scale
Reading
(5.5Gm)

5 —
6 —
7 —
8 —

I Minute

Postoperative peripheral iridectomy — No therapy
Applanation = 17   P$_o$ = 15   C = 0.18

Scale
Reading
(5.5Gm)

5 —
6 —
7 —
8 —
9 —

I Minute

Fig. 29-12. Peripheral iridectomy in chronic angle-closure glaucoma. This 72-year-old white female had recurrent attacks of angle-closure glaucoma. She refused surgery and was maintained on pilocarpine and acetazolamide. When first seen in the tonography laboratory, she had been on this regimen for over one year. She had extensive peripheral anterior synechias, and at the time of the initial tonogram the angle appeared completely occluded. She was admitted to the hospital for surgery. Prior to the operation urea was given intravenously. Her pressure fell to the range of 17 to 24 mm Hg. Operation was therefore delayed for 24 hours. The tonogram at that time is demonstrated in the second tracing with pressure of 17 mm Hg and facility of 0.20. Although gonioscopy failed to reveal any change in the status of the angle, because of the reasonable outflow facility a peripheral iridectomy was done. The last tracing demonstrates the status of control eighteen months after surgery and on no therapy.

This case illustrates the possibilities of functioning trabecular meshwork even in eyes with repeated attacks and considerable synechias. It also demonstrates the value of tonography in the prognosis of peripheral iridectomy for angle-closure glaucoma.

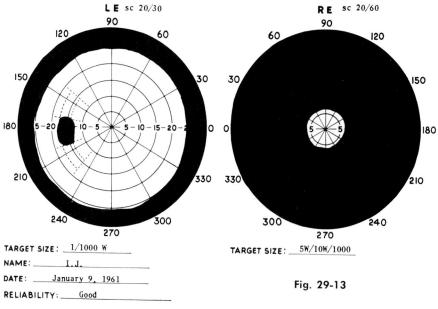

LE sc 20/30

TARGET SIZE: 1/1000 W
NAME: I.J.
DATE: January 9, 1961
RELIABILITY: Good

RE sc 20/60

TARGET SIZE: 5W/10W/1000

Fig. 29-13

Figs. 29-13 and 29-14. Iridectomy in advanced angle-closure glaucoma. A 44-year-old black woman was first examined in the Washington University Ophthalmology Clinic on January 9, 1961. A diagnosis of glaucoma had been made one year previously, and the patient had been on miotic therapy since that time. She had noted occasional halos around lights despite the use of medication.

Examination revealed the following visual acuities: right eye, 20/60; left eye, 20/30. The anterior chambers were shallow, and the cornea and lens were clear in both eyes. The right optic disc showed advanced cupping. The left optic disc appeared to be normal, and there were minimal pigmentary degenerative changes in the left macula. Central visual fields showed marked constriction on the right down to the seven-degree isopter, with a 10 mm white test object at 1 M. The left field was entirely normal to a 1 mm white test object at 1 M (Fig. 29-13). Schiøtz tensions were right eye, 4/10 = 43 mm Hg and left eye 3/5.5 = 24 mm Hg. Gonioscopy showed that both angles were completely occluded.

The patient refused surgery and was maintained on varying combinations of medications during the subsequent nineteen months. The right eye was poorly controlled during this entire period, with tensions ranging from 17 to 45 mm Hg. The visual fields remained stable. Tonography on August 13, 1962, on 4% pilocarpine (each eye every 6 hours) and acetazolamide (250 mg every 6 hours) showed the following: right eye, P_0 34, C = 0.02 (Fig. 29-14); left eye P_0 17, C = 0.04.

Bilateral peripheral iridectomies were performed—the right eye on August 14, 1962, and the left eye on August 17, 1962. A small hyphema was noted in the right eye on the first postoperative day. It cleared completely after one week. The left eye had an uneventful postoperative course. There has been no evidence of subconjunctival filtration in either eye.

The patient was maintained on no medication since surgery. On January 17, 1963, tonography showed the following: right eye, P_0 17, C = 0.27 (Fig. 29-14); left eye, P_0 15, C = 0.21.

Gonioscopic examination revealed extensive peripheral anterior synechias in both eyes, producing occlusion of approximately 80% of the right angle and 50% of the left angle. The visual acuities, visual fields, and optic nerve heads were unchanged as compared with the initial examination on January 9, 1961.

To determine the responsiveness of this patient to topical corticosteroids, the left eye was subjected to 0.1% dexamethasone four times daily. After three months tonography was as follows: right eye, applanation 17, P_0 16, C = 0.21; left eye, applanation 17, P_0 15, C = 0.20. Steroids were discontinued.

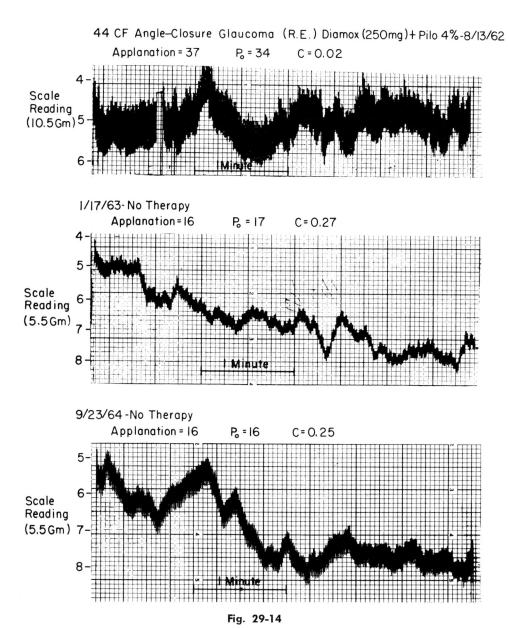

44 CF Angle–Closure Glaucoma (R.E.) Diamox (250mg)+ Pilo 4%-8/13/62
Applanation = 37 P_o = 34   C = 0.02

Scale Reading (10.5 Gm)

1/17/63- No Therapy
Applanation = 16 P_o = 17   C = 0.27

Scale Reading (5.5 Gm)

9/23/64 -No Therapy
Applanation = 16 P_o = 16   C = 0.25

Scale Reading (5.5 Gm)

Fig. 29-14

Follow-up examination on September 23, 1964, was as follows: right eye, applanation 16, P_o 16, C = 0.25 (Fig. 29-14); left eye, applanation 17, P_o 17, C = 0.25. The angles remain largely occluded, and visual acuities, cupping, and fields are unchanged.

This is a case of bilateral chronic angle-closure glaucoma with very extensive synechia formation. The preoperative outflow facilities were greatly diminished in spite of administration of pilocarpine and acetazolamide. Nevertheless the tonographic tracings have been entirely normal with *no medication* for a period of over two years after peripheral iridectomies. In spite of prior outflow impairment and obvious synechias, no pressure response whatsoever was noted to topical dexamethasone, even after three months. (Fig. 29-13 from Forbes, M., and Becker, B.: Amer. J. Ophthal. **57**:57, 1964.)

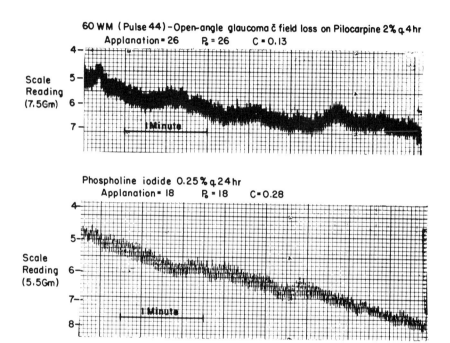

Fig. 29-15. Excellent response to echothiophate iodide (Phospholine iodide) in a patient no longer responsive to pilocarpine. This 60-year-old white male was referred for surgery because of progressive loss of visual field on 2% pilocarpine every 4 hours. The patient was known to have had glaucoma for five years and had been controlled on pilocarpine until the last 6 months. The upper tracing demonstrates his status while on pilocarpine. The control was inadequate, with a pressure of 26 mm Hg and an outflow facility of 0.13. Note the patient's slow pulse (approximately 44 per minute) due to heart block. Pilocarpine therapy was stopped, and the patient was placed on 0.25% echothiophate iodide every night. The second tracing demonstrates the excellent response to this medication, with pressure falling to 18 mm Hg and a facility of 0.28. The patient has been maintained on echothiophate iodide for over two years without further loss of visual field.

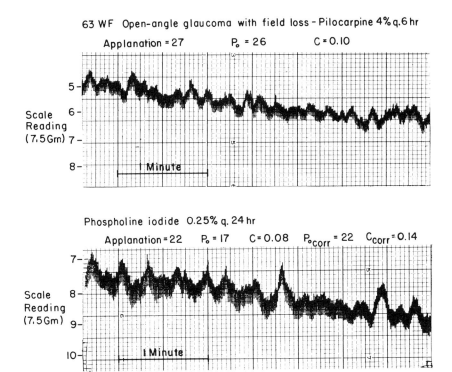

63 WF Open-angle glaucoma with field loss - Pilocarpine 4% q.6 hr

Applanation = 27   P₀ = 26   C = 0.10

Phospholine iodide 0.25% q. 24 hr

Applanation = 22   P₀ = 17   C = 0.08   P₀corr = 22   Ccorr = 0.14

Fig. 29-16. Decreased ocular rigidity after echothiophate iodide. This 63-year-old white female was referred for consultation because of inadequate glaucoma control and progressive field loss on 4% pilocarpine every 6 hours. The upper tracing demonstrates her status of control at that time. She was placed on 0.25% echothiophate iodide every night. A tonogram obtained one week later is illustrated in the lower tracing. The Schiøtz reading of 17 mm Hg suggested excellent control. However, the uncorrected outflow facility of 0.08 indicated either that the control was inadequate or that ocular rigidity might be abnormal. The applanation reading of 22 mm Hg confirmed the abnormally low ocular rigidity. When the tracings were corrected for ocular rigidity, the values were a pressure of 22 mm Hg and a facility of 0.14. Thus this patient was inadequately controlled on echothiophate iodide.

This case illustrates the reduction in ocular rigidity that often follows the use of strong miotics. Unless this is appreciated by applanation readings or by the flat tonographic tracing, the physician may misinterpret the Schiøtz reading as excellent control.

Fig. 29-17. Responsiveness to pilocarpine after resistance to echothiophate iodide. This 62-year-old white female had a diagnosis of open-angle glaucoma in 1958. As demonstrated in the first tracing, her pressures at the time were in the high thirties, with decreased outflow facility. She was placed on 2% pilocarpine every 6 hours and responded dramatically to this therapy. Pressures remained in the midteens, with outflow facilities of 0.25 to 0.30. In February, 1960, she was referred again to the tonography laboratory because of progressive elevation of intraocular pressures. This time the second tracing illustrated was obtained and demonstrated glaucoma that was out of control on pilocarpine therapy. Pilocarpine was therefore discontinued, and the patient was placed on 0.25% echothiophate iodide every 24 hours. She responded well to this medication, and a tonogram obtained in March, 1960, demonstrated excellent control on echothiophate iodide. The condition remained under excellent control until January, 1961, when she again demonstrated borderline to increased intraocular pressures and progressive reduction in outflow facility. The fourth tracing illustrates her status on February 2, 1961, with a pressure in the midtwenties and the facility reduced to 0.13. These tracings were obtained while she was taking echothiophate iodide. During the preceding week the drug had been increased to every 12 hours. The echothiophate iodide was therefore discontinued, and the patient was started on 2% pilocarpine every 6 hours. She again responded well to pilocarpine. The last tracing illustrates her status of February 16, 1961, with a pressure of 17 mm Hg and a facility of 0.22. This patient still demonstrated no cupping or field loss.

This case illustrates the importance of discontinuing medications such as pilocarpine when they are no longer effective and when one is starting a "strong" miotic. The interval of one year on no pilocarpine permitted reestablishment of responsiveness to the drug. This patient also illustrates the fact that eyes which have become resistant to the so-called stronger miotics can still be responsive to the "weaker" miotics.

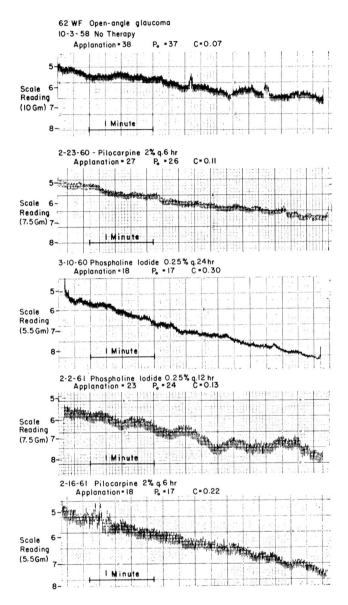

62 WF Open-angle glaucoma
10-3-58 No Therapy
    Applanation = 38 P_o = 37   C = 0.07

Scale
Reading
(10 Gm)

2-23-60 - Pilocarpine 2% q.6 hr
    Applanation = 27 P_o = 26   C = 0.11

Scale
Reading
(7.5 Gm)

3-10-60 Phospholine Iodide 0.25% q.24 hr
    Applanation = 18 P_o = 17   C = 0.30

Scale
Reading
(5.5 Gm)

2-2-61 Phospholine Iodide 0.25% q.12 hr
    Applanation = 23 P_o = 24   C = 0.13

Scale
Reading
(7.5 Gm)

2-16-61 Pilocarpine 2% q.6 hr
    Applanation = 18 P_o = 17   C = 0.22

Scale
Reading
(5.5 Gm)

Fig. 29-17

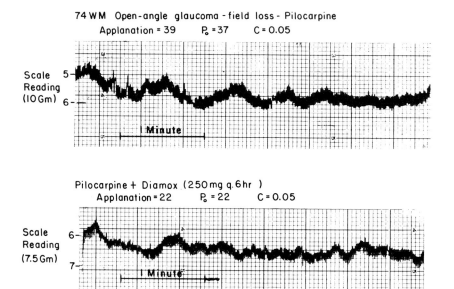

74 W M   Open-angle glaucoma - field loss - Pilocarpine
Applanation = 39 P_o = 37   C = 0.05

Scale   5
Reading
(10 Gm) 6

| Minute

Pilocarpine + Diamox (250 mg q. 6 hr)
Applanation = 22 P_o = 22   C = 0.05

Scale   6
Reading
(7.5 Gm) 7

I Minute

Fig. 29-18. Typical response to carbonic anhydrase inhibitors. This 74-year-old white male
was referred for consultation because of glaucoma inadequately controlled by pilocarpine.
The upper tracing demonstrates the elevated pressures and reduced outflow facility at the
time of referral. The patient was placed on acetazolamide, 250 mg every 6 hours, without changing his pilocarpine medication. The repeat lower tracing illustrates the fall in
intraocular pressure from 39 to 22 mm Hg without change in outflow facility, presumably
by inhibiting aqueous secretion by some 55% to 60%.

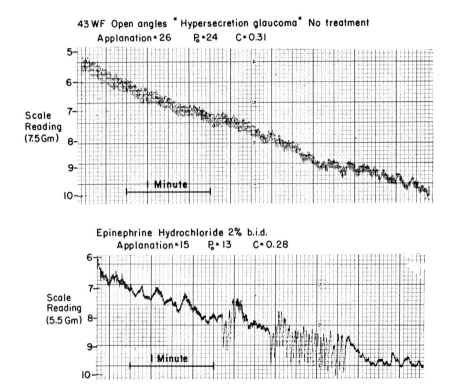

Fig. 29-19. Cardiac irregularity with topical epinephrine. This 43-year-old white female had a diagnosis of hypersecretion, as illustrated in the upper tracing. She had no field loss or cupping. She was placed on 2% epinephrine twice a day with an excellent response, as demonstrated in the lower tracing. Pressures were lowered from the midtwenties to the midteens. Outflow facility remained approximately the same. The lower tracing was obtained after one week of therapy. Note the cardiac irregularity demonstrated in the tracing. Because of this finding, an electrocardiogram was done simultaneously with a repeat tonogram. This confirmed the premature ventricular contractions.

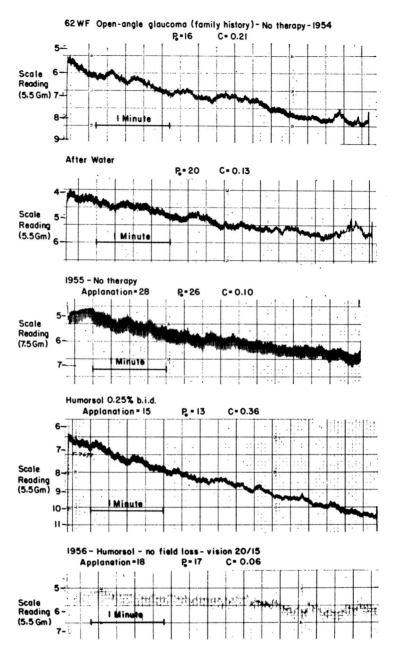

Fig. 29-20. Repeated tonograms over a period of six years. This 62-year-old white female was referred because of a family history of open-angle glaucoma. It will be noted that in 1954 without therapy the patient had a normal tonogram. However, after water drinking the pressure rose to 20 mm Hg, with a facility of 0.13. The patient was maintained without therapy and in 1955 for the first time demonstrated an abnormal tonogram even before water drinking. She was placed on 0.25% demecarium bromide twice a day, with a dramatic response and normalization of intraocular pressure and a high outflow facility. Note that ocular rigidity was somewhat reduced on initial therapy with demecarium bromide. After one year of demecarium bromide therapy, a progressive decline in outflow facility without pressure elevation was noted. Because there were no pressure elevations at office visits, therapy was not altered. In 1957 she was found to have a Bjerrum's scotoma, and at this time on demecarium bromide therapy her pressure was in the low forties, with a flat tonographic tracing. She was unable to tolerate carbonic anhydrase inhibitors,

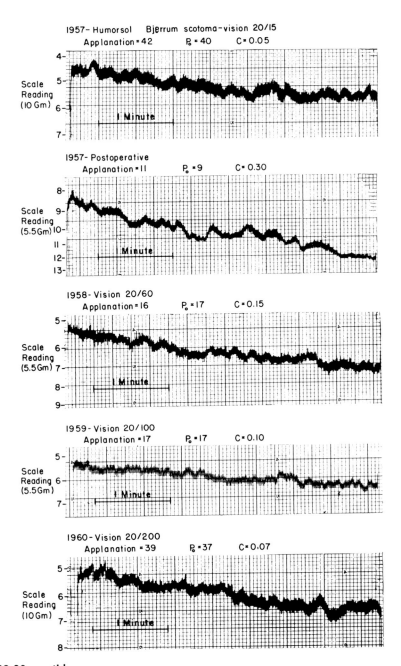

Fig. 29-20, cont'd.

and because of progression of the Bjerrum's scotoma an iridencleisis was done. A successful filtering bleb was obtained, with applanation pressure of 10 to 11 mm Hg and outflow facility of 0.30 or better. Some three months after the iridencleisis her vision, which had been 20/15, was reduced to 20/30. This was explained on the basis of lens changes. In 1958 her vision was reduced to 20/60. At this time her pressures were running in the midteens. Outflow facility was reduced to 0.15, the first evidence of impending scarring down of the bleb. In 1959 her vision was reduced to 20/100. Although her pressures still remained in the 15 to 19 mm Hg range, her outflow facility was further reduced to 0.10. At this time it became apparent that the bleb was nonfunctional. In 1960 her vision was reduced to 20/200, and for the first time pressure elevations were noted to the middle to high thirties, with reduced outflow facility. Subsequently she has had a cataract extraction and now remains in borderline control on echothiophate iodide.

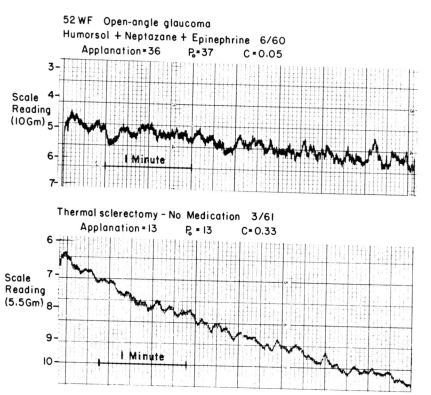

52 WF   Open-angle glaucoma
Humorsol + Neptazane + Epinephrine   6/60
Applanation = 36 P_o = 37   C = 0.05

Scale
Reading
(10 Gm)

I Minute

Thermal sclerectomy – No Medication   3/61
Applanation = 13 P_o = 13   C = 0.33

Scale
Reading
(5.5 Gm)

I Minute

Fig. 29-21. Successful filtering operation. This 52-year-old white female with open-angle glaucoma was followed for a number of years. In the early part of 1960, in spite of strong miotics, carbonic anhydrase inhibitors, and topical epinephrine, the glaucoma remained out of control, and she showed progressive loss of visual field. The upper tracing demonstrates her status preoperatively. Thermal sclerostomy was done in the beginning of June, 1960. Since the operation she has had excellent filtration and has maintained pressures in the low teens without medication. The lower tracing made in March, 1961, shows excellent outflow facility. She has maintained vision and fields to date.

Figs. 29-22 to 29-26. Examples of artifacts in the tonographic tracing.

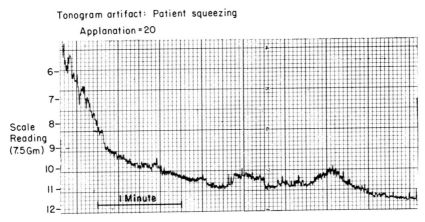

Fig. 29-22. The patient is squeezing for the first 30 to 40 seconds of the tonogram. No valid conclusions can be drawn as to the presence or absence of glaucoma from tracings such as these.

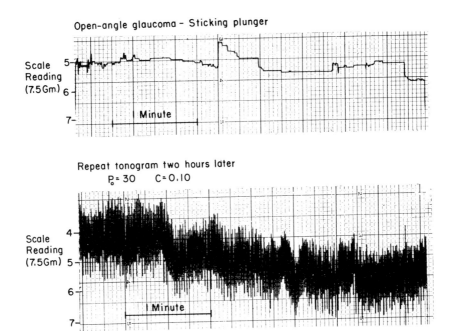

Fig. 29-23 illustrates a sticking plunger. This patient had open-angle glaucoma. After the plunger was cleaned, a repeat tonogram was obtained 2 hours later and is illustrated in the lower tracing.

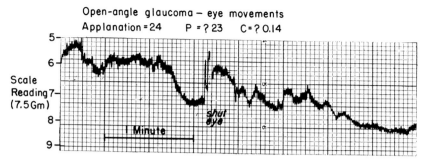

Fig. 29-24 demonstrates the effect of eye movements. The patient with known glaucoma moved her eye in the tonogram at the point indicated. This type of tracing is difficult to interpret, and tonography should be repeated at a later time. One may guess from the tracing that the condition is inadequately controlled.

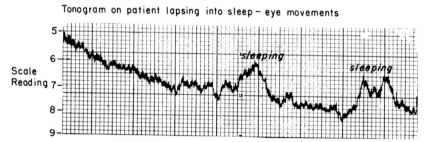

Fig. 29-25 is a tonogram of a patient who was falling asleep during the procedure. Note the artifacts in the tracing as the eyes move with the patient lapsing into sleep.

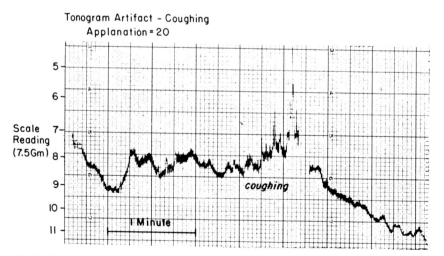

Fig. 29-26 illustrates an unsatisfactory tracing obtained from a patient who had a bout of coughing during the procedure. The tracing cannot be interpreted.

30

Gonioscopic examples

This series of goniophotographs is presented to help clarify the diagnostic use of gonioscopy. Stereophotographs of the illustrations are also presented in the stereo reels attached to the inside back cover. The case histories were particularly selected to demonstrate the manner in which gonioscopy is helpful to clinicians. The color stereoscopic goniophotographs were taken from Shaffer's *A Stereoscopic Manual of Gonioscopy,* St. Louis, 1962, The C. V. Mosby Co.

Fig. 30-1 (Reel I-1). Grade 3 to 4, open angle; iris processes; blood in Schlemm's canal. Shown here is the open angle of a brown-eyed 21-year-old patient. Schwalbe's line, *SL,* is easily identifiable. Brown iris processes, *IP,* bridge or run around the Grade 3 to 4 angle and extend over the scleral spur, *SS,* in a number of tendrils. All iris processes run around or bridge the angles recess, unlike peripheral anterior synechias, which are formed by the direct attachment of the peripheral iris to the angle wall. Iris processes do not decrease aqueous outflow. The filtering portion of the trabecular meshwork is manifest by the red streak produced by blood in Schlemm's canal, *SC.* Blood mixed with the aqueous in the canal is often found in normal eyes and in many inflamed eyes, especially if the intraocular pressure is not increased. The presence of blood is evidence against a diagnosis of glaucoma. Increasing the episcleral venous pressure by the edge of the contact lens, jugular compression, or Valsalva's maneuver or in pathologic states such as arteriovenous fistulas will allow blood to be forced into the canal. Blood is also usually found in the canal when the intraocular pressure of the eye is suddenly decreased, as by a paracentesis or injury.

Fig. 30-2 (Reel I-2). Slitlike narrow angle; closure imminent. The eye shown here has normal tension and facility of outflow, but the angle is critically narrowed. The trabecular meshwork and the angle recess, *AR,* can be seen only in the thin slitlike opening, *TR,* between the iris and Schwalbe's line, *SL.* An attack of angle closure could easily be precipitated by pupillary dilation.

Usually the occlusion of an angle like this is abrupt and total, resulting in a rapid rise in pressure with symptoms of blurred vision, halos, pain, and nausea and vomiting if the attack persists. The frequent accompanying dilation of the pupil may break the pupillary block and permit the angle to reopen. This is the usual pattern in prodromal attacks. In some eyes the iris may gradually occlude more and more of the circumference of the angle, resulting in a slow rise in pressure. When this occurs over a period of months or years, it is known as chronic angle-closure glaucoma. If the trabecular meshwork permits a normal facility of outflow, almost two thirds of the angle can be occluded before a definite increase in intraocular pressure will occur.

It must be remembered that an eye like this may have a damaged trabecular meshwork and a decreased facility of outflow. Such damage may have been caused by repeated episodes of subacute angle closure, or this could be a chronic, simple open-angle glaucoma that happened to occur in an eye with a shallow chamber and a narrow angle. Such an eye may have an acute attack of angle closure cured by iridectomy, but the open-angle component will continue to hinder the outflow of aqueous, resulting in a chronic glaucoma. Such coexisting types of glaucoma are known as combined- or mixed-mechanism glaucoma.

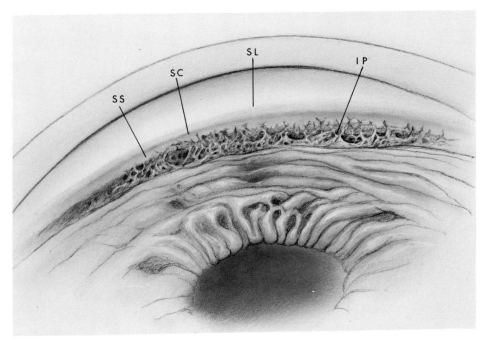

Fig. 30-1

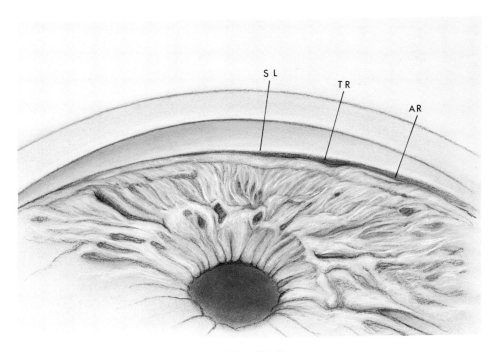

Fig. 30-2

Fig. 30-3 (Reel I-3). Grade 3, peripheral anterior synechias. This 65-year-old patient had had a cataract extracted. During the postoperative period the anterior chamber was collapsed for 2 days. In the area shown here, broad peripheral anterior synechias, *PAS,* extend up to Schwalbe's line, *SL.* Just above this point is the cataract incision line marked by a light dusting of pigment, *P.* To the left the synechias come anteriorly to attach at the incision line, whereas to the right the synechias extend only as high as the scleral spur, *SS.* Aqueous is able to reach the trabecular meshwork, *TR,* behind some of these synechias and has free access to the wide open angle at the right of the drawing. Synechias in the area of the angle recess, *AR,* have no effect on the facility of aqueous outflow.

This patient still has normal intraocular pressure and a normal facility of outflow because of the adequacy of the remaining meshwork. If the permeability of the latter were not normal, the obstruction of some of the meshwork by the peripheral anterior synechias may have been enough to result in glaucoma. Approximately one half of the normal angle can be occluded without an elevation in tension. If two thirds is blocked, a rise in pressure is to be expected. Anterior synechias are caused by iris being pushed up against the meshwork, as in pupillary block or in collapse of the anterior chamber, ciliary body tumors, etc. They may also be caused by iris being pulled up to the meshwork by shrinkage of inflammatory residue or fibrovascular membranes, as in iridocyclitis or rubeosis iridis. Only if Descemet's membrane has been injured or diseased will the iris stick to it. Consequently anterior synechias are usually attached on the roughened surface of the uveal meshwork at varying heights up to Schwalbe's line.

The longer the iris is against the trabecular meshwork, the more probable it is that a permanent peripheral anterior synechia will be formed. If the eye is never congested, the iris may remain for months and occasionally years without sticking. This apposition seems to lead to a decrease in permeability and a permanent decrease in the facility of aqueous outflow. Inflammation produces a fibrinous exudate that will quickly glue the iris permanently to the meshwork. Because of this, it is vital to re-form anterior chambers and relieve pupillary block promptly. The more inflamed the eye, the more urgently this is needed.

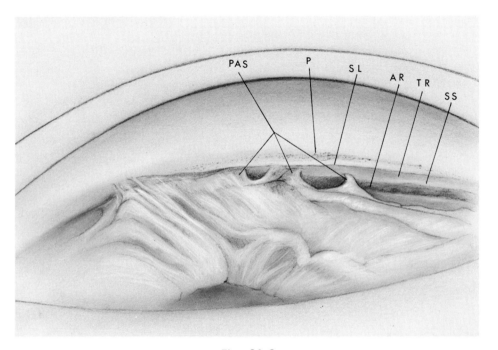

Fig. 30-3

Fig. 30-4 (Reel I-4). Closed angle preceding iridectomy. This 45-year-old woman gave a history of two episodes of blurred vision of the right eye with colored rings around light. The first attack was noted after watching television in a dimly lit room; the other was noted after a quarrel. In each instance there was a slight discomfort and fullness about the eye but no real pain. The anterior chambers were noted to be extremely shallow. Tension was 20 mm Hg in the right eye and 15 in the left eye by applanation. Gonioscopically, the right angle was noted to be almost closed, with only a few slitlike areas nasally and below to provide access of aqueous to the meshwork. The only visible angle structures are Schwalbe's line, *SL,* and a glimpse of the meshwork, *TR.* The left eye was only slightly less critically narrowed. The facility of outflow was 0.18 in the right eye and 0.30 in the left eye. The convexity of the iris-lens diaphragm is less marked through this direct contact lens (Koeppe) than through the Goldmann lens.

Because of the history typical of acute glaucomatous prodromal attack, the dangerous narrowing of the angle, and the differential in tension and facility of outflow, it was believed that there was more than enough evidence to warrant surgery without taking the considerable risk involved in even a dark room test. Preoperatively, 1% pilocarpine solution was administered every 8 hours. It was recognized that the miosis would increase the pupillary block and perhaps precipitate an attack. Actually, the slits opened slightly after the use of the pilocarpine. A peripheral iridectomy through a 1 mm ab externo incision with a McLean suture closure was performed uneventfully in the right eye, followed 2 days later by a similar procedure in the left eye.

Fig. 30-5 (Reel I-5). Opened angle following iridectomy. Postiridectomy photograph of the angle shown in Fig. 30-5 (Reel III-3). In both of these eyes there was a gratifying opening of the angles after the iridectomy. This could be seen by operating room gonioscopy. This technique is seldom necessary since intravenous urea and mannitol became available to lower tensions and often to open angles preoperatively.

The iridectomy, *IR,* can be seen on the right. The angle has dropped open beautifully without any peripheral anterior synechias. The angle opening would be called Grade 2, which is the usual degree to which a narrow angle can open. Schwalbe's line, *SL,* the trabecular meshwork, *TR,* and the angle recess, *AR,* are plainly visible. Tensions have been approximately 15 mm Hg, and the facility of outflow has been over 0.30 in each eye for the past four years without therapy.

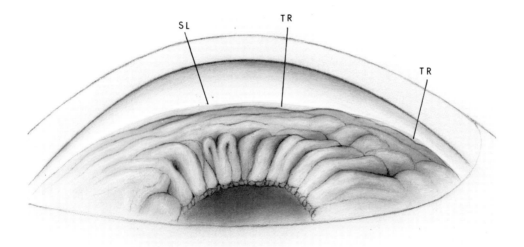

Fig. 30-4

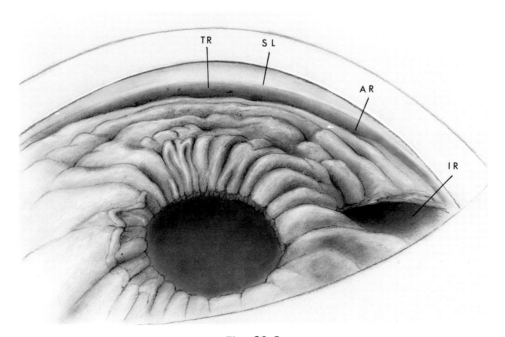

Fig. 30-5

Fig. 30-6 (Reel I-6). Iridocyclitis; Grade 3; small peripheral anterior synechias (PAS). This 36-year-old patient had recurrent nongranulomatous iridocyclitis. The angles were wide open, Grade 3, with the exception of a few small areas where shrinkage of cyclitic exudates have pulled the iris up onto the trabecular surface, forming peripheral anterior synechias, *PAS.* The central synechia is in front of the blood-filled Schlemm's canal, *SC,* but the others are no higher than the scleral spur, *SS,* and would have no influence on the facility of outflow. If the facility of outflow were decreased in such an eye, it would be on the basis of damage to the trabecular meshwork rather than to angle closure.

In the patients checked in the Uveitis Clinic of the University of California, peripheral anterior synechias were rare in those with acute iridocyclitis. They were much more common in patients with the granulomatous type of chronic uveitis. Blood was frequently seen in Schlemm's canal. A decreased facility of outflow was a frequent finding. Elevation of tension was infrequent because aqueous production was reduced by the cyclitis. Schwalbe's line, *SL,* is ledged. Iris processes, *IP,* can be seen in the angle recess, *AR,* and extending up onto the trabecular surface above the spur.

Fig. 30-7 (Reel I-7). Iridocyclitis; partial angle closure by peripheral anterior synechias (PAS). This patient had active granulomatous iridocyclitis. Large, irregular peripheral anterior synechias, *PAS,* have formed that are quite different from the flat-topped synechias caused by primary angle closure. Pigment, *P,* can be seen above Schwalbe's line, *SL.* Some pigment dusts the trabecular meshwork, *TR,* above the scleral spur, *SS.* The peripheral anterior synechias, *PAS,* to the right of the photograph cover only the angle recess, *AR.*

The patient had a facility of outflow of 0.11, but tension was 10 mm Hg by applanation. This low tension is caused by the low production of aqueous by the diseased ciliary body. Glaucoma may suddenly ensue if the ciliary body recovers without a corresponding improvement in the facility of outflow.

It is often said that the glaucoma of iridocyclitis is better tolerated than that of primary open-angle glaucoma. This is not strictly true. The tension rise in uveitis with secondary glaucoma tends to be erratic and variable. If the uveitis increases, aqueous production decreases and the tension drops, providing a respite for the optic disc. It probably takes approximately ten years of moderate pressure increases to produce the cupped disc and field defect of chronic open-angle glaucoma. A similar length of time may be needed in iritic glaucoma. Therefore any patient with severe uveitis should be periodically checked for glaucoma, even many years after subsidence of the original inflammation, if there is evidence of a decreased facility of aqueous outflow.

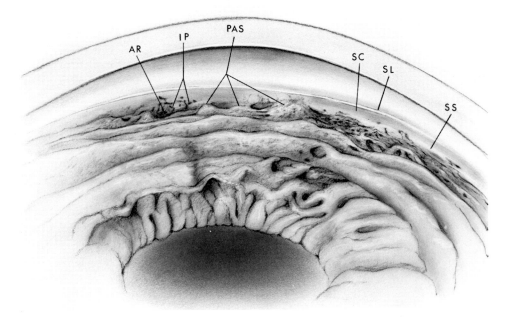

Fig. 30-6

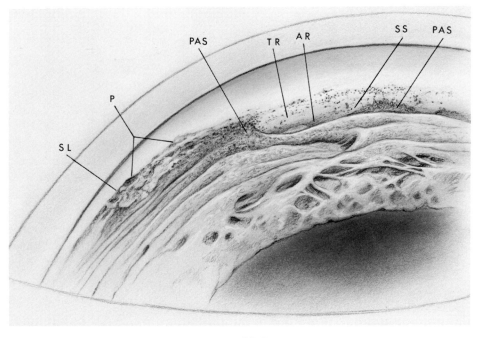

Fig. 30-7

Fig. 30-8 (Reel II-1). Acute granulomatous iridocyclitis. This 30-year-old black woman developed an acute granulomatous iridocyclitis of undetermined etiology. As is frequently seen in iridocyclitis, blood is partially filling Schlemm's canal, *SC,* which is just above the scleral spur, *SS.* Iris processes, *IP,* bridge and wrap around the angle recess, *AR.* The granulomatous type of keratic precipitates, *KP,* is prominently visible on the posterior cornea and on the meshwork, especially at Schwalbe's line, *SL.* When such precipitates touch both the meshwork and the iris, pillarlike synechias can be formed during their shrinkage and absorption. At the same time, similar inflammatory products are being deposited in the pores of the trabecular meshwork, resulting in an interference with the facility of aqueous outflow. The intraocular pressure is usually low because the diseased ciliary body is producing little aqueous humor.

Fig. 30-9 (Reel II-2). Rubeosis iridis; anterior synechias. In this advanced case of rubeosis the secondary glaucoma is caused by the total closure of the angle as high as Schwalbe's line, *SL.* In the first stages of a rubeosis, a network of newly formed blood vessels can be seen running over the trabecular meshwork from the region of the ciliary body. Similar neovascularization appears on the surface of the iris. This fibrovascular network then shrinks, pulling the peripheral iris up over the meshwork and closing the angle in a zipperlike fashion. The uveal ectropion, *EC,* is due to a similar shrinkage of the network on the iris surface. Rarely does either medical or surgical therapy provide any lasting relief from this condition.

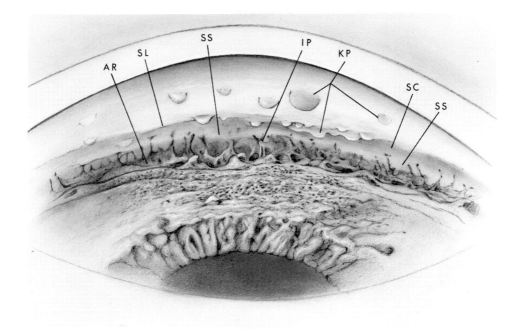

Fig. 30-8

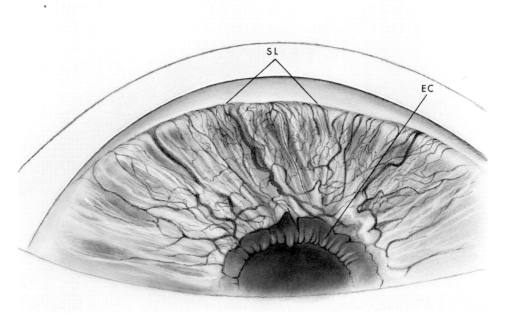

Fig. 30-9

Fig. 30-10 (Reel II-3). Essential iris atrophy; anterior synechias. This angle picture was taken through the mirror of the Goldmann lens and shows the iris hole through which the ciliary body, *CB,* can be seen. Peripheral anterior synechias, *PAS,* are forming, and the iris root has been pulled up onto the endothelium even above Schwalbe's line, *SL.* The mechanism of this synechia formation is not known. Since there is no known mechanism by which this iris can be pushed up onto the cornea, it must be pulled up by shrinkage of a theoretical edema residue.

The angle recess, *AR,* is visible on either side. At the time this photograph was taken, tension was normal and facility of outflow was normal, but as the meshwork was blocked by increasing peripheral anterior synechias in the next two years, an intractable glaucoma ensued, which was only partially controlled by cyclodialysis and intensive medical therapy. A successful sclerectomy held the pressure at a level of 10 to 12 mm Hg. At this tension the cornea remains clear.

Fig. 30-11 (Reel II-4). Exfoliation syndrome. In this brown eye, exfoliative material, *CE,* is visible in the angle. The focal point of the picture is on these deposits, leaving the Grade 3 angle structures slightly out of focus. It can be seen that there is a dense trabecular pigment band, *SC,* in the front of Schlemm's canal above the scleral spur, *SS,* and a dusting of pigment, *P,* on the peripheral cornea, *C.* Heaviest deposits are found on the back of the iris, on the underlying lens capsule, and on the ciliary body. Fragments can be seen on the zonules, the iris, and the angle of the anterior chamber.

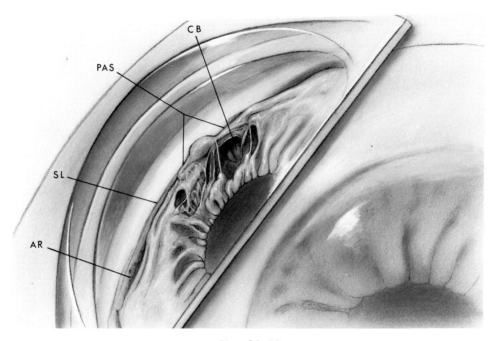

Fig. 30-10

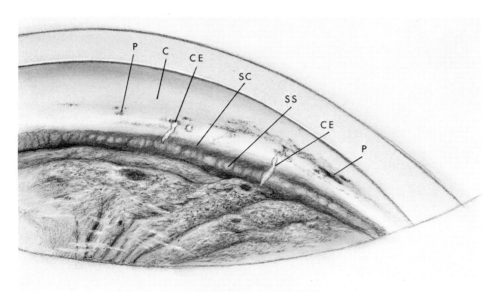

Fig. 30-11

Fig. 30-12 (Reel II-5). Krukenberg's spindle; pigmentary glaucoma. Pigmentary glaucoma is usually seen in young adults who have a moderate myopia. There is a loss of pigment from the pigment epithelium of the iris. With continuing loss, the iris may show areas that can be transilluminated. The pigment is carried forward by aqueous humor flow, where it is deposited in the trabecular meshwork in front of Schlemm's canal. Some of the pigment may stick to the corneal endothelium in the spindlelike pattern illustrated. The unwary ophthalmologist may interpret this Krukenberg spindle, *P,* as pigmented keratic precipitates, and when he sees floating pigment granules in the aqueous, he may misdiagnose the condition as iritis. Gonioscopy is diagnostic, since iritis seldom produces so dark a trabecular pigment band.

Fig. 30-13 (Reel II-6). Pigmentary glaucoma. This 32-year-old man came to the ophthalmologist complaining of seeing rainbow-colored rings around lights several times a week, each episode lasting 1 or 2 hours. The intraocular pressure was found to be 45 mm Hg, and the facility of outflow was 0.10. The patient had marked diurnal variations in pressure from 20 to 50 mm Hg. Corneal edema was produced at pressures above 40 mm Hg. It was at such times that halos could be observed.

Pilocarpine, 2%, controlled the tension but produced intolerable blurring during the working day. Satisfactory control was achieved by 0.125% echothiophate iodide (Phospholine iodide) at bedtime and 1:100 epinephrine hydrochloride each morning. The facility of outflow was improved to 0.20. Interestingly, the patient's father has been under treatment for several years for chronic open-angle glaucoma with little pigmentation of the angle.

The scleral spur, *SS,* the trabecular meshwork, *TR,* Schwalbe's line, *SL,* and the iris are speckled with pigments, *P.* In front of Schlemm's canal, *SC,* a dense trabecular pigment band can be seen.

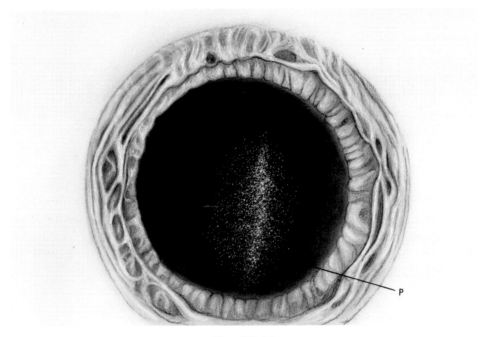

Fig. 30-12

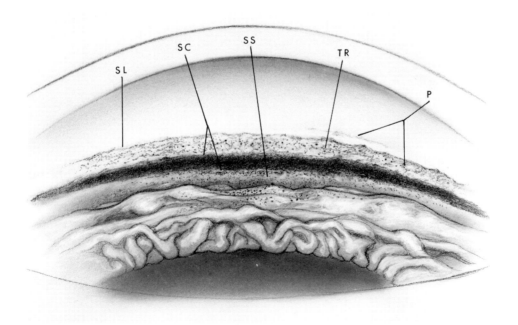

Fig. 30-13

Fig. 30-14 (Reel II-7). Infantile glaucoma. The gonioscopic findings in infantile glaucoma cannot be considered strictly diagnostic, since the angle frequently resembles some angles of the anterior chamber present in normal full-term infants. In all infant eyes the trabecular meshwork has a dimpled, glistening surface similar to the appearance of stippled cellophane, and its tissues are far more translucent than those of adults. Although an angle recess is often visible at birth in normal infants, it is never seen in infantile glaucoma. The meshwork itself appears a bit thicker than usual. Through its translucent tissues the dark color of the ciliary body, *SC,* is visible. The anterior iris stroma is hypoplastic in an arcadelike pattern. The iris pigment layer, *P,* is exposed peripherally. The iris blood vessels, *BV,* are largely unprotected by stroma and run on the iris to its junction with the trabecular meshwork, *TR.* Here the vessels rise slightly and then turn backward toward the ciliary body. The anterior insertion of the iris on the meshwork is rarely obvious with ordinary illumination, and it does not conceal Schlemm's canal when the latter is filled with blood and thus made visible. Schwalbe's line, *SL,* can be plainly seen.

The patient was 10 weeks old when his parents noted a gray hazing of the right cornea. Previous to this observation they had noted that the baby disliked bright lights and had considerable epiphora, especially in the right eye. The corneas measured 13.5 mm in the right eye and 13 mm in the left eye. The right cornea was hazy, and one rupture of Descemet's membrane was seen centrally. The tension was 40 mm Hg in the right eye and 32 mm Hg in the left eye. The optic discs were normal. Goniotomy of the nasal third of each eye was performed under contact lens visualization. Since then, the corneas have remained clear. Tension has been 14 to 17 mm Hg. There has been no epiphora or photophobia. Although the glaucoma is presumed to be cured, the child must be rechecked periodically throughout life.

Fig. 30-15 (Reel III-1). Aniridia. This 16-year-old black boy had aniridia without glaucoma. A 1½ mm fringe of peripheral iris can be seen gonioscopically, but when the iris is viewed without a lens, it is largely hidden by the limbus. The iris seems to run directly toward the angle, and then it turns abruptly up onto the meshwork in a solid sheet of iris processes, *IP,* behind which the ciliary body, *CB,* can be glimpsed. Congenital cataracts, *CAT,* are present in the lens, *L.* Schwalbe's line, *SL,* is easily recognized.

The patient's mother also has aniridia and an advanced glaucoma, demonstrating the dominant genetic pattern of this anomaly. The boy should be examined yearly for the possible onset of glaucoma, which frequently is found in young adulthood.

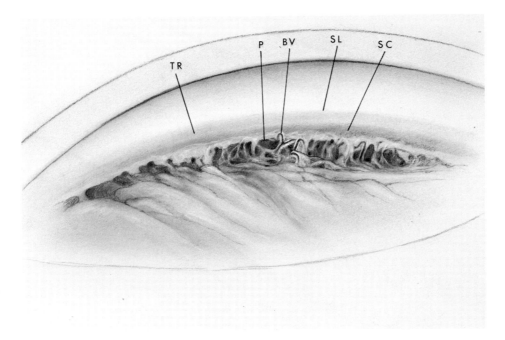

Fig. 30-14

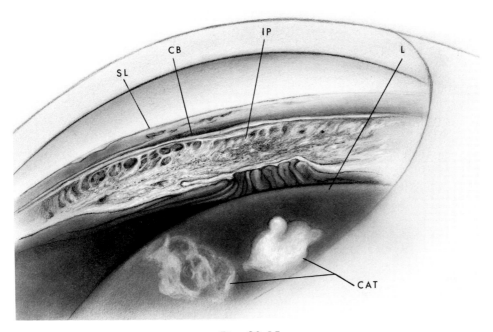

Fig. 30-15

Fig. 30-16 (Reel III-2). Axenfeld's syndrome. The gonioscopic view clearly shows the detached Schwalbe's line, *SL.* On it can be seen iris processes, *IP,* and tissue which resembles iris. It is thought that this represents an incomplete cleavage of iris from the cornea during embryologic development. The resulting stretching of iris, *I,* can form partial holes in the iris stroma. Iris processes may crowd the angle, or they may be sparse and fragmented as may be seen at the left of this picture. They always run up to Schwalbe's line, which forms an abnormally prominent ridge at the anterior end of a long trabecular meshwork. The trabecular meshwork, *TR,* and the angle recess, *AR,* can be seen behind the iris processes.

Fig. 30-17 (Reel III-3). Melanoma of iris. The angle recess of this eye is narrowed by the presence of a nevus, *N,* extending over the anterior ciliary body to the scleral spur, *SS.* Its nodular surface replaces the iris in this sector. Schwalbe's line, *SL,* and the trabecular pigment band, *SC,* as well as the whole trabecular surface, *TR,* have increased pigmentation. The lesion has been increasing in size. It interferes with the motility of the iris. All these characteristics make it probable that the lesion is a malignant melanoma of the iris. Fortunately, such iris melanomas rarely metastasize, and the prognosis is much better than in malignant melanomas of the ciliary body or choroid.

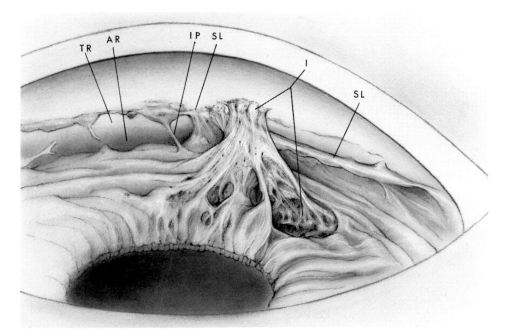

Fig. 30-16

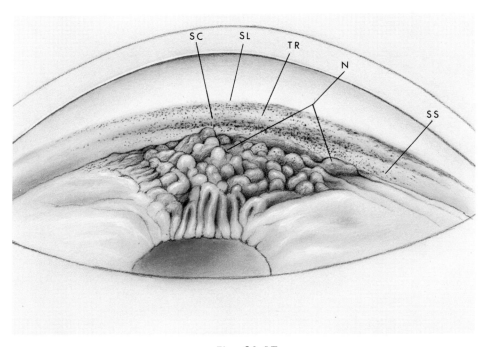

Fig. 30-17

Fig. 30-18 (Reel III-4). Pigment cyst of iris. A rounded swelling, *CY*, lifts the peripheral iris of this eye against the trabecular meshwork, *TR*, as high as Schwalbe's line, *SL*. Several similar elevations could be seen in other areas of the angle of both this and the other eye. When the pupil was dilated widely, it could be seen that the iris was lifted by thin-walled cysts on its peripheral undersurface. Occasionally such cysts may be so numerous as to produce angle closure and may then require surgical excision. Iris processes, *IP*, are visible to the right where the angle appears normal.

Fig. 30-19 (Reel III-5). Foreign body. Mild chronic iritis was found to be due to the presence in the angle of a foreign body, *FB*, with a white patch of exudate on its surface. No follow-up history could be obtained in this patient. In similar cases the surgical removal of the foreign body has resulted in cure of the iritis. Schwalbe's line, *SL*, is easily seen. The angle recess, *AR*, is beyond the focal point of the camera.

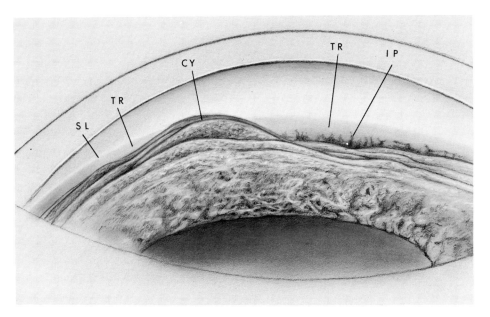

Fig. 30-18

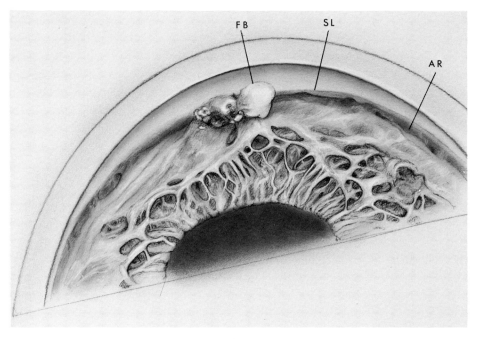

Fig. 30-19

Fig. 30-20 (Reel III-6). Cyclodialysis. Two years after a cyclodialysis, an excellent cleft, *CD,* extends from the anterior chamber into the suprachoroidal space. The inner surface of the sclera can be seen beyond the scleral spur, *SS,* which stands out clearly where the ciliary body attachment has been stripped away. There is a moderate amount of pigment, *P,* on the meshwork, *TR,* below Schwalbe's line, *SL.*

A wide open communication to the suprachoroidal space such as this usually guarantees a low intraocular tension for an indefinite time. Sometimes an apparent cleft is present, but accurate gonioscopy will reveal a reattachment of the ciliary body to the sclera at some point behind the spur. This forms a mere pocket communicating with the anterior chamber and is ineffective in reducing intraocular pressure.

Fig. 30-21 (Reel III-7). Detached Descemet's membrane. After iridectomy and synechialysis in this patient with neglected angle-closure glaucoma, Descemet's membrane, *DM,* was detached in the area of the iridectomy. It usually forms such a scroll-like roll. The ciliary body, *CB,* is visible. The irregular white flecks on the lens, *L,* are the *Glaukomflecken* of Vogt, *GL,* which are often seen after a prolonged attack of acute glaucoma. Over the area of a Descemet's detachment, the cornea can imbibe aqueous, causing corneal haze and bullous keratopathy. This haze, plus the sharp line of demarcation at the end of the detached membrane, can be misdiagnosed as an epithelial downgrowth. Dehydration of the epithelium with glycerin and careful examination by slit-lamp microscopy and gonioscopy should resolve the differential diagnosis. Eventually a new Descemet's membrane may grow over the denuded cornea, which can clear almost completely.

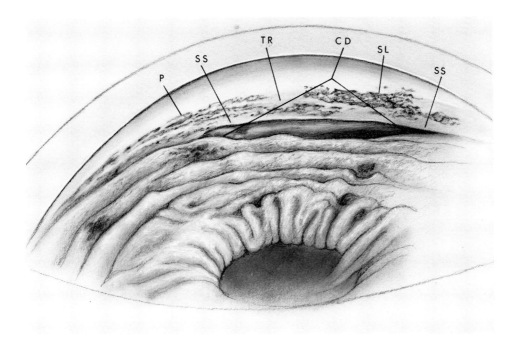

Fig. 30-20

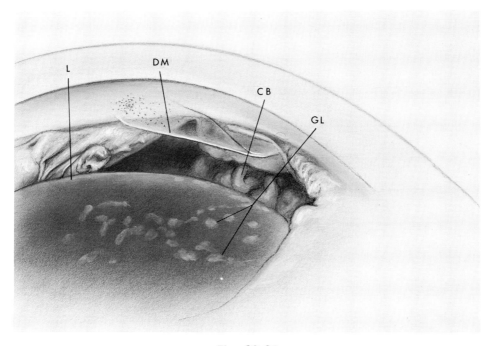

Fig. 30-21

INDEX

510